T0259451

Biologic Response Modifiers in Infectious Disease

Guest Editor

NANCY MISRI KHARDORI, MD, PhD

INFECTIOUS DISEASE CLINICS OF NORTH AMERICA

www.id.theclinics.com

Consulting Editor
ROBERT C. MOELLERING Jr, MD

December 2011 • Volume 25 • Number 4

SAUNDERS an imprint of ELSEVIER, Inc.

W.B. SAUNDERS COMPANY
A Division of Elsevier Inc.
1600 John F. Kennedy Blvd., Suite 1800, Philadelphia, PA 19103-2899.
http://www.theclinics.com

INFECTIOUS DISEASE CLINICS OF NORTH AMERICA Volume 25, Number 4
December 2011 ISSN 0891–5520, ISBN-13: 978-1-4557-1027-0

Editor: Stephanie Donley
Developmental Editor: Teia Stone

Infectious Disease Clinics of North America (ISSN 0891–5520) is published in March, June, September, and December by Elsevier Inc., 360 Park Avenue South, New York, NY 10010-1710. Periodicals postage paid at New York, NY and additional mailing offices. Subscription prices are $251.00 per year for US individuals, $435.00 per year for US institutions, $124.00 per year for US students, $297.00 per year for Canadian individuals, $538.00 per year for Canadian institutions, $355.00 per year for international individuals, $538.00 per year for international institutions, and $171.00 per year for Canadian and international students. To receive student rate, orders must be accompanied by name of affiliated institution, date of term, and the *signature* of program/residency coordinator on institution letterhead. Orders will be billed at individual rate until proof of status is received. Foreign air speed delivery is included in all *Clinics* subscription prices. All prices are subject to change without notice. **POSTMASTER**: Send address changes to *Infectious Disease Clinics of North America,* Elsevier Health Sciences Division, Subcription Customer Service, 3251 Riverport Lane, Maryland Heights, MO 63043. **Customer Service: 1-800-654-2452 (US). From outside of the US and Canada, call 1-314-447-8871. Fax: 1-314-447-8029. E-mail: JournalsCustomerService-usa@elsevier.com (print support) or JournalsOnlineSupport-usa@elsevier.com (online support).**

Infectious Disease Clinics of North America is also published in Spanish by Editorial Inter-MÅdica, Junin 917, 1er A 1113, Buenos Aires, Argentina.

Reprints. For copies of 100 or more, of articles in this publication, please contact the Commercial Reprints Department, Elsevier Inc., 360 Park Avenue South, New York, New York 10010-1710. Tel. (212) 633-3812, Fax: (212) 462-1935, E-mail: reprints@elsevier.com.

Infectious Disease Clinics of North America is covered in *MEDLINE/PubMed (Index Medicus), Current Contents/Clinical Medicine, Science Citation Alert, SCISEARCH,* and *Research Alert.*

Printed and bound by CPI Group (UK) Ltd, Croydon, CR0 4YY

Transferred to Digital Print 2011

Contributors

CONSULTING EDITOR

ROBERT C. MOELLERING Jr, MD
Shields Warren-Mallinckrodt Professor of Medical Research, Harvard Medical School; Department of Medicine, Beth Israel Deaconess Medical Center, Boston, Massachusetts

GUEST EDITOR

NANCY MISRI KHARDORI, MD, PhD, FACP, FIDSA
Professor of Medicine, Microbiology and Molecular Cell Biology, Division of Infectious Diseases, Eastern Virginia Medical School, Norfolk, Virginia

AUTHORS

HOWARD AMITAL, MD, MHA
Department of Medicine D, Zabludowicz Center for Autoimmune Diseases, Sheba Medical Center, Sackler Faculty of Medicine, Tel Aviv University, Ramat Aviv, Tel-Hashomer, Israel; Head of Internal Medicine B, Sheba Medical Center, Tel Hashomer, Israel

SCOTT J. BERGMAN, PharmD, BCPS
Assistant Professor, Department of Pharmacy Practice, Southern Illinois University Edwardsville School of Pharmacy, Edwardsville, Illinois; Division of Infectious Diseases, Southern Illinois University School of Medicine, Springfield, Illinois

MCKENZIE C. FERGUSON, PharmD, BCPS
Department of Pharmacy Practice, Southern Illinois University Edwardsville School of Pharmacy, Edwardsville, Illinois

JENNIFER L. HSU, MD
Instructor, Division of Infectious Disease, University of Wisconsin School of Medicine and Public Health, Madison, Wisconsin

VIVEK KAK, MD, FACP
Infectious Diseases, Allegiance Health, Jackson, Michigan

NANCY MISRI KHARDORI, MD, PhD, FACP, FIDSA
Professor of Medicine, Microbiology and Molecular Cell Biology, Division of Infectious Diseases, Eastern Virginia Medical School, Norfolk, Virginia

ROMESH KHARDORI, MD, PhD, FACP, FACE
Professor of Medicine Division of Endocrinology & Metabolism, Eastern Virginia Medical School, Norfolk, Virginia

JANAK KOIRALA, MD, MPH, FACP, FIDSA
Associate Professor of Medicine, Chief, Division of Infectious Diseases, Southern Illinois University, School of Medicine, Springfield, Illinois

W. CONRAD LILES, MD, PhD
Professor and Vice-Chair of Medicine, Canada Research Chair in Inflammation; Director, Division of Infectious Diseases, Department of Medicine; SA Rotman Laboratories, McLaughlin-Rotman Centre for Global Health, Toronto General Hospital, University Health Network, University of Toronto, Toronto, Ontario, Canada

K. NOEL MASIHI, PhD
Robert Koch Institute, Berlin, Germany

JIGNESH MODI, MD
Fellow (PGY-1), Division of Infectious Diseases, Southern Illinois University School of Medicine, Springfield, Illinois

PRAVEEN K. MULLANGI, MD
Clinical Assistant Professor, Division of Infectious Diseases, Springfield Clinic, Springfield, Illinois

ANDREA V. PAGE, MD
Division of Infectious Diseases, Department of Medicine; SA Rotman Laboratories, McLaughlin-Rotman Centre for Global Health, Toronto General Hospital, University Health Network, University of Toronto, Toronto, Ontario, Canada

HEMDA ROSENBLUM, MD
Department of Medicine B, Zabludowicz Center for Autoimmune Diseases, Sheba Medical Center, Sackler Faculty of Medicine, Tel Aviv University, Ramat Aviv, Tel-Hashomer, Israel

ROBERT RZEPKA, MD
Fellow (PGY2), Division of Infectious Diseases, Southern Illinois University School of Medicine, Springfield, Illinois

NASIA SAFDAR, MD, PhD
Assistant Professor, Division of Infectious Disease, University of Wisconsin School of Medicine and Public Health, Madison, Wisconsin

CATHY SANTANELLO, PhD
Department of Pharmaceutical Sciences, Southern Illinois University Edwardsville School of Pharmacy, Edwardsville, Illinois

HUBERT SCHÄFER, PhD
Robert Koch Institute, Berlin, Germany

LOKESH SHAHANI, MD
Resident, Department of Internal Medicine, Southern Illinois University School of Medicine, Springfield, Illinois

YEHUDA SHOENFELD, MD, FRCP
Zabludowicz Center for Autoimmune Diseases, Sheba Medical Center, Sackler Faculty of Medicine, Tel Aviv University, Ramat Aviv, Tel-Hashomer, Israel

CRISTIAN SPEIL, MD
Assistant Professor, Division of Infectious Diseases, Southern Illinois University School of Medicine, Springfield, Illinois

VIDYA SUNDARESHAN, MD, MPH
Assistant Professor, Division of Infectious Diseases, Southern Illinois University School of Medicine, Springfield, Illinois

JAN ter MEULEN, MD, DTM&H
Executive Director, Vaccine Research, Merck Research Laboratories, Sumneytown Pike, West Point, Pennsylvania

ROBERT S. WALLIS, MD, FIDSA
Department of Specialty Care, Pfizer, Groton, Connecticut

Contents

> Biologic response modifiers (BRMs) are substances that occur naturally in the body. They can also be manufactured in the laboratory and then administered as targeted therapy. Undoubtedly BRMs will find expanded role in terminal illness like cancer where other therapies have failed. However, great caution must be exercised in prescribing these agents in chronic indolent diseases where potential for ultimate harm might outweigh short-term benefits.

> The conventional treatment of infectious agents is increasingly encountering antimicrobial resistance. This resistance has led to an intense search for novel treatment modalities for infectious diseases. Elucidation of the mechanisms underlying the inhibitory activity of chemokines has been instrumental in the rational design of anti–human immunodeficiency virus chemokine drugs. The immune-based therapies, in combination with antimicrobial drugs, for viral hepatitis have attracted much attention. Recognition of toll-like receptors by synthetic immunomodulators is used for certain viral infections. New methodologies have the potential to identify novel targets and foster the development of individually tailored immunomodulatory drug treatments.

> Biologic response modifiers (BRMs) interact with the host immune system and modify the immune response. BRMs can be therapeutically used to restore, augment, or dampen the host immune response. Although they have been used for decades, their clinical applications have been expanded in the past decade for diagnosis and treatment of many diseases including cancers, immunologic disorders, and infections. This article discusses endogenous biological response modifiers (ie, naturally occurring immunomodulators as a part of the host immune system), which play vital roles as regulators of both innate and adaptive immune responses.

> Vaccines have been used successfully for many years to prevent death and morbidity from infectious diseases. In the last two decades major

advances in the fields of genetics and immunology have allowed a significant increase in the use of immunomodulatory drugs in a broad range of pathologic conditions. This article reviews several uses of immunomodulating properties of vaccines, both old and new, with a focus on cancer and autoimmune diseases. Special emphasis is placed on the historical aspects and current applications of the bacillus Calmette-Guérin vaccine, the first vaccine to be used in cancer immunotherapy.

Jennifer L. Hsu and Nasia Safdar

Immunoglobulin therapy has a rich history of use in preventing and treating infectious diseases; however, clinical data on the efficacy of immunoglobulin is lacking for many infectious diseases. Immunoglobulin therapy is routinely used in postexposure prophylaxis for bacterial infections, including tetanus, botulism, and diphtheria, and viral infections, including hepatitis A and B and varicella. Immunoglobulin therapy has also been used in many severe and life-threatening infections where treatments are limited, including toxic shock syndrome, respiratory syncytial virus infection, and cytomegalovirus infection. The authors review the evidence for the use of immunoglobulin therapy in common adult infectious diseases.

Jan ter Meulen

Of the more than 20 monoclonal antibodies (mAbs) generated to combat infectious diseases (ID) that are in clinical development in 2011, most are in phase 1 or 2 and are directed against either viruses or bacterial toxins. Several high-profile anti-ID mAbs have recently failed in clinical trials. Despite the advancement in recombinant engineering technologies, anti-ID mAbs have yet to deliver on their promise as "magic bullets," especially against nosocomial infections. A paradigm shift in favor of developing mAb combinations, which act synergistically with each other or with small molecule drugs, may be required to move the field forward.

Andrea V. Page and W. Conrad Liles

Colony-stimulating factors (CSFs) are attractive adjunctive anti-infective therapies. Used to enhance innate host defenses against microbial pathogens, the myeloid CSFs increase absolute numbers of circulating innate immune effector cells by accelerating bone marrow production and maturation, or augment the function of those cells through diverse effects on chemotaxis, phagocytosis, and microbicidal functions. This article summarizes the evidence supporting the accepted clinical uses of the myeloid CSFs in patients with congenital or chemotherapy-induced neutropenia, and presents an overview of proposed and emerging uses of the CSFs for the prevention and treatment of infectious diseases in other immunosuppressed and immunocompetent patient populations.

This article explains the rationale for development of interferons as therapeutic agents, and describes commercial products available today. It also provides a summary of studies that have been performed with interferons for use as exogenous biological response modifiers in viral infections. Overall, the best data exist for treatment of viral hepatitis B and C, for which interferons are a cornerstone of therapy. Although infections with human papillomavirus and common cold viruses sometimes respond favorably to interferons, their outcomes are far from ideal. Finally, the role of interferons as vaccine adjuvants is still being explored but could be promising.

The systemic inflammatory response syndrome, the host's response to infection involves a series of cascading events that mobilize a series of mediators involving the immune system, complement, and the coagulation cascade. Although the initial focus of mediators is to limit infection, this cascade may run amok and cause the development of hypotension, vascular instability, and disseminated intravascular coagulation, leading to morbidity and mortality in the host. Several therapeutic trials have focused on the modulation of these mediators, but use of recombinant human activated protein C in patients with severe sepsis is the only one that has shown a benefit in clinical trials.

Chronic fatigue syndrome (CFS) is characterized by unexplained fatigue that lasts for at least 6 months with a constellation of other symptoms. Most cases start suddenly, and are usually accompanied by a flu-like illness. It is a symptom-based diagnosis of exclusion, the pathogenesis of which is unknown. Studies have examined and hypothesized about the possible biomedical and epidemiologic characteristics of the disease, including genetic predisposition, infections, endocrine abnormalities, and immune dysfunction and psychological and psychosocial factors. Recently, the AISA (autoimmune/inflammatory syndrome induced by adjuvants) syndrome was recognized, indicating the possible contribution of adjuvants and vaccines to the development of autoimmunity.

With increasing use of biological response modifiers (BRMs) for various systemic inflammatory diseases there is a need to be vigilant about complications with the use of these therapies. It is important to have appropriate screening for the infections in patients requiring BRMs. However, many studies have reported benefits of certain BRMs in the treatment of infections such as tuberculosis as adjuncts. Continued research and technical advances in immunogenetics helps understand complex mechanisms in the usage of the BRMs. This article summarizes the different aspects of the relationship between mycobacterial infections and the use of various BRMs for inflammatory conditions.

In the decade since tumor necrosis factor α (TNF-α) antagonists were first approved for clinical use, they have proven invaluable for the treatment of specific types of chronic inflammation. Currently licensed TNF blockers fall into two classes, monoclonal antibody (or antibody fragments) and soluble receptor. Although they are equally effective in rheumatoid arthritis and psoriasis, important differences have emerged with regard to efficacy in granulomatous inflammation and risks of granulomatous infections, particularly tuberculosis. This article focuses on recent studies that inform prevention and management of infections in this susceptible patient population.

VISIT THE CLINICS ONLINE!
Access your subscription at:
www.theclinics.com

Preface

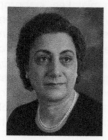

Nancy Misri Khardori, MD, PhD, FACP, FIDSA
Guest Editor

Biological response modifiers (BRMs) are often discussed with a narrow focus on the "biological therapies," ie, the pharmacologically administered form of cytokines, eg, interferon or antagonists of cytokines, eg, tumor necrosis factor blocking agents. In conceptualizing this issue of *Infectious Diseases Clinics of North America*, my focus was first and foremost, to make available to the readers a reference with up-to-date information on the endogenously produced BRM and their role in disease pathogenesis as well as in host defense, both of which determine the outcomes. These have been covered very well Khardori; Masihi and Schäfer; Mullangi and colleagues; and Sundareshan and colleagues. The second focus was on broadening the definition of BRMs particularly from the infectious diseases point of view. Historically, vaccination and administration of "anti-sera" raised in animals were the first and second attempts at modifying the interaction with microbial agents by augmenting the natural defenses. Speil and Rzepka discusses the role of vaccines and vaccine adjuvants not only in infectious diseases but more recently also in cancers and autoimmune disorders. Hsu and Safdar takes the readers from the early (pre-antibiotic) days of antitoxin sera raised in animals injected with the toxin to the current uses of polyclonal and hyperimmune globulins in the prevention and management of infectious diseases. This is followed by the discussion on the use of monoclonal antibodies in infectious diseases. In addition, Jan ter Meulen has provided extremely useful information on the pipeline of these agents for clinical use as of 2011.

The third focus was on detailing the use of BRM therapies in infectious disease as Vivek Kak discusses the failures of various immunologic biological response modifiers in sepsis and the modest if any improvement in outcome by the only clinically available agent, ie, recombinant activated protein C. Although this therapeutic agent provides triple intervention in the form of profibrinolytic, anticoagulant, and anti-inflammatory actions, the stage at which it is currently given is perhaps the stage of "no return". Rosenblum and colleagues highlights the complex interactions between infections, vaccines, vaccine adjuvants, and syndromes of unclear etiology. The last two articles discuss the fourth and the final focus, which is the fact that therapeutic BRMs are a two-edged sword. Their use involves evaluation of risk-benefit ratio and pre- and posttherapy preventive measures.

doi:10.1016/j.idc.2011.07.011
0891-5520/11/$ – see front matter © 2011 Elsevier Inc. All rights reserved.

id.theclinics.com

It seems every day more and more BRMs are being identified. The complexity and diversity of their interactions with the host continue to unravel. The following quote describes it all "I suspect that the host is caught up in mistaken, inappropriate and unquestionably self destructive mechanisms by the very multiplicity of defenses available to him, defenses which do not seem to have been designed to operate in net coordination with each other. The end result is not defense, it is an agitated 'committee directed, harum-scarum effort to make war'" (Louis Thomas, *The Immunopathology of Infection*, 1971). However, as in life in general, it seems most of the real work is done outside the "committees," which explains the success stories outnumbering adverse outcomes in infectious diseases. Human ingenuity made it possible that the prevention and management of infectious diseases contributed the most to the current state of human health and longevity.

It is obvious that this issue was made possible and of the highest quality because of the contributions made by the authors. However, I owe special thanks to Mrs Nancy Mutzbauer for the assistance she provided me in bringing this issue of *Infectious Disease Clinics of North America* to fruition.

Nancy Misri Khardori, MD, PhD, FACP, FIDSA
Division of Infectious Disease
Eastern Virginia Medical School
825 Fairfox Avenue
Norfolk, VA 23507, USA

E-mail address:
nkhardori@gmail.com

Biologic Response Modifiers: Relevance & Repercussions

Romesh Khardori, MD, PhD[a],*, Nancy Misri Khardori, MD, PhD, FIDSA[b]

KEYWORDS

- Biologic response modifiers • Terminal illness • Chronic illness

A defining characteristic of any living organism is the ability to react to its environment and readjust responses to bring itself back state of physiologic stability, loosely defined as homeostasis (*Greek: standing still*), a concept dating back to Claude Bernard in 1865 when explaining how blood glucose concentration stays within certain limits.[1] The term, however, was coined by WB Cannon, in 1926.[2] As a matter of fact, this reactive behavior is a biologic imperative to preserve the architecture and integrity of tissues in response to provocative stimuli. Nature of biologic response is often determined by the instigating stimulus. Response may be as simple as retraction of a podocyte in a unicellular organism to complex and well-coordinated electrophysiologic response that translates into release/secretion of products locally, as well as their transportation to distant sites for effects elsewhere in mulicellular species such as people. Electrophysiologic responses such as membrane depolarization leading to changes in action potential were studied long before secretory responses could be confirmed and quantified. It was the refinements in clinical chemistry/immunochemistry that led to current appreciation of how an organism reacts to external or internal threats by orchestrating a well-coordinated response that hinges vastly upon recruitment of various cellular components, secretion of various peptides, cytokines, chemokines, and induction of various protein kinases leading to shifts in balance of immunoregulatory cells depending up on the nature of threat. The products of this host and environment interaction that can be measured in blood and other biologic secretions are defined as biologic markers.

Average human body comprises of approximate 10^{13} eukaryotic cells with a microbial load of 10^{14}. Thus human body has to work continuously to maintain a state of homeostasis, which favors survival, averting threats that could potentially cause tissue damage or death.

[a] Division of Endocrinology & Metabolism, Eastern Virginia Medical School, 825 Fairfax Avenue, Norfolk, VA 23507, USA
[b] Division of Infectious Diseases, Eastern Virginia Medical School, 825 Fairfax Avenue, Norfolk, VA 23507, USA
* Corresponding author. 808 Wythe Road, Springfield, IL 62702.
E-mail address: rkhardori@gmail.com

Infect Dis Clin N Am 25 (2011) 719–722
doi:10.1016/j.idc.2011.07.001
0891-5520/11/$ – see front matter © 2011 Elsevier Inc. All rights reserved.

This effort involves several networks that lead to local and global response. Global response requires transportation of cells and cellular products through vast network of large and small blood vessels (capillaries). These blood vessels are not mere passive conduits. They allow diffusion of cells across their walls at the sites of injury to deliver the types of cells needed to contain the assault. A critical role is now being assigned to the blood volume, which is considered crucial in determining expression/repression of certain genes in the vessel wall and their products such as protein kinases that would affect/modify the immunoregulatory response downstream (*SAPK's* stretch activated protein kinases). The endothelial lining of blood vessels serve as repository of vast numbers of products that have important role beyond ensuring patency or activating cascade of coagulation when necessary. Throughout this issue elaborate lists are provided of various cytokines, chemokines and kinases, with assigned roles in biologic response (activating, modulating, suppressing). These mediators that affect/modify the cellular or humoral response are known as the biologic response modifiers (BRMs). They serve a purpose that is largely pro-survival. Therefore, neutralizing them by agents such as antibodies, kinase inhibitors, and immunosuppressants needs to be weighed carefully in any clinical decision-making. They have already entered therapeutic arena largely due to interest in containing disabling damages in certain autoimmune diseases such as rheumatoid arthritis, psoriasis, inflammatory bowel disease, and deadly cancers that have failed to respond to conventional chemotherapy.

Whenever there is a shift in equilibrium due to simple injury, infections, or emergence of mutant clones of cells, the immediate response is predictable. This typically involves an inflammatory response. It is essentially also a repair mechanism geared toward ensuring abrogation of the injury-provoking process that involves killing of pathogens, elimination of cells harboring pathogens, recruitment of stem cells to replace dead cells, and clearing debris. This repair process helps maintain cellular architecture that is both fresh and durable. A certain minimal degree of reparative process/inflammation may be an entirely desirable mechanism that keeps tissues healthy and protects against senescence. Thus the minimal normal reparative process permits constant turnover of cells, and this works quite favorably in maintaining skeletal health. If this process were to be suppressed, leading to an dynamic state, risk of spontaneous or even minimal trauma fractures would increase. Furthermore, this process allows for natural sculpting of bones favoring attributes such as certain architecture of cheek bones, shape of nose, and many other facial features that are considered desirable in certain cultures.

However, benefits of controlled low-grade inflammation would be offset if the response were exaggerated, leading to excessive elaboration of mediators (endogenous BRMs) that would hamper repair process and lead to undesirable outcomes. On the other hand, it would be equally damaging if exogenous agents (exogenous BRMs) were introduced too early in the process to suppress or neutralize endogenous mediators. Additionally, in states where intrinsic modifiers have an important role in containing a process in coexisting latent infection (such as granuloma formation or walling off in tuberculosis [TB]), exogenous BRM therapy is certainly fraught with reactivation of latent infection. Exogenous BRMs would have a definite role if they exclusively served the sole purpose of only suppressing the further amplification of endogenous response process. At present it is not clear when the process of repair changes to state of despair. If it were possible to know when this watermark is reached, use of BRMs would become more rational.

While the scope of identifying biomarkers has greatly expanded, and commercial assays are being introduced at a rapid pace, fundamental uncertainties exist in the interpretation and utility of these markers as therapeutic targets. A classical case would be the C-reactive protein (CRP). It was discovered by Tillett and Francis in 1930 as an acute-phase reactant that reacted with polysaccharide of *Pneumococcus*.[3] It is primarily produced in liver, and its circulating levels correspond to the severity of injury/infection. Its production correlates with concentrations of interleukin (IL)-6, a secretory product of macrophages as well as adipocytes. CRP binds to phospho-choline on microbes. It assists in complement binding to damaged cells and foreign proteins, assisting phagocytosis by macrophages that express a distinct CRP receptor. It also has a role in innate immunity as an early defense against infections. However, it has been viewed as collaborator in atherogenesis and diabetes and hence linked to cardiovascular disease/complication. This issue is far from settled, and the best evidence linking it to pathogenesis of diabetes and cardiovascular disease is still lacking. It has been proposed that higher concentrations of CRP might be patholog-ically intrinsic BRMs, a concept forwarded in the Justification for the Use of Statins in Primary Prevention: An Intervention Trial Evaluating Rosuvastatin trial, where patients with higher CRP concentration benefited the most with statin therapy in the absence of hyperlipidemia (statins are known to lower CRP concentration).[4] A subse-quent trial, however, failed to find any useful role for CRP in determining statin benefit.[5]

Nevertheless, study of BRMs and their therapeutic applications are not without merit. One area that has a proliferation of such agents in clinical therapeutics is oncology. Indeed an oncologist, William B. Coley, is considered father of BRMs based on his observation in 1893 that many cancer patients recovered after developing postopera-tive infections.[6] He concluded that fever/infection upregulated the immune system that recognizes and destroys cancer cells. Formally BRMs were first studied for cancer treatment in 1960 when bacillus Calmette-Gurrin and *Cornybacterium parvum* were used to boost immune system in cancer patients.[7] No one denies how the use of tyrosine kinase inhibitors in patients with chronic myeloid leukemia (CML) has changed the land-scape of this disease. Similarly, use of interferons in hairy cell leukemia, cutaneous T-cell lymphoma, and renal cell carcinoma has resulted in impressive outcomes.[8] However, interferon therapy has also been associated with development of thyroiditis, and there-fore warrants careful monitoring. Monoclonal antibodies used as BRMs are also not without risks. Discussion of these side effects is outside the scope of this article. Mono-clonal antibodies used as BRMs have found an increasing market share in treatment of rheumatoid arthritis, even when concern has been expressed about reactivation of latent infections. Thus, despite impressive clinical benefits in certain categories of patients who would otherwise suffer disabling complications, it remains to be resolved when is it most opportune to use these agents without risking adverse effects.

Limitations to use BRMs on a large scale include reactivation of dormant or latent infec-tions, interference with normal reparative processes, and unusually high cost of available agents. A recent meta-analysis of cost-effectiveness of BRMs compared with disease-modifying antirheumatic drugs (DMARDs) revealed that biologics are not cost-effective in adults at a cost-effectiveness threshold of $50,000 per quality-adjusted life-year (QALY).[9] However, this analysis is hindered by lack of data regarding long-term response and its consequences on downstream health care use and productivity.

Interest in BRMs has spawned interest in nutrients where deficiencies evoke a certain cascade of biologic response that is amenable to modification by correcting nutrient deficiencies. In this context, vitamins, particularly vitamins E and D seem to have generated buzz.

Again this research is still evolving, and at this writing vitamin D appears to be of greater interest.

Vitamin D deficiency has been linked to type-1 diabetes, and it is claimed that supplementation with vitamin D would be helpful in prevention efforts. The active metabolite of vitamin D, calcitriol, acts immunomodulator, which would in turn dampen autoimmune assault on the beta cell of pancreas. Calcitriol is also reported to play an important role in intracellular bacillary killing via induction of reactive oxygen species. The polymorphism of vitamin D receptor determines efficacy of calcitriol in this context.[10] This new role for vitamin D in intracellular bacillary killing puts recommending sanatoria for people with TB in perspective, where exposure to plenty of sunlight, fresh air, and adequate nutrition were highly emphasized.

SUMMARY

BRMs are substances that occur naturally in the body, such as cytokines, chemokines and antibodies, that help fight disease. BRMs can also be manufactured in the laboratory and then administered as targeted therapy. Given an important role for a reparative, low-grade inflammatory process in controlling undesirable growth of cells as well as elimination of pathogens, a balance needs to be struck such that unintended reactivation of diseases like TB does not occur. Undoubtedly BRMs will find expanded role in terminal illness like cancer where other therapies have failed. However, great caution must be exercised in prescribing these agents in chronic indolent diseases where potential for ultimate harm might outweigh short-term benefits. In the future, selective modulators with restricted activity would have to be designed so that impact is not felt beyond where target of therapy is located.

REFERENCES

1. Cannon WB. Physiological regulation of normal states: some tentative postulates concerning biological homeostasis. In: Pettit A, editor. A Charles Richet: ses anims, ses collegues, ses elves. Paris: editions Medicales; 1926. p. 91.
2. Cannon WB. Organization for physiological homeostasis. Physiol Rev 1929;9: 399–431.
3. Tillett WS, Francis T. Serological reactions in pneumonia and nonprotein somatic fraction of pneumococcus. J Exp Med 1939;52(4):561–85.
4. Ridker PM, Danielson E, Fonseca FA, et al. Rosuvastatin to prevent vascular events in men and women with elevated C-reactive protein. N Engl J Med 2008;359(21):2195–207.
5. HPS Collaborative Group. C-reactive protein concentration and the vascular benefits of statin therapy: an analysis of 20536 patients in heart protection study. Lancet 2011;377:469–76.
6. Bisht M, Bist SS, Dhasmana DC. Biologic response modifiers: current use and future prospects in cancer therapy. Indian J Cancer 2010;47:443–51.
7. Oettgen HF, Old LJ. The history of cancer immunotherapy. In: DeVita VT Jr, Hellman S, Rossenberg SA, editors. Biologic therapy of cancer. Philadelphia: Lippincott; 1991. p. 81–101.
8. Steiner A, Wolf C, Pehamberger H. Comparison of the effects of three different regimens of recombinant interferons(r-IFNa, r-IFNg, and r-IFNa + cimetidine) in disseminated malignant melanoma. J Cancer Res Clin Oncol 1987;113:459–65.
9. van der velde G, Machado M, Leraci L, et al. Cost-effectiveness of biologic response modifiers compared to disease modifying antirheumatic drugs for rheumatoid arthritis: a systemic review. Arthritis Care Res (Hoboken) 2011;63(1): 65–78.
10. Martineau AR, Timma PM, Botamley GH, et al. High-dose vitamin D3 during intensive phase antimicrobial treatment for pulmonary tuberculosis: a double blind randomized controlled trial. Lancet 2011;377:242–50.

Overview of Biologic Response Modifiers in Infectious Disease

K. Noel Masihi, PhD, Hubert Schäfer, PhD*

KEYWORDS

- Biological response modifiers • Immunomodulators
- Cytokines • Infections

Infectious diseases continue to impact human morbidity and mortality. The massive explosions of tourism, with an estimated 2 billion passengers each year on commercial airlines, and rapid globalization have facilitated the spread of disease-causing pathogens from one continent to another at unprecedented rates. According to the World Health Organization (WHO), at least 40 new diseases have emerged over the past 2 decades at a rate of 1 or more per year.

Antimicrobial drugs have been instrumental in saving the lives of millions of people worldwide. The effectiveness of many antibiotics is, however, being steadily eroded by the emergence of drug-resistant microorganisms,[1] with the WHO declaring that antibiotic resistance is among the 3 greatest challenges to human health. About 25,000 patients die each year in the European Union from infections with multidrug-resistant bacteria according to the European Medicines Agency causing extra health care costs and productivity losses of at least €1.5 billion each year. Crucial drug choices for the treatment of common infections by bacteria, viruses, parasites, and fungi are becoming limited and even nonexistent in some cases.[2] This development has not been paralleled by an effective increase in the discovery of new drugs for most pathogens, and the rate of new antimicrobials approvals is steadily dropping. The struggle to control infectious diseases, far from being over, has acquired a new poignancy. Novel concepts acting as adjunct to established therapies are urgently needed.

The immune system can be manipulated specifically by vaccination *or* nonspecifically by immunomodulation. Biologic response modifiers or immunomodulators include both immunostimulatory and immunosuppressive agents. This article concentrates on immunostimulatory agents capable of enhancing host defense mechanisms to provide protection against infections. Other synonymous terms for biologic response modifiers include immunostimulants, immunoaugmentors, or immunorestoratives.

The authors have nothing to disclose.
Robert Koch Institute, Nordufer 20, D-13353 Berlin, Germany
* Corresponding author.
E-mail address: schaeferh@rki.de

Infect Dis Clin N Am 25 (2011) 723–731
doi:10.1016/j.idc.2011.07.002
0891-5520/11/$ – see front matter © 2011 Elsevier Inc. All rights reserved.

Their modes of action include augmentation of anti-infectious immunity by the cells of the immune system encompassing lymphocyte subsets, macrophages, dendritic, and natural killer cells. Further mechanisms can involve induction or restoration of immune effector functions and tilting the balance toward cytokine pathways germane to protection. A diverse array of recombinant, synthetic, and natural immunomodulatory preparations for prophylaxis and treatment of various infections are available today.[3–6]

CYTOKINE IMMUNOMODULATORS

Cytokines, hormonelike polypeptides possessing pleiotropic properties, are crucial in orchestrating the appropriate immune responses critical for the outcome of an infection. Certain cytokines stimulate the production of other cytokines and interact in synergistic or antagonistic networks enabling manipulation of the host response to enhance overall immunogenicity and direct the nature of the response either toward type 1 or type 2 pathways. In the type 1 response, Th1 cells produce interferon (IFN)-γ, tumor necrosis factor (TNF), and interleukin (IL)-12 that are required for effective development of cell-mediated immune responses to intracellular microbes. In the type 2 response, Th2 cells produce IL-4, IL-5, and IL-13 that enhance humoral immunity to T-dependent antigens and are necessary for immunity to helminth infections. Recent studies have shown that toll-like receptors (TLR), mainly found on dendritic cells (DCs) and macrophages, are important in the transition from innate to adaptive immunity.

In humans, DCs are subdivided into plasmacytoid DCs, which secrete copious amounts of IFN-α, and myeloid DCs. Both subtypes of DCs recognize diverse microbial pathogens through specific TLR. Local and systemic effects of cytokines are, thus, intimately involved in the host control of infections. Several recombinant and natural cytokine preparations, such as interferons and granulocyte colony-stimulating factor, are already licensed for use in patients.

INTERFERONS AND COMBINATIONS

IFN was the first cytokine to be produced by the recombinant DNA technology. There are 2 classes of IFN: type I and type II. The type I IFN is produced in response to viral infection and includes IFN-α and IFN-β. Most of the IFN-α in humans is released by plasmacytoid dendritic cells, whereas IFN-β is produced by fibroblasts and many other cell types. The type II IFN is secreted by activated T cells and NK cells as IFN-γ, also known as immune interferon.

IFN-α is a clinically effective therapy used in a wide range of viral infections besides its application in malignant melanoma, basal cell carcinoma, and warts. Natural IFN-α obtained from human serum and leukocytes is currently licensed for the treatment of a rare form of cancer, hairy cell leukemia. Recombinant IFN-α2a is licensed for the treatment of chronic hepatitis B and hepatitis C virus infections.

Standard IFN-α has the drawbacks of a short serum half-life and rapid clearance. To overcome this problem, pegylated forms of IFN (PegIntron or Pegasys) have been developed and tested clinically. The greater polymer size of pegylated IFN acts to reduce glomerular filtration, markedly prolonging its serum half-life (72–96 hours) compared with standard IFN (6–9 hours).[7]

Hepatitis B virus (HBV) infection is widespread throughout the world, infecting around 400 million people and killing between 1.0 and 2.5 million people a year. The virus, transmitted by blood and body fluids, is up to 100 times more infectious than human immunodeficiency virus (HIV). Overall, 15% to 25% of HBV carriers die of chronic hepatitis, cirrhosis, or hepatocellular carcinoma (which accounts for up to 90% of all liver cancers).

At present, licensed therapies widely used for treating liver disease caused by HBV include IFN-α and the antiviral drugs lamivudine, adefovir, and entecavir.[8] Most of these therapies are limited in the clinic by a low response rate, with only a small subset of patients with hepatitis B attaining a long-term response.

Several promising studies have shown the effectiveness of pegylated interferon combination therapy with lamivudine or adefovir[9] with a better cost-benefit ratio. Interferon-α is also approved for treating condyloma acuminata caused by human papilloma virus and for Kaposi sarcoma in patients with HIV infection. Besides pegylated interferon, newer drug formulations demonstrated in clinical trials to be active against HBV include tenofovir, telbivudine, and clevudine.

Hepatitis C virus (HCV) is the major etiologic agent of posttransfusion and community-acquired non-A, non-B hepatitis infecting more than 200 million people worldwide. Combination therapy with pegylated IFN and ribavirin is the current standard of care for the treatment of chronic HCV infection. Recently, patients with a particular polymorphism of a gene called *IL28B* have been shown to respond more favorably to treatment.[10] The Food and Drug Administration (FDA) is expected to approve 2 protease inhibitors, telaprevir and boceprevir, in 2011 as the next generation of anti-HCV treatment.

IFN-β obtained from human FS-4 fibroblast cell lines is licensed for use in severe uncontrolled virus-mediated diseases in cases of viral encephalitis, herpes zoster, and varicella in immunosuppressed patients. A further indication is viral infection of the inner ear with loss of hearing. The standard treatment of multiple sclerosis, a disease without definitively elucidated etiology, is currently IFN-β.

IFN-γ is the major mediator of host resistance during the acute and chronic phases of infection and is pivotal in the protection against a variety of intracellular pathogens. Multicenter clinical trials have shown that sustained administration of IFN-γ to patients with chronic granulomatous disease markedly reduces the relative risk of serious infection. IFN-γ is licensed as a therapeutic adjunct for use in patients with chronic granulomatous disease for the reduction of the frequency of serious infections. Imukin and Actimmune are IFN-γ preparations marketed for chronic granulomatous disease, mycobacterial, and fungal infections. The major side effects of all interferon therapies include flulike syndromes, fever, myalgia, headache, and fatigue. Hypotension, granulocytopenia, and thrombocytopenia can also occur. Deleterious effects on the central nervous system, particularly at high doses, have been observed.

CYTOKINE INHIBITORS

Several host strategies exist for responding to infection. One mechanism by which the host attempts to restrain the infection is through the upregulation of cytokines. Some cytokines, such as IL-1, IL-6, IL-8, IL-18, and TNF, may worsen the disease in an effort to rid the host of infection. Overproduction of proinflammatory cytokines is thought to underlie the progression of many inflammatory diseases, including rheumatoid arthritis, Crohn disease, and sepsis syndrome. Many infectious diseases, including HIV, influenza H5N1, and malaria, can induce deleterious overproduction of proinflammatory cytokines.

Intense interest has been generated in developing agents that can block the activity of such cytokines. Inhibition of TNF activity has been singularly successful in the treatment of autoimmune diseases. Monoclonal antibodies, including adalimumab (Humira; Abbott), (Enbrel; Amgen/Wyeth), infliximab (Remicade; Centocor), and Certolizumab pegol, are used in the treatment of rheumatoid arthritis. An IL-1 receptor antagonist, Kineret, has also been licensed. Some of these monoclonal antibody products have shown promise for applications in disease management in patients with HIV/AIDS.[11,12]

Another potent TNF inhibitor, thalidomide, has been used in trials in patients with HIV.[13] More recently, thalidomide and its immunomodulatory imide analogues, such as Actimid, Lenalidomide, Pomalidomide and Revlimid, have been used as antiinflammatory drugs.

Pentoxifylline, a methylxanthine usually used in the treatment of peripheral arterial circulatory disorders, has been shown to inhibit TNF synthesis. Pentoxifylline has been used in patients with HIV for improving endothelial functions and reducing levels of vascular cell adhesion molecule-1 and IFN-γ–induced protein.[14] Currently, clinical trials are ongoing with phosphodiesterase inhibitors and small-molecule inhibitors of the TNF-converting enzymes that specifically interrupt the signaling pathways of TNF.

TNF plays an important role in the defense against bacterial and viral infections. Consequently, many patients on anti-TNF drug therapy have developed severe infections, such as tuberculosis.[15] A variety of opportunistic fungal infections, including *Candida*, *Aspergillus Pneumocystis*, *Coccidioides*, and *Histoplasma*, have also been reported in patients treated with anti-TNF monoclonals.[16]

Sepsis is one of the most common complications in surgical patients and one of the leading causes of mortality in intensive care units. Sepsis can be caused by infection with gram-negative bacteria, gram-positive bacteria, fungi, or viruses. Sepsis may, however, also occur in the absence of detectable bacterial invasion. In such cases, microbial toxins, particularly gram-negative bacterial endotoxin, and endogenous cytokine release have been implicated as initiators and mediators. Septic shock represents the most severe form of host response to infection. Despite recent progress in antibiotics and critical care therapy, sepsis is still associated with a high mortality rate ($\sim$40%–50%) and remains the 10th leading cause of death in Western countries. Several therapies delaying the onset or reducing the effects of proinflammatory cytokines induced during sepsis are under development. TAK-242 (resatorvid), a small molecule antagonist of TLR 4 signaling, reduces the lipopolysaccharide (LPS)-induced production of proinflammatory IL-1, IL-6, and TNF and is currently undergoing phase III evaluation.[17] Another compound, E5564 (eritoran), is a synthetic molecule derived from the nonpathogenic *Rhodobacter sphaeroides* and was observed to reduce TNF and IL-6 levels after LPS administration.[48,18] Eritoran is under evaluation in a phase III study in patients with severe sepsis.

CHEMOKINES AND CHEMOKINE MODULATORS

Chemokines have been historically regarded as leukocyte chemoattractants capable of regulating cellular trafficking into inflammatory sites. The sobriquet chemokine is abbreviated from *chemo*tactic cyto*kine*. The major classes of chemokines are constituted by the CXC or α chemokines, the CC or β chemokines, the C or γ chemokines, and the CX3C chemokines. The nomenclature of the chemokines is based on the spacing of 2 critical cystine residues near the amino terminus, indicating no (CC) or 1 (CXC) or 3 (CX3C) amino acids acids between the first 2 cysteines near the amino terminus. The chemokine family has expanded to 80 ligands, including CXCL; CCL; XCL; and CX3CL chemokines; and chemokine receptors, including CXCR, CCR, XCR, and CX3CR.

Many erudite reviews on the cause and manifestation of HIV/AIDS have been published, and these are not be dealt with here. It is noteworthy that currently there are more women worldwide who have been infected with HIV than men, and women account for nearly half of more than 40 million people living with HIV.[19] Women are more vulnerable to HIV infection than men, and their increased susceptibility has been linked to the use of hormonal contraceptives and sexually transmitted diseases. Also, susceptibility to HIV varies throughout a woman's reproductive life; adolescent girls seem to be most vulnerable to HIV because of high-risk sexual behavior and a not fully mature reproductive system. In addition, recent studies have indicated increases in the risk of acquiring HIV during pregnancy and during the early postpartum period, part of which could be attributed to higher levels of progesterone. Successful control of the HIV pandemic requires continuing focus on gender. Some of the fundamental issues of HIV transmission have been riddled with problems because it is neither feasible to obtain nor to examine relevant cells and tissue at the precise time of HIV acquisition.

The binding of the HIV envelope glycoprotein gp120 to CD4 and appropriate chemokine receptors triggers conformational changes facilitating the fusion of the viral and host cell membranes. Chemokine receptors (mainly CCR5 and CXCR4) have been discovered to be necessary as coreceptors for HIV entry.[20] HIV found in the vaginal and rectal mucosa is mainly CCR5 dependent. Macrophage-tropic (R5) HIV variants predominantly make use of the CCR5 coreceptors. The T cell–tropic (X4) and dual-tropic (R5X4) HIV strains, generally associated with the clinical manifestations of AIDS, emerge after a latency of several years; although pathogenesis of the central nervous system and related symptoms are normally associated with M-tropic (R5) HIV strains. X4 HIV infection augments the expression of chemokines, such as macrophage inflammatory protein-1α and RANTES (regulated upon activation normal T cell expressed and secreted).[21]

HIV infection can be inhibited by chemokines and chemokine-related molecules that are ligands for receptors that function as coreceptors. Chemokine receptors, thus, represent important targets for intervention in HIV, and search for molecules that have therapeutic potential as inhibitors of these receptors has been intense.[22] Intervention strategies based on chemokine antagonists that could be useful for the therapy for HIV include receptor-ligand interaction, prevention of the chemokine-glycosaminoglycan interaction, interfering with the signaling pathways that are induced upon receptor activation, and modification of receptor pathways.[23]

TARGETING CCR5 AND CXCR4

The chemokine receptors CXCR4 and CCR5 are the main coreceptors used respectively by T-cell–tropic (CXCR4-using, X4) and macrophage-tropic (CCR5-using, R5) HIV for cell entry. Several compounds targeting CXCR4 and CCR5 have been recently advocated. The idea for the drug class came from the observation that presence of mutated CCR5 can confer resistance to HIV infection, even after exposure to numerous high-risk sexual partners. Only around 2% of Caucasians carry such a mutation.

Modified chemokines with antiviral activity, several low-molecular weight CXCR4 and CCR5 antagonistic compounds, have been described. Maraviroc, developed by Pfizer as a CCR5 antagonist, was licensed in 2007 by the FDA for use in treatment-experienced patients with HIV harboring only R5 viruses. Another chemokine (CCR5) inhibitor, Aplaviroc or GSK 873,140, was developed by GlaxoSmithKline, but studies were discontinued because of liver toxicity concerns. Other companies working on CCR5 antagonists include Pfizer Inc and Schering-Plough Corporation.

Plerixafor (AMD3100, Mozobil), a bicyclam compound, targets CXCR4 and has a potent anti-HIV activity against T-tropic viruses. It is used in combination with granulocyte colony-stimulating factor (G-CSF) to enhance mobilization of hematopoietic stem cells in transplantation patients with non-Hodgkin lymphoma or multiple myeloma and has a good safety profile. It has marketing authorization in 33 countries worldwide, including the European Union and the United States, and is commercially available in 12 countries. A derivative AMD3451, pyridinylmethyl monocyclam, has been synthesized and reported to show dual CCR5/CXCR4 antagonistic activity against both X4 and R5 HIV strains.[24]

Most existing HIV drugs work inside the body's immune cells after the virus has infected and can cause anemia, diarrhea, and nerve pain. New drugs could provide an important treatment option for people with HIV/AIDS, by offering a different mode of action and an improved toxicity profile. Both CXCR4 and CCR5 chemokine receptor inhibitors may be needed in combination and even in combinations with antiviral drugs that also target other aspects of the HIV replication cycle to obtain optimum antiviral therapeutic effects.

COLONY-STIMULATING FACTORS

G-CSF preparations, such as filgrastim, can significantly enhance neutrophil functions. A high proportion of patients infected with HIV has neutropenia, which considerably increases the risk for bacterial and fungal infections. Filgrastim was granted license extension to cover the treatment of persistent neutropenia at an advanced stage of HIV infection.[25] In one study conducted at 27 European centers on patients with AIDS with cytomegalovirus infection, G-CSF (lenograstim) was found to be suitable for the treatment of ganciclovir-induced neutropenia.[26] Recently developed recombinant human G-CSF, pegfilgrastim, has been shown to be associated with a lower risk of neutropenia-related hospitalizations.[27]

G-CSF and granulocyte-macrophage colony-stimulating factor (GM-CSF) are used to reverse leukopenia as adjunctive therapy for HIV-associated infections. The GM-CSF preparation sargramostim helps overcome defects in neutrophil and macrophage function because of its broad range of effects on lymphocytes, macrophages, neutrophils, and dendritic cells. It enhances the antiretroviral activity of zidovudine and stavudine in macrophages and ameliorates the hematologic side effects of these agents. Multiple deficiencies are involved in the progression of fungal infections in patients with cancer with or without neutropenia. Although clinical experience is still limited, G-CSF, GM-CSF, and macrophage colony-stimulating factor show promise as adjuvant therapy for fungal infections.

SYNTHETIC IMMUNOMODULATORS

Microbial pathogens possess a variety of evolutionarily conserved structural motifs known as pathogen-associated molecular patterns (PAMPs). These PAMPS are recognized by a family of specific TLRs. Around 13 TLRs exhibiting distinct ligand specificities have been identified in humans. TLR2 recognizes bacterial peptidoglycan and lipopeptide, TLR3 recognizes double-stranded RNA, TLR4 binds to lipopolysaccharide, and TLR5 binds to flagellin that is part of the flagellum that propels many kinds of bacteria. TLR7 and TLR8 recognize imidazoquinoline compounds and single-stranded RNA from viruses, whereas TLR9 binds to unmethylated CpG DNA motifs frequently found in the genome of bacteria and viruses.

In humans, TLR7 and TLR9 are expressed on the plasmacytoid dendritic cells, which can rapidly synthesize large amounts IFN-α and IFN-β in response to viral infection. Interestingly, TLR7 recognizes synthetic immunomodulators, such as imiquimod (a fully synthetic immune response–enhancing imidazoquinoline amine),[28] that are used against viral infections. Imiquimod is marketed as Aldara for genital warts caused by the human papillomavirus subtypes number 6 and 11, but is widely used for basal cell carcinoma, actinic keratosis, and molluscum contagiosum. It has shown promise in lentigo maligna and cutaneous metastases of malignant melanoma.

Emerging Therapies with Synthetic Immunomodulators

Antimicrobial peptides

Antimicrobial peptides (AMPs), also known as host defense peptides, are mainly present in phagocytic cells of the immune system and are rapidly mobilized. AMPs demonstrate potent antimicrobial activity and can kill a wide array of gram-positive and gram-negative bacteria, enveloped viruses, fungi, and parasites through disruption of microbial membranes. Of clinical significance is the ability of AMPs to kill multidrug-resistant microorganisms.[29] Two AMPs have been shown in phase III clinical trials to be effective. Pexiganan has been developed for topical treatment of patients with mild diabetic foot infection and can cure approximately 90% of the patients. The other AMP, omiganan, has shown efficacy in preventing catheter-related infections.

Defensins

Defensins are polypeptides of the innate immune system produced in response to microbial infection in humans and animals. Recent reports have highlighted the anti-HIV activities of defensins, whose structure and charge resemble portions of the HIV-1 transmembrane envelope glycoprotein gp41. CD8 T cells from long-term non-progressors with HIV infection were found to secrete a cluster of proteins identified as α-defensin 1, 2, and 3. A study of seronegative women who were exposed constantly to HIV-1 demonstrated that their CD8$^+$ cells exhibit extensive α-defensin production at both peripheral and mucosal levels. The α-defensin expression level in these seronegative women was 10-fold higher than that of control subjects.[30] Likewise, overexpression of α-defensins in breast milk results in a low rate of HIV-1 transmission from mother to infant.[31]

HIV induces β-defensin-2 and 3 in human oral epithelial cells that exhibit strong anti-HIV activity because of the direct antiviral effect or competition for the chemokine receptors that HIV uses to enter the cell.[32] Mother-to-child transmission of HIV is the main source of pediatric AIDS. There is a significant relationship between genetic variants of the β-defensin-1 gene, viral load, and mother-to-child transmission of HIV. In mothers, the -52GG genotype is associated with low levels of HIV plasma viremia and a lower risk of maternal HIV transmission.[33]

Defensins are known to exhibit inhibitory activity against several viruses. The α-defensins promote the uptake of the influenza virus by neutrophils, and human defensins 5 and 6 are effective in neutralizing the influenza virus.[34] The expression of murine β-defensin was enhanced in influenza-infected lungs, trachea, and nasal mucosa[35]; and the treatment of cell cultures with human neutrophil peptides soon after infection resulted in marked inhibition of influenza virus replication and viral protein synthesis.[36] BK virus is a polyomavirus that establishes a lifelong persistence in most humans. Studies have shown that human α-defensins can inhibit BK virus infection,[37] inhibit adenovirus infection,[38] and α-defensins and human β-defensin–inhibited herpes simplex virus infection.[39]

REFERENCES

1. Gottlieb T, Nimmo GR. Antibiotic resistance is an emerging threat to public health: an urgent call to action at the Antimicrobial Resistance Summit 2011. Med J Aust 2011;194:281–3.

2. Amyes SG. The rise in bacterial resistance is partly because there have been no new classes of antibiotics since the 1960s. BMJ 2000;320:199–200.
3. Hengel H, Masihi KN. Combinatorial immunotherapies for infectious diseases. Int Immunopharmacol 2003;3:1–9.
4. Kayser O, Masihi KN, Kiderlen AF. Natural products and synthetic compounds as immunomodulators. Expert Rev Anti Infect Ther 2003;1:319–35.
5. Masihi KN. Immunomodulatory agents for prophylaxis and therapy of infections. Int J Antimicrob Agents 2000;14:181–91.
6. Masihi KN. Fighting infection using immunomodulatory agents. Expert Opin Biol Ther 2001;1:641–53.
7. Luxon BA, Grace M, Brassard D, et al. Pegylated interferons for the treatment of chronic hepatitis C infection. Clin Ther 2002;24:1363–83.
8. Brunetto MR, Lok AS. New approaches to optimize treatment responses in chronic hepatitis B. Antivir Ther 2010;15:61–8.
9. Villa E, Lei B, Taliani G, et al. Pretreatment with pegylated interferon prevents emergence of lamivudine mutants in lamivudine-naive patients: a pilot study. Antivir Ther 2009;14:1081–7.
10. Wapner J. Gene variants affect hepatitis C treatment, but link is elusive. Science 2010;330:579.
11. Ting PT, Koo JY. Use of etanercept in human immunodeficiency virus (HIV) and acquired immunodeficiency syndrome (AIDS) patients. Int J Dermatol 2006;45:689–92.
12. Cepeda EJ, Williams FM, Ishimori ML, et al. The use of anti-tumour necrosis factor therapy in HIV-positive individuals with rheumatic disease. Ann Rheum Dis 2008;67:710–2.
13. Johnson L, Jarvis JN, Wilkins EG, et al. Thalidomide treatment for refractory HIV-associated colitis: a case series. Clin Infect Dis 2008;47:133–6.
14. Gupta SK, Johnson RM, Mather KJ, et al. Anti-inflammatory treatment with pentoxifylline improves HIV-related endothelial dysfunction: a pilot study. AIDS 2010;24(9):1377–80.
15. Strangfeld A, Listing J. Infection and musculoskeletal conditions: bacterial and opportunistic infections during anti-TNF therapy. Best Pract Res Clin Rheumatol 2006;20:1181–95.
16. Tsiodras S, Samonis G, Boumpas DT, et al. Fungal infections complicating tumor necrosis factor alpha blockade therapy. Mayo Clin Proc 2008;83:181–94.
17. Rice TW, Wheeler AP, Bernard GR, et al. A randomized, double-blind, placebo-controlled trial of TAK-242 for the treatment of severe sepsis. Crit Care Med 2010;38:1685–94.
18. Tidswell M, Tillis W, Larosa SP, et al. Phase 2 trial of eritoran tetrasodium (E5564), a toll-like receptor 4 antagonist, in patients with severe sepsis. Eritoran Sepsis Study Group. Crit Care Med 2010;38:72–83.
19. Quinn TC, Overbaugh J. HIV/AIDS in women: an expanding epidemic. Science 2005;308:1582–3.
20. Dragic T. An overview of the determinants of CCR5 and CXCR4 co-receptor function. J Gen Virol 2001;82:1807–14.
21. Wetzel MA, Steele AD, Henderson EE, et al. The effect of X4 and R5 HIV-1 on C, C-C, and C-X-C chemokines during the early stages of infection in human PBMCs. Virology 2002;292:6–15.
22. Lusso P. HIV and chemokines: implications for therapy and vaccine. Vaccine 2002;20:1964–7.

23. Proudfoot AE, Power CA, Rommel C, et al. Strategies for chemokine antagonists as therapeutics. Semin Immunol 2003;15:57–65.
24. Princen K, Hatse S, Vermeire K, et al. Inhibition of human immunodeficiency virus replication by a dual CCR5/CXCR4 antagonist. J Virol 2004;78:12996–3006.
25. Welch W, Foote M. The use of filgrastim in AIDS-related neutropenia. J Hematother Stem Cell Res 1999;8(Suppl 1):S9–16.
26. Dubreuil-Lemaire ML, Gori A, Vittecoq D, et al. Lenograstim for the treatment of neutropenia in patients receiving ganciclovir for cytomegalovirus infection: a randomised, placebo-controlled trial in AIDS patients. Eur J Haematol 2000; 65:337–43.
27. Tan H, Tomic K, Hurley D, et al. Comparative effectiveness of colony-stimulating factors for febrile neutropenia: a retrospective study. Curr Med Res Opin 2011; 27:79–86.
28. Stanley MA. Imiquimod and the imidazoquinolones: mechanism of action and therapeutic potential. Clin Exp Dermatol 2002;27:571–7.
29. Kruse T, Kristensen HH. Using antimicrobial host defense peptides as anti-infective and immunomodulatory agents. Expert Rev Anti Infect Ther 2008;6: 887–95.
30. Trabattoni D, Caputo SL, Maffeis G, et al. Human alpha defensin in HIV-exposed but uninfected individuals. J Acquir Immune Defic Syndr 2004;35:455–63.
31. Kuhn L, Trabattoni D, Kankasa C, et al. Alpha-defensins in the prevention of HIV transmission among breastfed infants. J Acquir Immune Defic Syndr 2005;39: 138–42.
32. Garzino-Demo A. Chemokines and defensins as HIV suppressive factors: an evolving story. Curr Pharm Des 2007;13:163–72.
33. Ricci E, Malacrida S, Zanchetta M, et al. Role of beta-defensin-1 polymorphisms in mother-to-child transmission of HIV-1. J Acquir Immune Defic Syndr 2009;51:13–9.
34. Doss M, White MR, Tecle T, et al. Interactions of alpha-, beta-, and theta-defensins with influenza A virus and surfactant protein D. J Immunol 2009;182:7878–87.
35. Chong KT, Thangavel RR, Tang X. Enhanced expression of murine beta-defensins (MBD-1, -2, -3, and -4) in upper and lower airway mucosa of influenza virus infected mice. Virology 2008;380:136–43.
36. Salvatore M, Garcia-Sastre A, Ruchala P, et al. Alpha-defensin inhibits influenza virus replication by cell-mediated mechanism(s). J Infect Dis 2007;196:835–43.
37. Dugan AS, Maginnis MS, Jordan JA, et al. Human alpha-defensins inhibit BK virus infection by aggregating virions and blocking binding to host cells. J Biol Chem 2008;283:31125–32.
38. Smith JG, Nemerow GR. Mechanism of adenovirus neutralization by Human alpha-defensins. Cell Host Microbe 2008;3:11–9.
39. Hazrati E, Galen B, Lu W, et al. Human alpha- and beta-defensins block multiple steps in herpes simplex virus infection. J Immunol 2006;177:8658–66.

Role of Endogenous Biological Response Modifiers in Pathogenesis of Infectious Diseases

Praveen K. Mullangi, MD[a], Lokesh Shahani, MD[b],
Janak Koirala, MD, MPH[c],*

KEYWORDS

- Biological response modifiers • Pathogenesis
- Immune response • Infection

Biological response modifiers (BRMs), or immunomodulators, are agents that interact with the host immune system and mediate various aspects of immune response.[1] BRMs have been used as a therapeutic modality for more than 40 years. The attenuated vaccine strain of mycobacteria (bacillus Calmette-Guerin [BCG]) was the first BRM used for bladder cancer.[2] Similarly, other bacteria and their derivatives, such as *Corynebacterium parvum* and lipopolysaccharides (LPSs), have been used as BRMs for their stimulatory effects on the immune system.[3] These BRMs are derived from the external environment and are therapeutically administered for their biological effects and therefore can be designated as exogenous BRMs. In contrast, the substances that are produced within the host's internal environment as a result of the natural immunologic response to various internal and external stimuli are referred to as endogenous BRMs. With the advances in immunology and better understanding of immunologic processes, various endogenous BRMs are being used and studied for the treatment of cancer, infections, and immunologic disorders. Common examples include interferon (IFN)-α, used for treatment of hepatitis B and C, and interleukin (IL)-2 for renal cancer and melanoma.

The authors have nothing to disclose.

[a] Division of Infectious Diseases, Springfield Clinic, 301 North 8th Street, Springfield, IL 62701, USA

[b] Department of Internal Medicine, Southern Illinois University, School of Medicine, PO Box 19636, Springfield, IL 62794-9636, USA

[c] Division of Infectious Diseases, Southern Illinois University, School of Medicine, PO Box 19636, Springfield, IL 62794-9636, USA

* Corresponding author.

E-mail address: jkoirala@siumed.edu

Infect Dis Clin N Am 25 (2011) 733–754
doi:10.1016/j.idc.2011.07.003
0891-5520/11/$ – see front matter © 2011 Elsevier Inc. All rights reserved.

id.theclinics.com

This article discusses various endogenous biological response modifiers produced during innate and adaptive immune responses, and describes 2 clinically important groups of BRMs (IFNs and ILs), and reviews the roles of BRMs in the pathogenesis of different types of infection.

BRMs AND INNATE IMMUNE RESPONSE

When exposed to external stimuli, such as microbial, toxin, or allergenic structures, the host's innate immune system initially recognizes the unique molecular patterns as foreign and responds by inducing a cascade of effector immune responses. Subsequently, the specific adaptive immune response occurs. The mediators of adaptive response are encoded by genes that are rearranged somatically to assemble antigen-binding molecules specific for individual antigenic structure. After the primary immune response, certain adaptive immune cells persist in a dormant form known as memory cells that are capable of responding rapidly during the subsequent exposure to the same antigens.[4]

The cellular components of the innate immune system consist of hematopoietic cells including macrophages, dendritic cells, neutrophils, eosinophils, mast cells, natural killer (NK) cells, and natural killer T (NK-T) cells. In addition, the epithelial linings of skin, respiratory tract, genitourinary tract, and gastrointestinal tract participate in the innate immune response. The humoral components of innate immunity consist of complement components, antimicrobial peptides (eg, defensins), pentraxins (eg, C-reactive protein [CRP] and PTX3), collectins, and ficolins.[5] The humoral innate immune system performs tasks such as activation and regulation of the complement cascade, agglutination and neutralization, facilitation of recognition via cellular receptors (opsonization), and regulation of the inflammatory response.[6]

The first challenge for the innate immune system is to recognize nonself molecular structures, for which it largely relies on the germline encoded receptors. These nonself, conserved molecular structures, also known as pathogen-associated molecular patterns (PAMPs), are present on a diverse group of microbes, toxins, and other antigens.[7,8] The Toll-like receptors (TLRs) present on human cells allow the innate system to recognize extracellular or engulfed (inside endocytic vesicles) pathogens and respond to microbial epitopes by inducing a cascade of effector immune responses.[5] Similarly, nucleotide oligomerization domain (NOD)–like receptors (NLRs) sense intracellular microbial products, such as peptidoglycans and metabolic stresses of infection and inflammation. These NLRs form large cytosolic complexes called inflammosomes, which result in proteolytic activation of the proinflammatory cytokines IL-1β and IL-18.[9] In addition to PAMPs, the innate immune system is also able to detect damage-associated molecular patterns (DAMPs). DAMP molecules are upregulated and released as a result of tissue damage during inflammation and infection. Examples of DAMPs include heat shock proteins, uric acid and endogenous alarmins such as high mobility group box-1 (HMGB-1).[5,8]

Deficiencies or functional impairment of TLR receptors and accessory molecules necessary for recognition by the innate immune system can result in impaired innate immune response. For example, a deficiency of TLR-adapter protein, myeloid differentiation primary response gene (MyD88), increases risks for pyogenic bacterial infections, such as Streptococcus pneumoniae, Staphylococcus aureus, and Pseudomonas aeruginosa.[5] Similarly, the role of TLR-4 is important in recognition of LPS during an acute infection by gram-negative bacteria. Deficiency of IL-1 receptor associated kinase 4 (IRAK4), which is important for TLR function, is associated with severely impaired immune response to viral and bacterial challenge.[10]

Immunomodulators, such as imiquimod and resiquimod, use TLRs (TLR 7 and TLR 7/8, respectively), activate innate immune cells to produce IFN-α and other cytokines, and induce antigen-specific cell-mediated immune responses.[11]

Antigen-presenting cells (APCs) functionally serve as a part of both innate and adaptive immune responses. Once the antigens are phagocytosed by the APCs, they are metabolized, inserted into MHC Class II complex proteins, and presented to the T-helper cells. In addition, the APCs also produce cytokines including tumor necrosis factor (TNF), IL-1, IL-6, IL-8 (CXCL8), IL-12, IL-15, IL-18, IL-23, IL-27, IL-32, and other chemokines which impact the adaptive immune response.[12] Cellular origins and biological functions of some of the important cytokines and their clinically relevant roles are listed in **Table 1**.

BRMs AND ADAPTIVE IMMUNE RESPONSE

In contrast to the innate immune system, the adaptive immune system has evolved to provide a more specific recognition of nonself antigens via a vast repertoire of lymphocyte receptor specificities (on both T and B cells) generated through somatic combination of gene segments. Adaptive immunity generates immunologic memory leading to a more rapid and effective response with the subsequent antigenic challenges, and requires a complex and robust regulatory system for such responses.[13]

Although T and B lymphocytes are the main players of the adaptive immunity, APCs are important in processing microbial proteins and presenting them to the T lymphocytes. The APCs are phagocytic cells of monocyte-macrophage lineage, such as dendritic cells in tissues, Kupffer cells in liver, Langerhans cells in skin, and microglial cells in the central nervous system. The T-cells survey infected host cells via MHC Class I + II molecules. These cellular surface glycoproteins are differentially expressed on host cells. Class I MHC molecules are synthesized within virtually all nucleated host cells and contain peptides from endogenous sources. Class II MHC molecules are selectively expressed primarily on B-cells, dendritic cells, monocytes and macrophages, all of which present antigens to T-helper cells. Class II proteins contain peptides derived from phagocytosed or endocytosed exogenous antigens to form a protein-peptide complex which is then delivered to the plasma membrane for recognition by T-helper (CD4$^+$) cells.[4]

T-helper (T$_H$) cells, bearing CD4$^+$ αβ receptors, are the most prominent group of T lymphocytes, and are functionally divided into several subclasses based on their repertoire of cytokines (**Fig. 1**). Undifferentiated T-helper cells (T$_H$0) differentiate into T$_H$1 cells under the influence of IL-12 and IFN-γ and subsequently produce IFN-γ and IL-2 on activation. These cytokines produced by T$_H$1 cells lead to activation of monocyte-macrophage lineage cells, NK cells, and cytotoxic T cells that help in killing and controlling cells harboring intracellular pathogens.[12] In contrast, the presence of IL-4 and transcription factor GATA-3 lead to development of T$_H$2 cells that produce IL-4, IL-5, IL-10, and IL-13.[12] The T$_H$2 cytokines play an important role in antibody production, hypersensitivity reactions, and immune response to parasites. The T$_H$2 cytokines are associated with eosinophilia, increased immunoglobulin E (IgE) levels, atopic dermatitis, and atopic asthma.[14,15]

Another important type of differentiation of T-helper cells is T$_H$17, which occurs in response to IL-23 production by APCs (see **Fig. 1**). The T$_H$17 cells produce IL-17A, IL-17F, IL-21, and IL-22, contributing to the production of other proinflammatory cytokines and chemokines such as IL-6, GCSF, GM-CSF, CXCL8, CXCL10, and TGF-β. These cytokines play an important role in neutrophil recruitment and fibroblast

Table 1
Functions and origins of important cytokines

Cytokine	Origin	Function	Clinical Role
IFN-α	Plasmacytoid dendritic cells	Induction of IFN-stimulated genes, activates cytotoxic T cells and NK cells, upregulates class I MHC proteins	Control of viral infections, mediates antitumor activity
IFN-γ	T_H1 cells, NK cells NK-T cells	Stimulates cell-mediated immunity (T_H1 pathway), inhibits T_H2 and T_H17 responses	Control of mycobacteria, fungi, and other intracellular pathogens
IL-1	Monocytes	Activates T lymphocytes	Produces fever, anorexia, lethargy
IL-2	T_H0 lymphocytes	Stimulates cell-mediated immunity, controls B lymphocytes, intensifies proliferation and activity of all cytotoxic cell clones, dendritic cell differentiation, control of cell growth including tumors	Hematopoietic cancers (leukemia and lymphomas), autoimmune diseases, AIDS, various solid tumors (ovarian, prostate, renal, pulmonary, melanoma), graft rejection
IL-4	T_H2 cells, NK-T cells, basophils, eosinophils, mast cells	B cell differentiation, IgM to IgE switch, antiinflammatory effect on mononuclear functions (inhibits IL-1, IL-6, TNF, T_H17 cells)	Control of parasitic infestations; role in allergy and autoimmune disorders
IL-6	Monocytes	B cell differentiation, induction of acute phase proteins, generation of T_H17 cells	Produced in parasitic infestations; role in allergy and autoimmune disorders
IL-12	Monocytes, dendritic cells	Induction of T_H1 pathway	Control of mycobacteria, fungi, and other intracellular pathogens
IL-17	T_H17 cells, NK cells, NK-T cells	Proinflammatory (production of IL-6, GCSF, TGF-β), neutrophil recruitment, induction of matrix destruction, synergy with TNF and IL-1	Control of extracellular pathogens; contributes to fibrotic autoimmune disease; possible roles in inflammatory bowel disease, multiple sclerosis, severe asthma
TNF	Monocytes, dendritic cells	Proinflammatory	Control of intracellular pathogens, granuloma formation

Abbreviations: AIDS, acquired immune deficiency syndrome; IgM, immunoglobulin M; T_H, T-helper.

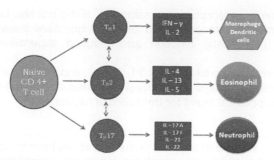

Fig. 1. Current understanding of T$_H$ cell differentiation and cytokine production. (*Data from* Miossec P, Korn T, Kuchroo VK. Interleukin-17 and type 17 helper T cells. N Engl J Med 2009;361(9):888–98; and O'Shea JJ, Paul WE. Mechanisms underlying lineage commitment and plasticity of helper CD4+ T cells. Science 2010;327(5969):1098–102.)

activation.[12,16] T$_H$17 differentiation and subsequent cellular immune response are important in the control of extracellular pathogens such as *S aureus* and *Candida* species, as shown by increased susceptibility to these organisms in animals with defective T$_H$17 response. They also have a role in the pathogenesis of fibrotic autoimmune disease, inflammatory bowel disease, multiple sclerosis, and severe persistent asthma (see **Table 1**).[12]

As shown in **Fig. 1**, more recent works have pointed away from this classic monolithic view and toward a more flexible differentiation of, and cytokine production by, T$_H$ cells.[17]

EXAMPLES OF ENDOGENOUS BRMs
Interferons

There are 3 classes of IFNs: types I, II, and III. Type I IFNs are IFN-α, IFN-β, IFN-ε, IFN-κ, and IFN-ω, which are produced by monocytes, macrophages, dendritic cells, B lymphocytes, and NK cells. In response to viral infections, plasmacytoid dendritic cells (PDCs) produce IFN-α, which plays an important role in inhibition of intracellular replication of virus by induction of IFN-stimulated genes (ISGs), which have direct antiviral effects.[18,19] The IFN-induced transmembrane proteins (IFITM 2 and 3), a type of ISGs, have been shown to restrict viral entry and significantly inhibit replication of influenza, West Nile, and dengue virus.[19] IFN-α also activates cytotoxic T lymphocytes and NK cells against infected cells, upregulates class I MHC proteins, and mediates antitumor activity.[12] Based on their antiviral and immunomodulatory properties, type I IFNs (IFN-α and IFN-β) have been successfully used in treatment of hepatitis B, hepatitis C, and multiple sclerosis.[20]

IFN-γ, the only member of type II IFNs, is produced by T$_H$1 cells, NK cells, and macrophages. IFN-γ is perhaps one of the most important immunomodulatory cytokine involved in regulation of various phases of immunity and inflammatory responses. IFN-γ is involved in expression of class I and II MHC molecules, antigen presentation, and cytokine production by APCs. IFN-γ is also responsible for macrophage activation, phagocytosis, and intracellular killing of pathogens.[21] IFN-γ plays a significant role in control of intracellular pathogens such as mycobacteria, fungi, intracellular bacteria, and viruses. It has been used as an adjuvant therapeutic agent for refractory mycobacterial diseases and fungal infections, and as a prophylactic agent for patients with chronic granulomatous disease.[22,23] It has also been used as an adjunct therapy for treatment of disseminated mycobacterial infections in patients with genetic defects of IFN-γ production or its receptor expression.[24–28] IFN-g has also been shown to be useful in the treatment of osteopetrosis, a rare childhood bone disease characterized by a defect in osteoclastic function and reduced superoxide generation in leukocytes.[28]

Type III IFNs consist of the IFN-λs (IFN-λ1, IFN-λ2, and IFN-λ3), which have similar intracellular response pathways and antiviral properties to IFN-α. IFN-λ3 is currently being studied as a potential agent for treatment of hepatitis C.[29]

Interleukins

IL-2 is derived from supernatants of cell cultures and has been used as lymphocyte-stimulating factor since 1960s, although the molecule was discovered in 1976 as T cell growth factor (TCGF). Its designation as IL-2, and further understanding of its structure, function, and characterization of its receptors, occurred only in the 1980s.[30,31] IL-2 is mainly synthesized and produced by the T-helper lymphocytes on activation by antigens or cytokines such as IL-2. In addition, it is produced by CD8$^+$ T lymphocytes, dendritic cells, and thymic regulatory T cells (Treg). IL-2 binds to its heterodimer receptor IL-2R, which has 3 subunits, on the surface of effector cells triggering intracellular signaling via Jak-STAT or another pathway involving a different set of molecules. As a result, the effector cells, for example T$_H$ (CD4$^+$) and cytotoxic (CD8$^+$) T cells proliferate and expand their clones.[31] Similarly, peripheral blood NK cells proliferate and produce IFN-γ, and also differentiate into cytotoxic cells and lymphokine-activated killer (LAK) cells. In the presence of IL-2, B lymphocytes differentiate, proliferate, and produce antibodies. IL-2 induces differentiation of mononuclear cells into macrophages and dendritic cells, enhances phagocytosis and intracellular killing, and enhances production of IL-1.[30,31] In 2 large clinical trials (INSIGHT and ESPRIT), a recombinant form of human IL-2 (rhIL-2) was studied in patients infected with human immunodeficiency virus (HIV) and -receiving antiretroviral therapy, which led to a sustained increase in CD4$^+$ counts but failed to show any clinical or survival benefits.[32] IL-2 has also been used as an adjuvant therapeutic agent in renal cell cancer, melanoma, and acute leukemia. Although its cytotoxic effect helps in prolongation of clinical remission, its use is limited by toxicities. Combination proteins, also known as fusokines, such as IL-2 plus IL-18 or IL-2 plus GM-CSF, are also being studied for immunotherapy.[33,34]

The IL-12 family of cytokines consist of IL-12, IL-23, and IL-27, which all share homology at the subunit, receptor, and signaling levels, and are produced by activated APCs, including monocytes, macrophages, and dendritic cells. IL-12 is composed of p35 and p40 subunits, whereas IL-23 is a heterodimeric cytokine composed of a novel p19 subunit in addition to the p40 subunit. These 3 cytokines, which share homologous receptor components, activate similar members of the JAK/STAT signaling pathways leading to activation and differentiation of T cells. IL-12 enhances IFN-γ production and induction of T$_H$1 cell differentiation, whereas IL-23 is associated with induction of the T$_H$17 cells and IL-27 with production of T$_H$1 cells from naive T cells.[35,36] Animal experiments have shown that IL-23 administration in mice with cryptococcal infection reduced fungal burden and prolonged survival but was inferior compared with IL-12.[37] Clinical application of these cytokines deserves further exploration.

Chemokines

Chemokines are a large family of proteins that are chemotactic cytokines and play importants role in modulating immune responses to infections (**Fig. 2**). Chemokines are normally produced transiently in response to an inducing stimulus and

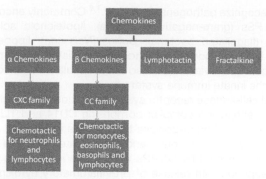

Fig. 2. The chemokine family.

subsequently are downregulated rapidly. They induce changes in the target cell membrane protein composition, thereby enhancing chemotaxis of leukocytes through the vascular endothelium into inflamed tissues. They play an important role in directed cellular migration, cellular activation, and differentiation. Chemokines are broadly categorized as the CXC or CC families (**Fig. 2**). The CXC chemokines are chemotactic for neutrophils. The CC family of chemokines attracts and activates monocytes/ macrophages, lymphocytes, NK cells, and dendritic cells. Chemokine receptors are expressed on different types of leukocytes; some are constitutively expressed and some are inducible. They can be upregulated or downregulated, allowing for a channeled and directed response to an infective agent. Receptor activation leads to a cascade of events including generation of inositol triphosphate, release of intracellular calcium, and activation of protein kinase C. It also activates the guanosine triphosphate–binding proteins of the Rho and Ras families (C1-25). Rho proteins are involved in cell motility through regulation of actin-dependent processes such as membrane ruffling, pseudopod formation, and assembly of focal adhesion complexes. Chemokines interact with nonsignaling molecules like DARC (duffy antigen receptor for chemokines) on erythrocytes, which clears them from circulation. Chemokines bind to heparan sulfate proteoglycans in the extracellular matrix and on the surface of endothelial cells, a process that helps to establish a concentration gradient from the point source of chemokine secretion. The main stimuli for chemokine production are early proinflammatory cytokines such as IL-1, TNF-α, viral infections, and bacterial products such as LPS (C1-7).

ROLE OF BRMs IN INFECTIONS

This article discusses the pathogenesis of various infections to explain the roles of endogenous BRMs. Understanding these mechanisms can help in identifying appropriate molecular targets and designing response-modifying molecules.

Sepsis Syndrome

Severe sepsis is one of the leading causes of morbidity and mortality among hospitalized patients.[38] Systemic inflammatory response syndrome (SIRS), a term that signifies nonspecific, systemic activation of the innate immune system and proinflammatory cascade, is generally a hallmark of sepsis syndrome. The early induced but nonadaptive responses to infection and tissue injury involve a wide variety of effector mechanisms directed at distinct classes of pathogens.[39–42] As described earlier, the innate immune system detects pathogens via pattern-recognition receptors (PRRs), which are able to recognize pathogens via PAMP.[7,8] Commonly encountered bacterial PAMPs include LPSs (gram-negative bacteria), lipoteichoic acid (gram-positive bacteria), flagellin (flagellated bacteria), porins (Neisseria), lipopeptides, peptidoglycan, and CpG DNA.[8] In addition, pathogen-associated inflammation and tissue injury triggers danger signals via DAMP, also known as alarmins, which are also recognized by PRRs of the innate immune system.[8]

A well-described cell-surface receptor system for recognition by the innate immune system is the LPS recognition complex comprising CD14 and TLR type 4 (TLR-4). Similarly, peptidoglycans of gram-positive bacteria are recognized by TLR-2. Potent APCs, such as dendritic cells, recognize and are activated by these bacterial PAMPs. In addition, they are activated by DAMPs from tissue injury. As a result, the innate immune system responds with release of proinflammatory cytokines including IL-1 and TNF-α. These cytokines upregulate adhesion molecules in neutrophils and endothelial cells, resulting in phagocytosis and antimicrobial killing, nitric oxide (NO) release and vasodilatation, and tissue injury leading to increased vascular permeability and pulmonary edema.[43] They also increase body temperature, reduce the host's spontaneous activity, and induce behavioral changes (sickness syndrome).

The primary cytokines secreted by the phagocytes in response to infection are IL-1, IL-6, IL-8, IL-12, and TNF-α. Phagocytes also release a variety of other molecules such as free oxygen radicals, peroxides, NO, and other mediators of inflammation such as prostaglandin and leukotrienes. Activation of the complement pathway contributes inflammatory mediators such as C5a and C3a. C5a has been shown to inhibit neutrophil apoptosis in a dose-dependent and time-dependent manner.[44] Neutrophil apoptosis has been considered an important mechanism for eliminating activated neutrophils from inflamed tissues and preventing release of toxic cellular products from the necrotic neutrophils.

TNF-α, as well as IL-1, causes vasodilation and increased vascular permeability leading to loss of plasma volume and ultimately shock. Disseminated intervascular coagulation (DIC) is also triggered by TNF-α, leading to fibrin deposition in small vessels and ischemic injury to various organs.

The proinflammatory cytokines and other molecules produced during sepsis stimulate coagulation and downregulate anticoagulation, whereas coagulation can also modulate inflammation.[45] In recent years, much attention has been focused on the role of protease-activated cell receptors (PARs) in linking coagulation and inflammation.[46] The PARs are located on the surface of vascular endothelial cells, mononuclear cells, platelets, fibroblasts, and smooth muscle cells. Current evidence suggests that activation of PAR-1 is harmful during the early phases of sepsis because it facilitates pulmonary leakage and DIC.[47] This vascular permeability is regulated by thrombin, activated protein C (APC), and its receptor endothelial protein C receptor (EPCR) in sepsis.[46]

Bacterial Infections

Periodontal infections are chronic inflammatory diseases characterized by destruction of tooth-supporting structures. The presence of periodontopathogens is required but not sufficient for disease development. Association between persistent host inflammatory immune response against these pathogens and destruction of the periodontal tissue has been shown.[48,49] The innate host system plays a significant part in recognizing microbial pathogens such as Actinobacillus actinomycetemcomitans, Porphyromonas gingivalis and Tananerella forsythensis. TLR-2 and TLR-4 are key components in recognizing the periodontal pathogens with subsequent production of inflammatory mediators.[50,51] TNF-α plays a central role in inflammatory reaction, alveolar bone resorption, and loss of connective tissue attachment.[48,52] It upregulates the production of other classic proinflammatory cytokines such as IL-1β and IL-6, which have been associated with inflammatory cell migration and osteoclastogenesis.[48,53] IFN-γ is present in high levels in periodontal lesions.[54,55]

Helicobacter pylori infection induces an innate immune response mediated by the TLR-2 receptors resulting in production of IL-8, IL-12, IL-17, and IL-23.[56–58] Cytotoxin-associated gene A (Cag A), a virulence factor of *H pylori*, is associated with higher rates of ulcers, precancerous changes, and gastric cancer. The local gastric mucosal layer of these patients produces higher levels of IL-17 and IL-8, leading to local neutrophil infiltration and chronic inflammation that is believed to predispose to gastric cancer.[58,59]

The immune response plays an important role in the pathogenesis of bacterial meningitis. Several TLRs, known to recognize bacterial factors, are expressed on and can activate microglial cells. Once activated, release of chemokines/cytokines promotes leukocyte migration into the nervous system and perpetuates the production of pro-inflammatory cytokines and other free radicals. This process leads to arterial vasculitis and cerebral venous thrombosis, further leading to secondary ischemia and cytotoxic and vasogenic brain edema.[60]

Viral Infections

Viral infections are known for activation of the innate immune system and recruitment of effector cells including monocytes and macrophages, dendritic cells (DC), NK cells, and NK-T cells. The most studied innate immune receptors involved in viral infections are TLRs, retinoic acid-inducible gene I (RIG-I), and NOD-like receptors (NLRs).[61] The TLRs, NK cell receptors, and mannose-binding receptors recognize viral PAMPs including CpG DNA, dsDNA, and viral proteins.[62] For example, it has been shown that TLR9 recognizes and binds to unmethylated CpG DNA present in bacteria and DNA viruses. CpG DNA present in human and other vertebrate cells is methylated and suppressed.[63] Activation of these receptors triggers production of proinflammatory cytokines, generates signals that recruit and activate cells involved in inflammation, and induce adaptive immunity. These phagocytic cells in turn release a range of molecules including cytotoxic cytokines, cationic proteins, lipid mediators, metalloproteinases, and by products of the oxygen burst responses. The reactive oxygen species accumulate in the mitochondria, leading to killing of virus-infected cells and contributing to tissue damage. The adaptive immune effector cells further contribute to tissue damage. For example, CD8+ cytotoxic T cells destroy virus-infected cells and release cytokines such as TNF that can produce tissue damage. Destruction of infected cells in hepatitis B or C infections by the cytotoxic (CD8+) T cells contribute to hepatic damage.[61] Antibody response to the viral infection also contributes to tissue damage by activation of classical complement cascade and further recruitment of inflammatory cells. Antibody-mediated inflammatory reactions involve toxicity following engagement of immunoglobulin G (IgG) with Fc receptors in inflammatory cells, which causes inflammatory mediator release.[64]

The major immunogenic epitopes of hepatitis C virus (HCV) include the core proteins NS3, NS4B, and NS5A.[65] Dendritic cells release IL-12 and IL-15 in response to viral infection, which stimulate NK cell function and elaboration of IFN-γ to mediate antiviral effects. Viral clearance depends on a rapid expansion and persistence of HCV-specific CD4+ and CD8+ T cells, and elaboration of IFN-γ. However, HCV develops mechanisms to decrease release of IFNs and cytotoxic granules by NK cells via E2 protein that binds to the NK81 receptor. It also depresses function and numbers of dendritic cells and increases Tregs further decreasing NK cell functions.[66,67] In both acute and chronic hepatitis C infection, the frequency of plasmacytoid dendritic cells (PDCs) is decreased, they are immature, and produce reduced amounts of IFN-α compared with healthy controls.[67]

Human papilloma virus (HPV) infection is known to elicit a robust production of inflammatory cytokines and components in the microenvironment that have been shown to play a role in tumor development.[68,69] HPV infection has been shown to be associated with the release of several inflammatory cytokines from keratinocytes and skin fibroblasts. Proinflammatory cytokines such as ILs and TNF are important mediators of skin and mucosal inflammation.[68]

Heterologous immunity is a phenomenon by which exposure to one pathogen generates immune response against numerous antigenic epitopes derived from that pathogen. Some of these may cross-react with epitopes from other pathogens. When an infection with the second pathogen occurs later, the cross-reactive memory cells expand rapidly and dominate the overall response. This mechanism has been shown to be instrumental in the occurrence of severe disease such as dengue hemorrhagic fever (DHF). DHF usually occurs in patients who are immune to one dengue strain and later get infected with a heterologous strain.[61]

HIV

The mechanism by which HIV causes immune dysfunction has been an area of interest since the discovery of the virus. It is well known that HIV infection causes destruction of T_H cells, which is followed by decline in mononuclear-macrophage functions as a result of reduction in IL-12 and IFN-γ production. In untreated HIV cases, while the T_H1 function continues to decline, occurrence of concurrent, persistent immune activation has been shown, leading to further dysregulation of immune function.[21] In a large randomized clinical trial, the Strategic Management of Antiretroviral Therapy (SMART) study, investigators found that patients with HIV had increased levels of IL-6, CRP, and D-dimer. These inflammatory and coagulopathy biomarkers were found to be associated with subsequent development of opportunistic infections and all-cause mortality among HIV-infected individuals.[70,71] A multifactorial cause for the immune activation has been described.[72] Innate and adaptive immune activation occur directly in response to viral proteins. For example, binding of the HIV envelope protein gp120/160 to CD4 and CCR5 receptors leads to intracellular signaling triggering immune response.[73–75] HIV-associated immune activation is also caused in part by translocation of microbial products, such as bacterial LPS and DNA, from the intestinal lumen to the systemic circulation where they can activate the immune system by binding various TLRs.[76,77] The microbial translocation occurs as HIV infection causes rapid and severe depletion of CD4[+] T cells, monocytes, and macrophages from gut associated lymphoid tissue (GALT) as a result of the direct cytopathic effect of the virus.[72,78] When translocated bacterial LPS binds with TLR-4, soluble CD14 (sCD14) is secreted into the plasma. The increase of sCD14, a biomarker of monocyte activation, is associated with activation of CD8[+] T cells and increased mortality in HIV-infected patients.[79] In addition, an increased production of proinflammatory cytokines such as TNF-α, IL-1, and IL-18 cause a non–antigen-specific bystander activation of the T and B lymphocytes.[72] This might involve upregulation of the apoptosis-related molecules on the surface of T cells making them prone to activation-induced cell death.[74,80–85] Depletion of the CD4 regulatory T cells that normally suppress the immune activation via mechanisms involving direct cell-to-cell contact, production of cytokines, and inhibition of dendritic cell activity could be another factor contributing to this immune activation.[72] The inflammatory cytokine IL-1 has been linked to

HIV-associated dementia, and IL-18 has been suggested to play an important role in the development of progressive immunodeficiency.[86]

HIV is known to replicate more efficiently in activated CD4$^+$ T lymphocytes and this immune activation could provide available targets for HIV replication.[87] This could result in killing of the HIV-specific CD4$^+$ T cells and contribute to the failure of the CD8-mediated cytotoxic T lymphocyte responses to the virus.

Sexually transmitted infections (STIs) have been known to increase the transmission of HIV infection. STI pathogens interact directly with langerin (CD207), a type II transmembrane glycoprotein, and compete for HIV-1 binding and hence increase the HIV-1 infection of Langerhans cells via CD4 and CCR5 receptors.[88] STIs increase the production of proinflammatory cytokines that affect the susceptibility of Langerhans cells to HIV-1 transmission. TNF-α enhances HIV-1 infection of Langerhans cells, which increases HIV-1 transmission to CD4$^+$ cells.[89]

HIV and Immune Reconstitution Inflammatory Syndrome

Antiretroviral therapy (ART) for patients with HIV results in significant reduction in viral load followed by immunologic recovery.[90] However, a subgroup of patients experience clinical deterioration secondary to immune reconstitution inflammatory syndrome (IRIS).[91–94] Different types of IRIS have been described, including infective (either unmasking or paradoxic type), autoimmune, and malignant forms.[95] IRIS manifests as an inflammatory reaction to the replicating organisms unmasking untreated or undertreated infection. The paradoxic form is a response to the dead or dying organisms. A common example of the autoimmune form includes recurrence of Graves disease, usually after a median duration of 2 years after starting ART.[96] Kaposi sarcoma associated with HIV responds partially or completely to ART alone.[97,98] However, a minority of patients develop Kaposi sarcoma–related IRIS after commencing ART and present with new or enlarged lesions.[99]

IRIS is caused by a rapid restoration of a dysregulated immune function characterized by innate and adaptive immune responses to replicating or dead pathogens and release of cytokines and chemokines. Increased IL-6 production leading to induction of inflammatory molecules, such as CRP, have been observed in IRIS. The types of BRMs (chemokines and cytokines) may vary depending on the type of pathogens. For example, in IRIS related to tuberculosis (TB) and cryptococcal infections, increased T$_H$1 response is shown by increased production of IFN-γ and IL-18, whereas chemokines such as CXCL10 help in recruiting T cells and NK cells to the sites of inflammation.[94,100] Defective or inappropriate regulatory T cell function in HIV infection has also been proposed as a predisposition toward uncontrolled antigen-specific response.[101] HIV infection affects both the plasmacytoid dendritic cell (pDC) and myeloid dendritic cells (mDC). ART has been shown to partially reverse pDC count and increase mDC activity.[102–104] This differential recovery may influence IRIS because the mDC subset is responsible for exaggerating the Th1 response.

Fungal Infections

Cell-mediated immunity is a crucial line of defense against fungal infections. Cell-mediated phagocytosis is the initial event after the breach of the first line of defense. A complex array of intercellular signals and various chemicals and receptors play a final role in the control and prevention of infections. Cells of the innate immune system rapidly release cytokines in response to fungal products and/or binding of opsonized fungi. Depending on the type of stimulation, APCs activate and recruit lymphocytes, which develop into distinct types of T-helper cells, including T$_H$1, T$_H$2, or T$_H$17.[105] Activation of T$_H$1 leads to production of TNF-α and IFN-γ, activation and recruitment of macrophages, phagocytosis, and control of fungi, whereas T_H2 activation results in allergy and relapse of fungal infections. The T_H17 cells perform important effector and regulatory functions at the mucosal level but also promote inflammation. For example, T_H17 is important in controlling mucosal colonization with *Candida* species.[106] IL-22, a member of the IL-10 cytokine family, plays an important role via IL-23/IL-22 axis, controls the initial fungal growth, and prevents tissue damage.[105]

Phagocytic cells are an important source of TNF-α, IL-12, macrophage inflammatory protein-1α (MIP-1α), and IL-1. NK cells and $\gamma\delta$ T cells can synthesize IFN-γ. TNF-α, an early response cytokine, plays a critical role during fungal infections. IFN-γ is a potent activator of fungicidal activity for cells of the innate immune system and it also drives the T_H1 responses to fungal infections.[107] CC chemokines modulate the development of antifungal adaptive immunity.

In infections caused by *Candida*, T_H cells play a pivotal role in the regulation of phagocytosis. Once *Candida* is recognized by polymorphonuclear leukocytes and dendritic cells, they produce IL-12, which in turn activates T_H1 cells. The activated T_H1 cells then secrete INF-γ and IL-12, which stimulate phagocytic cells. Once phagocytosed, myeloperoxidase, hydrogen peroxide, superoxide anion system, and chymotrypsinlike cationic proteins all play an important role in intracellular killing of the *Candida*. A dysfunction of the lymphocyte system results in chronic mucocutaneous candidiasis as seen in patients with acquired immune deficiency syndrome (AIDS), severe combined immunodeficiency, hyperimmunoglobulin E syndrome, or more recently described genetic causes related to IL-17 defect. The genetic causes may be related to a deficiency of IL-17F or its receptor IL-17RA.[108,109] Components of complement factors like C3b, along with IgG antibody, are also necessary for optimal opsonization of *Candida* blastospores.

Recognition of *Aspergillus* motifs by TLRs (TLR-2 and TLR-4) and dectin-1 results in activation of intracellular pathways leading to the release of proinflammatory cytokines, such as TNF-α and IL-8.[94] Various fungal epitopes may have different immunomodulatory effects on the cellular immunity.[110] T_H cytokines have vital role in innate and adaptive defense against *Aspergillus*. Although a T_H1 response to infection with production of IFN-γ, IL-12, and IL-18 is favorable and protective, a T_H2 response characterized by release of cytokines IL-4 and IL-10 contributes to progression of infection. Allergic bronchopulmonary aspergillosis (ABPA) and allergic fungal sinusitis are examples of T_H2 response.[111–114] Pulmonary macrophages are a major line of defense, and they are capable of ingesting and killing *Aspergillus* conidia. Complement and other molecules such as mannose–binding protein (MBP) and surfactant proteins enhance opsonization.

The cryptococcal capsule is the key virulence factor of the organism. It is composed of 2 types of polysaccharides, namely glucuronoxylomannan (GXM) and galactoxylomannan (GalXM), and a smaller proportion of mannoproteins (MP).[115] Once cryptococci enter the alveoli, they elicit a T_H1 response similar to *Aspergillus*. Complement receptors 1, 3, and 4 (CR1, CR3, and CR4) can mediate the uptake of opsonized cryptococcus. The presence of CR3 is important for resistance to cryptococcal infection. PRRs like mannose and β-glucan receptors also aid in phagocytosis of fungi by recognizing and binding to mannan/mannoproteins and glucan, respectively, on the fungal capsule and cell wall.[107] MPs have been shown to shift the balance toward a T_H1 protective response. Cryptococcus is able to evade the host immune defense system because its polysaccharide capsule's component (eg, GXM) drives a nonprotective T_H2 response and promotes IL-10 secretion, which leads to downregulation of T_H1 cytokines.[116,117]

Similarly, T cells are pivotal in clearance of *Histoplasma capsulatum*. IFN-γ, TNF-α, and IL-12 have been shown to exhibit survival benefit in mice.[118] *Histoplasma* binds and colonizes the host using its cell wall carbohydrates, such as glucans, which can also activate the innate response. The α-1,3-glucan in *H capsulatum* is associated with virulence and it contributes to the establishment of intracellular latency, regulates proliferation of *Histoplasma* inside the host macrophages, and protects it inside phagolysosomes. It may also block innate immune recognition of the *Histoplasma* yeast and suppress TNF-γ production by phagocytes. However, β-1,3-glucan is immunogenic and triggers an innate immune response releasing proinflammatory cytokines, NO synthase, TNF-α, and macrophage inflammatory protein-2 (MIP-2).[119,120] Although infections caused by *Histoplasma* are limited by cell-mediated immunity, tissues are not sterilized altogether. Reactivation of infection may occur several years later, as seen in individuals who move from endemic to nonendemic areas. TNF-α and IFN-γ facilitate generation of granulomas, thereby containing the fungal growth. Aberrations in the cell-mediated response and cytokine production can result in extremes of infection, either progressive disseminated histoplasmosis, in which there is no significant T cell–mediated response, or excessive granuloma formation and fibrosis with exaggerated response.

Mycobacteria

In mycobacterial infections, macrophages constitute the initial line of defense. They phagocytose and kill the inhaled mycobacteria and activate T cells, generating a T_H1 type of response. IL-12 plays an important role in producing mycobacterial antigen–specific T lymphocytes. It induces differentiation of T_H1 lymphocytes and production of IFN-γ. It upregulates antimycobacterial processes and antigen presentation by macrophages. Both IFN-γ and TNF-α play important roles in the formation of granuloma and protection against TB. More recent work suggests that mycobacteria release early secretory antigen-6 (ESAT-6) at the initial site of infection and stimulate bystander epithelial cells on the periphery of the infection site to produce matrix metalloproteinase-9 (MMP-9). The MMP-9 attracts and recruits macrophages that become infected, resulting in bacterial proliferation and granuloma expansion.[121,122] *M tuberculosis* infection and expression of ESAT-6 in the macrophages stimulate caspase-1 activity, promoting IL-1β secretion.[123] After the aerosol of *M tuberculosis* gets deposited in the alveoli, it takes about 20 days for an adequate number of antigen-specific IFN-γ–producing T cells to accumulate in the lung to inhibit bacterial growth. The infected dendritic cells produce IL-23, which in turn induces T_H17 differentiation and IL-17 production. The main role of IL-17 is induction of chemokine expression and recruitment of neutrophils, but, unlike the T_H1 response, their role in providing protective immunity is limited.[124] T_H1 cytokines and mononuclear cells play a major role in controlling mycobacteria other than TB (MOTT) including *Mycobacterium avium* complex (MAC). Inborn or acquired deficiency of IFN-γ or its receptors has been associated with disseminated mycobacterial infections.[17] IFN-γ and its inducer, IL-12, have been used as adjunct therapies in the treatment of disseminated MAC infections in immunocompromised hosts, patients with AIDS and idiopathic CD4 lymphocytopenia, and patients with genetic defects of either IFN-γ production or IFN-γ receptors expression.[24–27,125,126]

Chemokines also play an important role in the host immune response to *M tuberculosis*. CXCL8 helps in recruiting inflammatory cells to the site of infection and facilitates elimination of microorganisms by enhancing nonoxidative mechanisms and increasing efficiency of bactericidal activity.[127] CXCL8 is the most potent attractant and activating factor for lymphocytes. In addition, CXCL8 activates neutrophils, inducing degranulation, calcium mobilization, shape change, respiratory burst, upregulation of receptors, and changes in phagocytic activity. CXCL 10 stimulates NK cell and T cell migration in tuberculosis.[127]

Parasitic Infections

A T_H2 response is the major immune mechanism involved in helminth infection. The helminthic PAMPs are recognized by pattern-recognition receptors (PRRs) expressed on DCs, leading to differentiation of DCs with suppressed expression of TLRs and elaboration of T_H2 and Treg lymphocytes.[128] More recently, IL-25, IL-33, and thymic stromal lymphopoietin have been proposed as the link between the pathogen recognition by DCs and T_H-2 cell action.[129] This T_H2 differentiation enhances production of IL-4, IL-5, and IL-13, contributing to production of eosinophils, basophils, mast cells, and goblet cells.[128,130] IL-4 induces B cell switch to produce IgE, whereas IL-13 is mainly involved in inflammation and fibrosis. The T_H2 response also contributes to expulsion of parasites and the healing process of tissue damage sustained from helminthic infections. The Treg cells produce IL-10 and TGF-β, which are antiinflammatory cytokines.[131] This combination of T_H2/Treg helps in downregulation of immune response leading to both reduced host tissue damage and persistence of the parasites. Although T_H2 is the predominant form of immune response in helminthic infections, T_H1 response may also occur in the presence of tissue invasion, giving rise to significant tissue damage and clinical manifestations of systemic inflammation.[131] For example, in schistosomiasis, the eggs induce a strong T_H2 response that orchestrates granuloma formation, limiting associated lethal inflammation. In leishmania infections, IFN-γ activates macrophages, and induces nitric oxide synthase expression and NO production, thereby promoting parasite killing.

IL-12 plays a central role in initiating protective immune responses against intracellular parasites. IL-12 production by macrophages, dendritic cells stimulated by parasitic infection, activates NK cells to produce IFN-γ, which in turn leads to Th-1 response. TNF-α and IL-1 are important cofactors for IL-12–induced NK cell production of IFN-γ.[111] CD 8+ T cells survey and recognize intracellular infections in the context of MHC class I expressed on all cell surfaces. This action is helpful in controlling intracellular pathogens like *Trypanosoma cruzi* and *Toxoplasma*.

Plasmodium vivax and *Plasmodium knowlesi* gain entry into erythrocytes by binding specifically to DARC.[132] *P vivax* may evade host immunity by indirectly downregulating humoral responses against erythrocytic invasion and development through DARC.[133] Individuals with a DARC mutation or lack of expression of DARC on erythrocytes are protected from these infections. Immunity to *Plasmodium* seems to be complex and stage specific. IFN-γ produced by CD8+ and CD4+ cells plays a role in the response to hepatic stages. Antiplasmodial antibody is the primary protective mediator against erythrocytic stages of infection.[107]

Interestingly, Patients with parasitic infections tend to have lower prevalence of allergic and immunologic disorders, which are also mediated by T_H2 cells. In addition to adaptive cellular immune responses, soluble innate mechanisms help control parasitic infections. Alternate and mannose-binding lectin pathways of complement activation are two of the oldest, first line defenses against extracellular parasites. Lectin present on the parasite activates the complement and leads to C3b deposition on the parasite surface leading to membrane attack complex and lysis or opsonization.

AUTOIMMUNITY

Autoimmunity occurs when the immune system recognizes and attacks the host tissue. Environmental triggers, especially infectious agents, are thought to play a major role in the pathogenesis of certain autoimmune diseases. Multiple mechanisms have been postulated by which infection could lead to autoimmunity.[134]

Molecular mimicry is the most accepted mechanism in which the T or B cells activated in response to the pathogen cross-react with the self-antigen and cause destruction the tissue. The initial expansion of the T cells requires activation of the T cell receptor by the MHC-bound peptides.[135] Rheumatic heart disease following infection with *Streptococcus pyogenes* infection is a common example of this type of autoimmunity. Common antigenic determinants have been shown between streptococcal proteins and heart autoantigens,[136] and T cell response to these determinants leads to the appearance of antiheart autoimmunity. Similarly, intestinal infection with *Campylobacter jejuni* has been associated with Guillain-Barré syndrome. Antibodies cross-reacting with *C jejuni* and peripheral nerve gangliosides are detected in the serum of patients with Guillain-Barré syndrome.[137]

The epitope-spreading model postulates immune response to a persisting pathogen or direct lysis by the persisting pathogen causing damage to self-tissue. The antigens released from the damaged tissue are taken up by the APCs, leading to initiation of a self-specific immune response. Coxsackie virus B (CVB) infection in the chronic phase is characterized by mononuclear cell infiltration into the myocardium and production of antibodies to the cardiac myosin. Lysis of cardiac myocytes results in myocarditis by the epitope-spreading mechanism.

The other known mechanism is bystander activation, in which host tissue damage occurs as a result of local production of cytokines during viral infection. Cytosolic receptors and TLRs play an important role in detecting viral nucleic acid and activating the IFN-mediated antiviral response.[138] The acute phase of infection with *T cruzi* is characterized by parasitemia in the heart muscle cells leading to inflammatory infiltration. Bystander tissue destruction mediated by inflammatory cytokines, especially IFN-γ, leads to irreversible cardiomyopathy in the chronic phase of the disease. Similarly, patients with untreated Lyme disease have a high likelihood of developing arthritis by bystander inflammatory response to *Borrelia burgdorfeii*.

Viruses and bacteria could act as superantigens and bind to a variety of MHC class II molecules, leading to activation of large numbers of T cells. Herpes simplex virus (HSV) leads to infection of the corneal epithelial cells with production of proinflammatory cytokines IL-1 and IL-6, leading to influx of neutrophils into the corneal stroma. Furthermore, after 10 days of infection, a second wave of infiltration occurs, leading to production of IFN-γ and stromal keratitis.[134] The peak of HSV keratitis occurs 5 to 7 days after the infectious virus is typically detectable, which is suggestive of its autoimmune nature.[139]

Innate inflammation, originally known to provide protection against bacterial infections, has been shown to play an important role in the pathogenesis and progression of atherosclerosis, plaque rupture, thrombosis, and stroke. Multiple chronic infections have been associated with increased risk of atherosclerosis and stroke. Acute infections, particularly of the respiratory tract, have also been found to serve as precipitants of stroke in various epidemiologic studies.[140] This could have future clinical implications in the role of infection and immune response in the pathogenesis of stroke.

SUMMARY

Recent advances in molecular biology and immunology have increased the understanding of immunopathology of infectious diseases. Cytokines (such as IFNs and ILs) and their receptors, chemokines, pattern-recognitions receptors (such as TLRs), and other intracellular mediators play vital roles in the defense against microorganisms. These protective mechanisms can be modulated or augmented with the help of endogenous biological response modifiers. Some of these endogenous BRMs are already in clinical use as adjunct or primary therapy. Others have been found useful as diagnostic tools. Many endogenous BRMs are being genetically engineered and are undergoing evaluation for wider and safer clinical applications, including treatment of infectious diseases, cancers, genetic disorders of immunity, and autoimmune disorders. As technology advances, it will also be possible to genetically regulate BRMs and the immune response in a desirable manner (ie, switch it off and switch it on).

REFERENCES

1. Tzianabos AO. Polysaccharide immunomodulators as therapeutic agents: structural aspects and biologic function. Clin Microbiol Rev 2000;13(4):523–33.
2. Bast RC Jr, Zbar B, Borsos T, et al. BCG and cancer (first of two parts). N Engl J Med 1974;290(25):1413–20.
3. Chang CC, Naiki M, Halpern GM, et al. Pharmacological regulation of the immune system. J Investig Allergol Clin Immunol 1993;3(1):8–18.
4. Chaplin DD. Overview of the immune response. J Allergy Clin Immunol 2010; 125(2 Suppl 2):S3–23.
5. Turvey SE, Broide DH. Innate immunity. J Allergy Clin Immunol 2010; 125(2 Suppl 2):S24–32.
6. Bottazzi B, Doni A, Garlanda C, et al. An integrated view of humoral innate immunity: pentraxins as a paradigm. Annu Rev Immunol 2010;28:157–83.
7. Si-Tahar M, Touqui L, Chignard M. Innate immunity and inflammation–two facets of the same anti-infectious reaction. Clin Exp Immunol 2009;156(2):194–8.
8. Anas AA, Wiersinga WJ, de Vos AF, et al. Recent insights into the pathogenesis of bacterial sepsis. Neth J Med 2010;68(4):147–52.
9. Martinon F, Mayor A, Tschopp J. The inflammasomes: guardians of the body. Annu Rev Immunol 2009;27:229–65.
10. Zhu J, Mohan C. Toll-like receptor signaling pathways—therapeutic opportunities. Mediators Inflamm 2010;2010:781235.
11. Miller RL, Meng TC, Tomai MA. The antiviral activity of Toll-like receptor 7 and 7/8 agonists. Drug News Perspect 2008;21(2):69–87.
12. Commins SP, Borish L, Steinke JW. Immunologic messenger molecules: cytokines, interferons, and chemokines. J Allergy Clin Immunol 2010;125(2 Suppl 2):S53–72.
13. Bonilla FA, Oettgen HC. Adaptive immunity. J Allergy Clin Immunol 2010;125(2):S33–40.
14. Lloyd CM, Hessel EM. Functions of T cells in asthma: more than just T(H)2 cells. Nat Rev Immunol 2010;10(12):838–48.
15. Datta S, Milner JD. Altered T-cell receptor signaling in the pathogenesis of allergic disease. J Allergy Clin Immunol 2011;127(2):351–4.
16. Miossec P, Korn T, Kuchroo VK. Interleukin-17 and type 17 helper T cells. N Engl J Med 2009;361(9):888–98.
17. O'Shea JJ, Paul WE. Mechanisms underlying lineage commitment and plasticity of helper CD4+ T cells. Science 2010;327(5969):1098–102.
18. Geissmann F, Manz MG, Jung S, et al. Development of monocytes, macrophages, and dendritic cells. Science 2010;327(5966):656–61.
19. Liu SY, Sanchez DJ, Cheng G. New developments in the induction and antiviral effectors of type I interferon. Curr Opin Immunol 2011;23(1):57–64.

20. Duddy M, Haghikia A, Cocco E, et al. Managing MS in a changing treatment landscape. J Neurol 2011;258(5):728–39.
21. Koirala J, Adamski A, Koch L, et al. Interferon-gamma receptors in HIV-1 infection. AIDS Res Hum Retroviruses 2008;24(8):1097–102.
22. Holland SM. The Interferons. In: Holland S, editor. Cytokine therapeutics in infectious diseases. 1st edition. Philadelphia: Lippincott Williams & Wilkins; 2001. p. 221–50.
23. Segal BH, Kwon-Chung J, Walsh TJ, et al. Immunotherapy for fungal infections. Clin Infect Dis 2006;42(4):507–15.
24. Sternfeld T, Nigg A, Belohradsky BH, et al. Treatment of relapsing. *Mycobacterium avium* infection with interferon-gamma and interleukin-2 in an HIV-negative patient with low CD4 syndrome. Int J Infect Dis 2010;14(Suppl 3):e198–201.
25. Rezai MS, Khotaei G, Mamishi S, et al. Disseminated bacillus Calmette-Guerin infection after BCG vaccination. J Trop Pediatr 2008;54(6):413–6.
26. Seneviratne SL, Doffinger R, Macfarlane J, et al. Disseminated *Mycobacterium tuberculosis* infection due to interferon gamma deficiency. Response to replacement therapy. Thorax 2007;62(1):97–9.
27. Kedzierska K, Paukovics G, Handley A, et al. Interferon-gamma therapy activates human monocytes for enhanced phagocytosis of *Mycobacterium avium* complex in HIV-infected individuals. HIV Clin Trials 2004;5(2):80–5.
28. Key LL Jr, Rodriguiz RM, Willi SM, et al. Long-term treatment of osteopetrosis with recombinant human interferon gamma. N Engl J Med 1995;332(24):1594–9.
29. Kelly C, Klenerman P, Barnes E. Interferon lambdas: the next cytokine storm. Gut 2011. [Epub ahead of print].
30. Miller KD, Kuruppu JC, Kovacs JA. Interleukin-2. In: Holland S, editor. Cytokine therapeutics in infectious diseases. 1st edition. Philadelphia: Lippincott Williams & Wilkins; 2001. p. 15–44.
31. Olejniczak K, Kasprzak A. Biological properties of interleukin 2 and its role in pathogenesis of selected diseases–a review. Med Sci Monit 2008;14(10):RA179–89.
32. INSIGHT-ESPRIT Study Group, SILCAAT Scientific Committee, Abrams D, Lévy Y, Losso MH, et al. Interleukin-2 therapy in patients with HIV infection. N Engl J Med 2009;361(16):1548–59.
33. Penafuerte C, Bautista-Lopez N, Boulassel MR, et al. The human ortholog of granulocyte macrophage colony-stimulating factor and interleukin-2 fusion protein induces potent ex vivo natural killer cell activation and maturation. Cancer Res 2009;69(23):9020–8.
34. Acres B, Gantzer M, Remy C, et al. Fusokine interleukin-2/interleukin-18, a novel potent innate and adaptive immune stimulator with decreased toxicity. Cancer Res 2005;65(20):9536–46.
35. Gee K, Guzzo C, Che Mat NF, et al. The IL-12 family of cytokines in infection, inflammation and autoimmune disorders. Inflamm Allergy Drug Targets 2009; 8(1):40–52.
36. Kleinschek MA, Muller U, Brodie SJ, et al. IL-23 enhances the inflammatory cell response in *Cryptococcus neoformans* infection and induces a cytokine pattern distinct from IL-12. J Immunol 2006;176(2):1098–106.
37. Kleinschek MA, Müller U, Schütze N, et al. Administration of IL-23 engages innate and adaptive immune mechanisms during fungal infection. Int Immunol 2010;22(2):81–90.
38. Parrillo JE, Parker MM, Natanson C, et al. Septic shock in humans. Advances in the understanding of pathogenesis, cardiovascular dysfunction, and therapy. Ann Intern Med 1990;113(3):227–42.

39. Brown E, Atkinson JP, Fearon DT. Innate immunity: 50 ways to kill a microbe. Curr Opin Immunol 1994;6(1):73–4.
40. Ezekowitz RA, Hoffmann JA. Innate immunity. Curr Opin Immunol 1996;8(1):1–2.
41. Fearon DT, Locksley RM. The instructive role of innate immunity in the acquired immune response. Science 1996;272(5258):50–3.
42. Oberholzer A, Oberholzer C, Moldawer LL. Cytokine signaling–regulation of the immune response in normal and critically ill states. Crit Care Med 2000; 28(Suppl 4):N3–12.
43. Russell JA. Management of sepsis. N Engl J Med 2006;355(16):1699–713.
44. Perianayagam MC, Balakrishnan VS, King AJ, et al. C5a delays apoptosis of human neutrophils by a phosphatidylinositol 3-kinasesignaling pathway. Kidney Int 2002;61:456–63.
45. Levi M, van der Poll T. Inflammation and coagulation. Crit Care Med 2010; 38(Suppl 2):S26–34.
46. Petäjä J. Inflammation and coagulation. An overview. Thromb Res 2011; 127(Suppl 2):S34–7.
47. Kaneider NC, Leger AJ, Agarwal A, et al. 'Role reversal' for the receptor PAR1 in sepsis-induced vascular damage. Nat Immunol 2007;8(12):1303–12.
48. Graves D. Cytokines that promote periodontal tissue destruction. J Periodontol 2008;79(Suppl 8):1585–91.
49. Liu YC, Lerner UH, Teng YT. Cytokine responses against periodontal infection: protective and destructive roles. Periodontol 2000;52(1):163–206.
50. Kikkert R, Laine ML, Aarden LA, et al. Activation of toll-like receptors 2 and 4 by gram-negative periodontal bacteria. Oral Microbiol Immunol 2007;22(3):145–51.
51. Nussbaum G, Ben-Adi S, Genzler T, et al. Involvement of Toll-like receptors 2 and 4 in the innate immune response to *Treponema denticola* and its outer sheath components. Infect Immun 2009;77(9):3939–47.
52. Graves DT, Cochran D. The contribution of interleukin-1 and tumor necrosis factor to periodontal tissue destruction. J Periodontol 2003;74(3):391–401.
53. Fonseca JE, Santos MJ, Canhão H, et al. Interleukin-6 as a key player in systemic inflammation and joint destruction. Autoimmun Rev 2009;8(7):538–42.
54. Garlet GP, Martins W Jr, Ferreira BR, et al. Patterns of chemokines and chemokine receptors expression in different forms of human periodontal disease. J Periodontal Res 2003;38(2):210–7.
55. Honda T, Domon H, Okui T, et al. Balance of inflammatory response in stable gingivitis and progressive periodontitis lesions. Clin Exp Immunol 2006;144(1):35–40.
56. Amedei A, Cappon A, Codolo G, et al. The neutrophil-activating protein of *Helicobacter pylori* promotes Th1 immune responses. J Clin Invest 2006;116: 1092–101.
57. Fischer W, Puls J, Buhrdorf R, et al. Systematic mutagenesis of the *Helicobacter pylori* cag pathogenicity island: essential genes for CagA translocation in host cells and induction of interleukin-8. Mol Microbiol 2001;42:1337–48.
58. Kabir S. The role of interleukin-17 in the *Helicobacter pylori* induced infection and immunity. Helicobacter 2011;16(1):1–8.
59. Weel JF, van der Hulst RW, Gerrits Y, et al. The interrelationship between cytotoxin-associated gene A, vacuolating cytotoxin, and *Helicobacter pylori*-related diseases. J Infect Dis 1996;173:1171–5.
60. Gerber J, Nau R. Mechanisms of injury in bacterial meningitis. Curr Opin Neurol 2010;23(3):312–8.
61. Rouse BT, Sehrawat S. Immunity and immunopathology to viruses: what decides the outcome? Nat Rev Immunol 2010;10(7):514–26.

62. Iannello A, Debbeche O, Martin E, et al. Viral strategies for evading antiviral cellular immune responses of the host. J Leukoc Biol 2006;79(1):16–35.
63. Chen J, Nag S, Vidi PA, et al. Single molecule in vivo analysis of toll-like receptor 9 and CpG DNA interaction. PLoS One 2011;6(4):e17991.
64. Tinoco R, Alcalde V, Yang Y, et al. Cell-intrinsic transforming growth factor-β signaling mediates virus-specific CD8+ T cell deletion and viral persistence in vivo. Immunity 2009;31:145–57.
65. Sillanpää M, Melén K, Porkka P, et al. Hepatitis C virus core, NS3, NS4B and NS5A are the major immunogenic proteins in humoral immunity in chronic HCV infection. Virol J 2009;6:84.
66. Nellore A, Fishman JA. NK cells, innate immunity and hepatitis C infection after liver transplantation. Clin Infect Dis 2011;52(3):369–77.
67. Dolganiuc A, Szabo G. Dendritic cells in hepatitis C infection: can they (help) win the battle? J Gastroenterol 2011;46(4):432–47.
68. Boccardo E, Lepique AP, Villa LL. The role of inflammation in HPV carcinogenesis. Carcinogenesis 2010;31(11):1905–12.
69. Balkwill F, Coussens LM. Cancer: an inflammatory link. Nature 2004;431(7007): 405–6.
70. Kuller LH, Tracy R, Belloso W, et al. Inflammatory and coagulation biomarkers and mortality in patients with HIV infection. PLoS Med 2008;5(10):e203.
71. Rodger AJ, Fox Z, Lundgren JD, et al. INSIGHT Strategies for Management of Antiretroviral Therapy (SMART) Study Group. Activation and coagulation biomarkers are independent predictors of the development of opportunistic disease in patients with HIV infection. J Infect Dis 2009;200(6):973–83.
72. Sodora DL, Silvestri G. Immune activation and AIDS pathogenesis. AIDS 2008; 22(4):439–46.
73. Ascher MS, Sheppard HW. A unified hypothesis for three cardinal features of HIV immunology. J Acquir Immune Defic Syndr 1991;4:97–8.
74. Herbeuval JP, Hardy AW, Boasso A, et al. Regulation of TNF-related apoptosis inducing ligand on primary CD4R T cells by HIV-1: role of type I IFN-producing plasmacytoid dendritic cells. Proc Natl Acad Sci U S A 2005;102:13974–9.
75. Sailaja G, Skountzou I, Quan FS, et al. Human immunodeficiency virus-like particles activate multiple types of immune cells. Virology 2007;362(2):331–41.
76. Brenchley JM, Price DA, Douek DC. HIV disease: fallout from a mucosal catastrophe? Nat Immunol 2006;7:235–9.
77. Brenchley JM, Price DA, Schacker TW, et al. Microbial translocation is a cause of systemic immune activation in chronic HIV infection. Nat Med 2006;12: 1365–71.
78. Nixon DE, Landay AL. Biomarkers of immune dysfunction in HIV. Curr Opin HIV AIDS 2010;5(6):498–503.
79. Sandler NG, Wand H, Roque A, et al. Plasma levels of soluble CD14 independently predict mortality in HIV infection. J Infect Dis 2011;203(6):780–90.
80. Estaquier J, Idziorek T, de Bels F, et al. Programmed cell death and AIDS: significance of T-cell apoptosis in pathogenic and nonpathogenic primate lentiviral infections. Proc Natl Acad Sci U S A 1994;91:9431–5.
81. Finkel TH, Tudor-Williams G, Banda NK, et al. Apoptosis occurs predominantly in bystander cells and not in productively infected cells of HIV- and SIV infected lymph nodes. Nat Med 1995;1:129–34.
82. Katsikis PD, Wunderlich ES, Smith CA, et al. Fas antigen stimulation induces marked apoptosis of T lymphocytes in human immunodeficiency virus-infected individuals. J Exp Med 1995;181:2029–36.

83. Muro-Cacho CA, Pantaleo G, Fauci AS. Analysis of apoptosis in lymph nodes of HIV-infected persons. Intensity of apoptosis correlates with the general state of activation of the lymphoid tissue and not with stage of disease or viral burden. J Immunol 1995;154:5555–66.

84. Gougeon ML, Lecoeur H, Dulioust A, et al. Programmed cell death in peripheral lymphocytes from HIV-infected persons: increased susceptibility to apoptosis of CD4 and CD8 T cells correlates with lymphocyte activation and with disease progression. J Immunol 1996;156:3509–20.

85. Badley AD, Pilon AA, Landay A, et al. Mechanisms of HIV-associated lymphocyte apoptosis. Blood 2000;96:2951–64.

86. Iannello A, Samarani S, Debbeche O, et al. Potential role of interleukin-18 in the immunopathogenesis of AIDS: involvement in fratricidal killing of NK cells. J Virol 2009;83:5999–6010.

87. Cullen BR, Greene WC. Regulatory pathways governing HIV-1 replication. Cell 1989;58:423–6, 3031.

88. de Witte L, Nabatov A, Pion M, et al. Langerin is a natural barrier to HIV-1 transmission by Langerhans cells. Nat Med 2007;13(3):367–71.

89. de Jong MA, de Witte L, Oudhoff MJ, et al. TNF-alpha and TLR agonists increase susceptibility to HIV-1 transmission by human Langerhans cells ex vivo. J Clin Invest 2008;118(10):3440–52.

90. Hammer SM, Squires KE, Hughes MD, et al. A controlled trial of two nucleoside analogues plus indinavir in persons with human immunodeficiency virus infection and CD4 cell counts of 200 per cubic millimeter or less. AIDS Clinical Trials Group 320 Study Team. N Engl J Med 1997;337(11):725–33.

91. Hirsch HH, Kaufmann G, Sendi P, et al. Immune reconstitution in HIV-infected patients. Clin Infect Dis 2004;38(8):1159–66.

92. French MA, Lanzo N, John M, et al. Immune restoration disease after treatment of immunodeficient HIV-infected patients with highly active antiretroviral therapy. HIV Med 2000;1(2):107–15.

93. Shelburne SA, Hamill RJ, Rodriguez-Barradas MC, et al. Immune reconstitution inflammatory syndrome: emergence of a unique syndrome during highly active antiretroviral therapy. Medicine (Baltimore) 2002;81(3):213–27.

94. Müller M, Wandel S, Colebunders R, et al. IeDEA Southern and Central Africa. Immune reconstitution inflammatory syndrome in patients starting antiretroviral therapy for HIV infection: a systematic review and meta-analysis. Lancet Infect Dis 2010;10(4):251–61.

95. Dhasmana DJ, Dheda K, Ravn P, et al. Immune reconstitution inflammatory syndrome in HIV-infected patients receiving antiretroviral therapy: pathogenesis, clinical manifestations and management. Drugs 2008;68(2):191–208.

96. French MA. Disorders of immune reconstitution in patients with HIV infection responding to antiretroviral therapy. Curr HIV/AIDS Rep 2007;4(1):16–21.

97. Cattelan AM, Calabro' ML, De Rossi A, et al. Long-term clinical outcome of AIDS-related Kaposi's sarcoma during highly active antiretroviral therapy. Int J Oncol 2005;27(3):779–85.

98. Holkova B, Takeshita K, Cheng DM, et al. Effect of highly active antiretroviral therapy on survival in patients with AIDS - associated pulmonary Kaposi's sarcoma treated with chemotherapy. J Clin Oncol 2001;19(18):3848–51.

99. Bower M, Nelson M, Young AM, et al. Immune reconstitution inflammatory syndrome associated with Kaposi's sarcoma. J Clin Oncol 2005;23(22):5224–8.

100. Sereti I, Rodger AJ, French MA. Biomarkers in immune reconstitution inflammatory syndrome: signals from pathogenesis. Curr Opin HIV AIDS 2010;5(6):504–10.

101. Ruhwald M, Ravn P. Immune reconstitution syndrome in tuberculosis and HIV-co-infected patients: th1 explosion or cytokine storm? AIDS 2007;21(7):882–4.
102. Finke JS, Shodell M, Shah K, et al. Dendritic cell numbers in the blood of HIV-1 infected patients before and after changes in antiretroviral therapy. J Clin Immunol 2004;24(6):647–52.
103. Chehimi J, Campbell DE, Azzoni L, et al. Persistent decreases in blood plasmacytoid dendritic cell number and function despite effective highly active antiretroviral therapy and increased blood myeloid dendritic cells in HIV-infected individuals. J Immunol 2002;168(9):4796–801.
104. Barron MA, Blyveis N, Palmer BE, et al. Influence of plasma viremia on defects in number and immunophenotype of blood dendritic cell subsets in human immunodeficiency virus 1 infected individuals. J Infect Dis 2003;187(1):26–37.
105. Zelante T, Iannitti R, De Luca A, et al. IL-22 in antifungal immunity. Eur J Immunol 2011;41(2):270–5.
106. van de Veerdonk FL, Kullberg BJ, Netea MG. Pathogenesis of invasive candidiasis. Curr Opin Crit Care 2010;16(5):453–9.
107. Kaufmann S, Sher A, Ahmed R. Immunology of infectious diseases. Washington, DC: ASM Press; 2002. p. 127–34.
108. Dominguez-Villar M, Hafler Immunology DA. An innate role for IL-17. Science 2011;332(6025):47 8.
109. Puel A, Cypowyj S, Bustamante J, et al. Chronic mucocutaneous candidiasis in humans with inborn errors of interleukin-17 immunity. Science 2011;332(6025):65–8.
110. Chai LY, Hsu LY. Recent advances in invasive pulmonary aspergillosis. Curr Opin Pulm Med 2011;17(3):160–6.
111. Phadke AP, Mehrad B. Cytokines in host defense against *Aspergillus*: recent advances. Med Mycol 2005;43(Suppl 1):S173–6.
112. Stevens DA, Moss RB, Kurup VP, et al. Allergic bronchopulmonary aspergillosis in cystic fibrosis—state of the art: cystic fibrosis foundation consensus conference. Clin Infect Dis 2003;37(Suppl 3):S225–64.
113. Meier A, Kirschning CJ, Nikolaus T, et al. Toll-like receptor (TLR) 2 and TLR4 are essential for *Aspergillus*-induced activation of murine macrophages. Cell Microbiol 2003;5:561–70.
114. Marr KA, Balajee SA, Hawn TR, et al. Differential role of MyD88 in macrophage-mediated responses to opportunistic fungal pathogens. Infect Immun 2003;71:5280–6.
115. Zaragoza O, Rodrigues ML, De Jesus M, et al. The capsule of the fungal pathogen *Cryptococcus neoformans*. Adv Appl Microbiol 2009;68:133–216.
116. Schop J. Protective immunity against *Cryptococcus neoformans* infection. McGill J Med 2007;10(1):35–43.
117. Vecchiarelli A, Retini C, Monari C, et al. Purified capsular polysaccharide of *Cryptococcus neoformans* induces interleukin-10 secretion by human monocytes. Infect Immun 1996;64(7):2846–9.
118. Deepe GS Jr, Seder RA. Molecular and cellular determinants of immunity to *Histoplasma capsulatum*. Res Immunol 1998;149:397–406.
119. Rappleye CA, Eissenberg LG, Goldman WE. *Histoplasma capsulatum* alpha-(1,3)-glucan blocks innate immune recognition by the beta-glucan receptor. Proc Natl Acad Sci U S A 2007;104(4):1366–70.
120. Gorocica P, Taylor ML, Alvarado-Vásquez N, et al. The interaction between *Histoplasma capsulatum* cell wall carbohydrates and host components: relevance in the immunomodulatory role of histoplasmosis. Mem Inst Oswaldo Cruz 2009;104(3):492–6.

121. Volkman HE, Pozos TC, Zheng J, et al. Tuberculous granuloma induction via interaction of a bacterial secreted protein with host epithelium. Science 2010; 327(5964):466–9.

122. Agarwal N, Bishai Microbiology WR. Subversion from the sidelines. Science 2010;327(5964):417–8.

123. Mishra BB, Moura-Alves P, Sonawane A, et al. *Mycobacterium tuberculosis* protein ESAT-6 is a potent activator of the NLRP3/ASC inflammasome. Cell Microbiol 2010;12(8):1046–63.

124. Khader SA, Cooper AM. IL-23 and IL-17 in tuberculosis. Cytokine 2008;41(2): 79–83.

125. Jacobson MA, Spritzler J, Landay A, et al. A phase I, placebo-controlled trial of multi-dose recombinant human interleukin-12 in patients with HIV infection. AIDS 2002;16(8):1147–54.

126. Greinert U, Ernst M, Schlaak M, et al. Interleukin-12 as successful adjuvant in tuberculosis treatment. Eur Respir J 2001;17(5):1049–51.

127. Mendez-Samperio. Expression and regulation of chemokines in mycobacterial infection. J Infect 2008;57(5):374–84.

128. Jackson JA, Friberg IM, Little S, et al. Review series on helminths, immune modulation and the hygiene hypothesis: immunity against helminths and immunological phenomena in modern human populations: coevolutionary legacies? [review erratum in: Immunology 2009 Mar;126(3):446]. Immunology 2009; 126(1):18–27.

129. Coffman RL. Immunology. The origin of TH2 responses. Science 2010; 328(5982):1116–7.

130. Carvalho L, Sun J, Kane C, et al. Review series on helminths, immune modulation and the hygiene hypothesis: mechanisms underlying helminth modulation of dendritic cell function. Immunology 2009;126(1):28–34.

131. Moreau E, Chauvin A. Immunity against helminths: interactions with the host and the intercurrent infections. J Biomed Biotechnol 2010;2010:428593.

132. Murdoch C, Finn A. Chemokine receptors and their role in inflammation and infectious diseases [review]. Blood 2000;95(10):3032–43.

133. Maestre A, Muskus C, Duque V, et al. Acquired antibody responses against *Plasmodium vivax* infection vary with host genotype for Duffy antigen receptor for chemokines (DARC). PLoS One 2010;5(7):e11437.

134. Ercolini AM, Miller SD. The role of infections in autoimmune disease. Clin Exp Immunol 2009;155(1):1–15.

135. Wucherpfennig KW. Mechanisms for the induction of autoimmunity by infectious agents. J Clin Invest 2001;108(8):1097–104.

136. Dale JB, Beachey EH. Epitopes of streptococcal M proteins shared with cardiac myosin. J Exp Med 1985;162:583–91.

137. Neisser A, Schwerer B, Bernheimer H, et al. Ganglioside-induced antiganglioside antibodies from a neuropathy patient cross-react with lipopolysaccharides of *Campylobacter jejuni* associated with Guillain-Barre syndrome. J Neuroimmunol 2000;102:85–8.

138. Stetson DB. Connections between antiviral defense and autoimmunity. Curr Opin Immunol 2009;21(3):244–50.

139. Bouley DM, Kanangat S, Wire W, et al. Characterization of herpes simplex virus type-1 infection and herpetic stromal keratitis development in IFN-gamma knockout mice. J Immunol 1995;155:3964–71.

140. Elkind MS. Impact of innate inflammation in population studies. Ann N Y Acad Sci 2010;1207:97–106.

Vaccines and Vaccine Adjuvants as Biological Response Modifiers

Cristian Speil, MD*, Robert Rzepka, MD

KEYWORDS

- Immunomodulatory drugs • Cytokines • Vaccine adjuvants

According to the *Concise Dictionary of Modern Medicine*, biological response modifiers (BRM) are "any of a broad family of natural or synthetic molecules that up- or down-regulate, or restore immune responsiveness."[1] Their immune modulatory properties are being used increasingly to selectively (or less so) manipulate parts of the immune system for the treatment of a variety of autoimmune, infectious, or neoplastic diseases. BRMs include a large variety of naturally occurring and synthetic molecules such as cytokine colony-stimulating factors (CSF), interferons (IFN), interleukins (IL), monoclonal antibodies, and receptor antagonists directed against proinflammatory cytokines, immunoglobulins, glucocorticoids, and anticoagulant proteins such as activated protein C (APC).[2]

VACCINES AND VACCINE ADJUVANTS

A "traditional" infectious disease vaccine is a preparation of a live attenuated, inactivated, or killed pathogen, a part of the pathogen's structure or products (toxins) that stimulates immunity against the pathogen by enhancing humoral and/or cellular immune response, but is not capable of causing significant infection.[3] Vaccines are designed to stimulate specific immune responses; however, they typically induce immunity against themselves and related antigens, being immunogenic rather than true immunomodulatory, and were not traditionally included in most classifications of BRMs. There is a notable exception: the antituberculous bacillus Calmette-Guérin (BCG) vaccine has been used extensively for 35 years (with good results) to stimulate local immunity against superficial bladder cancer, therefore acting as a true BRM.[4]

More recently, however, advances in basic sciences have been emphasizing the role played by infection, immunity, and inflammation in cancer biology, and there

The authors have nothing to disclose.
Division of Infectious Diseases, Southern Illinois University School of Medicine, 801 North Rutledge, PO Box 9636, Springfield, IL 62794, USA
* Corresponding author.
*E-mail address:*cspeil@siumed.edu

Infect Dis Clin N Am 25 (2011) 755–772
doi:10.1016/j.idc.2011.07.004
0891-5520/11/$ – see front matter © 2011 Elsevier Inc. All rights reserved.

id.theclinics.com

now is a tremendous interest in cancer immunotherapy, including different types of cancer vaccines.[5] Vaccines targeting viral agents involved in cancer pathogenesis, such as human papilloma virus (HPV) or hepatitis B virus (HBV), are already in use and may be regarded as prophylactic cancer vaccines. Looking at tumor growth from the perspective of immune surveillance failure, therapeutic cancer vaccines targeting tumor antigens certainly appear very promising.[6] There is significant ongoing research on the use of vaccines as immunotherapy for a variety of noninfectious conditions from autoimmune diseases to hypertension, diabetes mellitus, and Alzheimer disease.[5,7] One category of immunomodulatory vaccines directly targets endogenous or exogenous substances or metabolic products involved in disease pathogenesis, such as like tumor necrosis factor (TNF)-α in rheumatoid arthritis, IL-5 in asthma, β-amyloid in Alzheimer disease, and angiotensin I and II in hypertension. Another type of therapeutic vaccines inhibits the pathologic immune response directed against self-antigens, shifting the balance toward immunotolerance in autoimmune diseases such as myasthenia gravis, type 1 diabetes mellitus (DM1), and multiple sclerosis.[7]

Vaccine immunologic adjuvants are compounds incorporated into vaccines to enhance immunogenicity, and are an important part of immunomodulatory and cancer vaccines.[5,8] The term adjuvant was coined by Ramon in 1926 to designate substances he was using to increase immunogenicity of tetanus and diphtheria toxins.[9] Whereas the earlier vaccines using inactivated or attenuated whole cells were highly immunogenic by themselves, more recent vaccines using highly purified antigens may benefit even more from the use of adjuvants.[8] Nonspecific adjuvants, such as aluminum salts, increase the exposure of antigen-presenting cells (APCs) to the antigen by increasing the local antigen concentration, but also stimulate dendritic cells (DCs) and cytokine release.[10] The aluminum salts induce humoral immunity via a T-helper type 2 (Th2) response but have lesser effect on cell-mediated immunity, and therefore are not useful in vaccines directed against intracellular pathogens.[11] Aluminum salts have been in use for 80 years and were the first adjuvants approved by the Food and Drug Administration (FDA) for use in vaccines in the United States.[11] Incomplete Freund adjuvant (IFA) is made of paraffin oil combined with a surfactant. When combined with an antigen suspension, it forms a water-in-oil emulsion, the antigen being in the water phase.[12] Complete Freund adjuvant (CFA) is created by adding killed mycobacteria (traditionally *Mycobacterium tuberculosis*) to IFA.[12] Both are strongly immunogenic, but only CFA induces a T-helper type 1 (Th1) response, presumably because of the presence of mycobacterial antigens.[11] Freund adjuvants are not used clinically but they have been used in immunologic research for more than 75 years.[13] Another water-in-oil emulsion-based adjuvant (MF59) was recently approved for use in humans, and has replaced aluminum hydroxide in several influenza vaccines.[9] MF59 has been studied as an adjuvant for multiple other experimental vaccines, including human immunodeficiency virus (HIV), HBV, herpes simplex virus, and cytomegalovirus vaccines, and has shown significant immunogenicity and a good side-effect profile.[8] In contrast to aluminum salts, MF59 is capable of inducing a good Th1 response and to stimulate cellular immunity.[11] Saponins are naturally occurring steroid or terpenoid glycosides currently being researched as adjuvants in various types of vaccines.[14]

A different class of adjuvants directly stimulates the innate immune system via Toll-like receptors (TLRs), and includes many microbial-derived adjuvants such as cholera toxin, flagellin and, more recently, monophosphoryl lipid A (MPL).[8] TLRs are an important subclass of pattern recognition receptors (PRR) on phagocytes. TLRs are capable of recognizing and binding to pathogen-associated molecular patterns (PAMPs), and initiating a cascade that results in phagocytosis and activation of APCs that eventually triggers the adaptive immune response.[15] MPL is derived from the lipopolysaccharide (LPS) of *Salmonella minnesota* R595, and has strong immunogenic properties through activation of TLR-2 and TLR-4.[11,16] LPS induces a predominantly Th1 response, and is currently used in Cervarix, a prophylactic HPV vaccine.[17,18] It has also been used as an adjuvant in several therapeutic cancer vaccine trials, either alone or in combination with other adjuvants.[19] Cytokines, such as TNF-α, granulocyte macrophage CSF (GM-CSF), IL-12, and monoclonal antibodies, are being studied as adjuvants in cancer vaccines, but are not without risk.[5,20] A superagonist anti-CD-28 monoclonal antibody, with direct T-cell stimulatory properties, resulted in severe systemic reaction and shock when administered to healthy volunteers during a phase 1 trial.[20]

The remainder of this article discusses some of the uses of vaccines as immunomodulators, with emphasis on cancer and autoimmune diseases.

CANCER VACCINES

Cancer caused more than 500,000 deaths in the United States in 2007, being the second most frequent cause of death, very closely after cardiovascular diseases.[21] Traditional cancer therapies such as surgery, radiation, and chemotherapy are associated with significant side effects and often are not able to cure the disease. The important role played by the immune system in controlling the malignant cells, proved by the increased risk of cancer in immunosuppressed individuals such as those with HIV infection or in transplant recipients is well established. The first instance of successful cancer immunotherapy was the use of BCG vaccine in superficial bladder cancer, and for a long time it was the only application of vaccines in cancer treatment.[22] More recently, however, cancer immunotherapy has become a rapidly expanding field, and various types of cancer vaccines are currently under development.[23] Cancer vaccines may be prophylactic, directed against infectious agents known to cause or to be strongly associated with cancers such as HBV, Epstein-Barr virus (EBV), or HPV, or therapeutic, directed against tumor antigens. Simply stated, a therapeutic cancer vaccine has several components: a tumor antigen coupled to a delivery system, an adjuvant to increase immunogenicity, and an immunomodulatory molecule.[5,24] The tumor antigens may be tumor specific (such as mutated oncogene products or immunoglobulin idiotypes in hematological malignancies) or tumor-associated antigens, which may be shared by several different tumors.[24] The choice of antigen is paramount because the antigen determines the magnitude of immune response and the specificity of the vaccine. Given the large number of known cancer antigens, choosing the most appropriate target for a vaccine is a very complex task. The National Cancer Institute has published a ranking of cancer antigens using a list of "ideal" cancer antigen characteristics, including therapeutic function, immunogenicity, oncogenicity, specificity, expression level, and so forth.[25]

From the antigen delivery standpoint, cancer vaccines may belong to 1 of 3 categories:

1. Cellular vaccines (whole-tumor cells, DCs)
2. Protein-based vaccines
3. Vector-based vaccines (recombinant viruses, bacteria, yeast, or DNA)[26]

A promising new type of cellular vaccines is the dendritic cell (DC) vaccines. DCs are APCs strategically positioned at the skin and mucosal surfaces where they can come into contact with foreign antigens.[27] Together with neutrophils, macrophages, natural killer (NK) cells, and the complement system, they are part of the innate or nonspecific immune system that represents the body's first line of immunologic defense. DCs are able to initiate a primary immune response by processing and presenting foreign antigens and then migrating to the regional lymph nodes, where they interact with and activate antigen-specific T cells, thus being the main interface between the innate immunity and the more evolved adaptive immune system.[28] DCs cells are also capable of stimulating humoral immunity by direct interaction with B cells.[29] DCs can modulate the immune response, resulting in immunologic rejection or tolerance depending on the type of antigen being processed and the stage of maturation of DC presenting the antigen.[30] For example, antigen presentation by immature DCs is thought to be an important mechanism of inducing immunotolerance to self-antigens.[30] Their ability to activate T cells, B cells, and NK cells makes them ideal candidates as a cancer vaccine delivery platform.[31] Several approaches have used DCs in cancer vaccines. One approach is to generate DCs in vitro and use them as a delivery system for tumor antigens because of their ability to migrate to local lymphoid organs. Another strategy is to deliver tumor antigens directly to DCs in lymphoid organs by use of monoclonal or anti-DC antibodies.[27] Although DC vaccines are showing promising results, for better efficacy they may need to be combined with different types of immunotherapy, such as blocking antibodies or soluble receptors.[29] Combining cancer vaccines with chemotherapy or other standard treatments may also increase chances for a successful outcome. A DC-based vaccine targeting the mutated p53 gene significantly enhanced the response to subsequent chemotherapy in patients with advanced small-cell lung cancer.[32] In a phase 2 trial, a vaccine using autologous DCs incubated with tumor antigens in patients with advanced melanoma showed increased overall survival in responders.[33] In a subgroup analysis from the same trial, vaccination improved response to subsequent cancer therapy.[34] Another DC-based cancer vaccine (sipuleucel-T) was recently FDA-approved for prostate cancer therapy.[35]

Peptide vaccines are based on the ability of T cells to recognize small peptides resulting from the degradation of complex antigens and bound to HLA class I and II molecules.[36] These vaccines offer the advantage of a more specific immune response, thus decreasing the risk of cross-reactivity with self-antigens. On the down side, they are less immunogenic compared with more complex antigens, and various strategies are being employed to increase their immunogenicity, including coformulation with adjuvants, administration in combination with immunomodulatory cytokines, or using them in DC-based vaccines.[36] A gp-100 peptide vaccine has been studied in combination with the immunomodulatory molecule IL-2 or with ipilimumab, a monoclonal antibody that blocks cytotoxic T-lymphocyte–associated antigen 4 (CTLA-4) for melanoma therapy.[37]

New delivery systems based on recent advances in gene therapy and description of genes coding for tumor antigens for cancer vaccines involve plasmid DNA and viral vector vaccines.[36,38]

DNA vaccines typically involve insertion of the gene producing the antigen into bacterial plasmid DNA, which uses the host's cellular machinery to synthesize the antigen and induce an immune response.[39] This approach can be used for protein antigens, and has been studied in many cancers as well as autoimmune diseases such as rheumatoid arthritis and multiple sclerosis.[40,41] Advantages of DNA vaccines include safety, stability, and relative ease of production. The main disadvantage is lower immunogenicity in humans.[38] To overcome this disadvantage different approaches have been tried, including different routes of administration, plasmid design to maximize expression of encoded antigens, use of immunomodulatory molecules as adjuvants, and different prime-boost regimens. Ongoing clinical trials are studying DNA vaccines in cancer therapy, including treatment of lymphoma, melanoma, and breast, cervical, and prostate cancer.[38]

Vaccines using recombinant viruses as vectors are another type of gene therapy. Genes for tumor-associated antigens (TAA) are introduced into the viral genome of attenuated viruses that are lacking in in vivo replicative abilities. The most promising viral vectors are poxviruses, such as vaccinia virus, and adenoviruses.[36] A major disadvantage of this class of vaccine is the presence of neutralizing antiviral antibodies in the host, not an uncommon occurrence, giving repeated natural exposure to these viruses.[36] A promising prostate cancer vaccine involving a recombinant vaccinia virus (PROSTVAC VF) is currently undergoing clinical trials.[42]

Use of immunomodulatory substances in association with or included in cancer vaccines has led to good results in many clinical trials, and is now widely employed. Examples include costimulatory molecules B7-1, ICAM-1, and LFA-3 (TRICOM) in the recombinant poxvirus vector vaccine (PROSTVAC), or GM-CSF in a DC vaccine (sipuleucel-T), both used in the treatment of prostate cancer, and IL-2, used in combination with the gp209-2 M peptide vaccine in multiple myeloma.[35,43,44]

Selected Uses of Vaccines in Cancer Immunotherapy

BCG vaccine

BCG vaccine is one of the oldest vaccines still available, the original BCG vaccine being the first live vaccine of the twentieth century. It was developed by Albert Calmette and Camille Guérin in 1921 at l'Institut Pasteur in France from a virulent strain of *Mycobacterium bovis* attenuated by multiple passages (approximately 230) on bile, glycerin, and potato media.[45] The initial method of administration was oral, intradermal, and multiple puncture and scarification routes, being developed in 1927, 1939, and 1947, respectively.[45] In its long history, the BCG vaccine has been administered to billions of people with the goal of preventing tuberculosis.[46]

The original BCG strain, now lost, was initially maintained by serial passages at the Pasteur Institute then distributed to different laboratories for vaccine manufacture. Until lyophilization was developed as a storage method in 1961, each of these laboratories maintained their own strains by subculturing them in conditions possibly different from each other, resulting in BCG stocks different in terms of genetics, biochemical characteristics, virulence, and immunogenicity.[45,47] Numerous studies have shown different levels of efficacy of the vaccine in preventing tuberculosis in different populations.[46] While this may be at least partially related to varying potencies of different strains of BCG used for vaccines, it is still not clear whether and how the strains currently available differ in terms of preventing tuberculosis.[48]

The United States (besides the Netherlands) is one of the few countries in the world that has never instituted mandatory BCG vaccination. BCG vaccination is not routinely recommended in the United States because of the low risk of infection with *Mycobacterium tuberculosis*, the variable efficacy of the vaccine, and its interference with tuberculosis skin-test reactivity. The only indications for BCG vaccination in the United States are in children with a negative skin test who are continuously exposed and cannot be separated from adults with tuberculosis resistant to isoniazid (INH) and rifampin, and in health care workers caring for tuberculosis patients in whom there is a high prevalence of resistance to INH and rifampin in the community.[49]

Despite the variable efficacy in prevention of tuberculosis, the vaccine has since found widespread use as a nonspecific immunomodulatory agent, particularly in the treatment of superficial bladder cancer.

The beginnings may have been in a 1929 article called "Cancer and tuberculosis" by Raymond Pearl, based on 816 autopsies, showing that active tuberculosis patients were at lower risk of having malignant tumors. However, subsequent studies brought his results under scrutiny, particularly the selection of his controls.[50] The first big step in using BCG as immunotherapy for cancer actually came in 1971 when Zbar and colleagues[51] demonstrated that BCG injected into animals had local antitumor effects. Moreover, animals that showed inhibition of tumor growth with BCG showed a delayed sensitivity reaction when being rechallenged with tumor cells. In 1974, the same investigators proposed criteria for successful BCG therapy for bladder cancer.[52] In another case report from 1975, deKernion and colleagues[53] showed cure of a metastatic melanoma of the urinary bladder after intralesional BCG injection. In 1975, Bloomberg and colleagues[54] showed that BCG caused a marked inflammatory reaction when injected into the bladder of sensitized dogs. Following these initial results, Alvaro Morales, in a milestone study in 1976, showed that BCG administered intradermally and intravesically reduced tumor recurrence or cured existing disease in 7 patients.[22,52] Subsequent randomized control trials showed similar results, significantly decreasing tumor recurrence when added to standard therapy at that time, and paved the way for large-scale use of BCG vaccines in the treatment of superficial bladder cancer.[55,56]

The proposed antitumor action of BCG instilled intravesically is not through direct cytotoxic effect but via a delayed hypersensitivity reaction to the live mycobacteria.[51] BCG initially may attach to bladder mucosa via fibronectin receptors, followed by phagocytosis by macrophages that migrate to regional lymph nodes and trigger a cellular immune response by activated CD4+ lymphocytes, resulting in killing of BCG together with tumor cells and eventually granuloma formation.[57] The exact mechanism of action is not known, but it has been shown that live BCG induces a strong Th1 response.[58] A Th1 lymphocyte phenotype is associated with production of specific cytokines, including IL-2, TNF, and IFN-γ, which would be mostly effective against viruses and other intracellular pathogens and is also required for antineoplastic activity.[59,60] More recent research suggests that neutrophils also play an important role in BCG-induced tumor lysis via production of TNF-related apoptosis-inducing ligand (TRAIL).[59] TRAIL is a type II membrane protein related to the TNF family, capable of inducing apoptosis in neoplastic cells but not in normal cells.[61] Recent studies showed increased urine levels of TRAIL in patients who responded to BCG therapy, compared with nonresponders, suggesting a role for TRAIL in the antineoplastic effect of BCG.[62]

BCG is currently recommended by the American Urological Association guidelines on management of non–muscle-invasive bladder cancer as first-line treatment for carcinoma in situ, and as adjuvant therapy to prevent recurrences following transurethral resection of bladder tumor (TURBT) in intermediate-risk and high-risk patients.[63] Given the higher incidence of adverse reactions to BCG compared with intravesical chemotherapy, patients at low risk for recurrence are managed with surgery that may be followed by a single dose of chemotherapy.

Current recommendations for use of BCG in superficial (non–muscle invasive) bladder cancer are mainly based on studies comparing BCG with mitomycin C chemotherapy. Most data shows superiority of BCG but also a higher incidence of side effects.[64] Maintenance therapy with BCG has proved to be beneficial in terms of decreasing recurrence but without affecting 5-year survival, and is currently recommended only for high-risk patients.[65]

In a recent Cochrane review, adverse reactions associated with BCG use were common but self-limited and included cystitis (67%), hematuria (23%), fever (25%), and urinary frequency (71%). No BCG-related deaths were reported.[66] However, BCG is also a live vaccine capable of causing local and systemic infection in susceptible individuals, although the incidence of serious infectious complications is very low.[67] In a retrospective study of 2602 patients, the most common infectious complication was granulomatous prostatitis in 0.9%, and systemic infection was noted in

0.4%.[67] Because of the higher risk of local and systemic infection, BCG administration is usually withheld for 2 weeks after TURBT, and even longer if there is history of traumatic catheterization, urinary tract infection, or persistent hematuria. In addition, BCG administration is contraindicated in patients with active tuberculosis or significant immunosuppression who are at higher risk of developing systemic infection.[4] There was no significant difference between different strains of BCG in terms of efficacy or adverse reactions.[4]

Although BCG is highly effective as immunotherapy for bladder cancer (even more so than in preventing tuberculosis), side effects associated with therapy are common, and efforts have been made toward preventing or decreasing adverse reactions. Different strategies include dose reduction, addition of ofloxacin to decrease local reactions, use of other proinflammatory cytokines, and identification of mycobacterial components able to induce a strong immune response but with fewer side effects than the live mycobacteria.[59] IFN-α2b has been studied in both BCG-naïve and relapsing patients, and is showing promise although the results are still controversial.[68,69] Other cytokines being studied are GM-CSF and IL-2, all part of the cellular immune response induced by BCG.[59] Mycobacterial components, such as a cell wall extract of *Mycobacterium phlei*, have shown efficacy and a good safety profile in small studies.[70,71]

Novel and fascinating applications of BCG vaccine, based on its immunologic properties (strong immunogenicity and ability to replicate inside APC [macrophages and DCs]) have been studied recently. Variants of recombinant BCG are being researched as vectors for other vaccines, as improved vaccines against tuberculosis, and as potent immunomodulatory molecules engineered to express a specific cytokine profile.[72] In a study by Murray and colleagues,[73] mice injected with recombinant BCG strains secreting GM-CSF, IL-2, and IFN-γ showed an increased antigen-specific T-cell response, independent of the inoculation route. These recombinant strains that elicit long-lasting cellular immunity may have applications as novel tuberculosis vaccines, as vaccine vectors, or in tumor immunotherapy.

An exciting potential application of recombinant BCG is in breast cancer immunotherapy. Breast cancer is a worldwide leading cause of morbidity and cancer death, and the search for a candidate therapeutic cancer vaccine is rapidly expanding. Mucin1 (MUC1), a breast cancer tumor-associated antigen, is a potential target for immunotherapy.[74] In a recent study, immune-deficient mice were inoculated with MUC1(+) breast cancer cells and then injected with 3 different recombinant BCG strains. The vaccine strains were engineered to express one or multiple variable-number tandem repeat (VNTR) epitopes of MUC1 antigen, and also to secrete GM-CSF. Mice receiving the vaccine showed a lower incidence of breast cancer and lower mortality rate compared with controls. The investigators also noted that efficacy of the vaccines increased with the number of VNTR epitopes, which may correlate with a stronger immune response, because VNTR epitopes are important for induction of a cytotoxic T-cell response.[75]

Sipuleucel-T

Prostate cancer is one of the most common cancers and the second most common cause of cancer death in men in the United States.[76] Sipuleucel-T is an autologous DC-based therapeutic vaccine targeting prostatic acid phosphatase (PAP), a tumor antigen present in 95% of prostatic adenocarcinomas.[77] A recombinant fusion protein (PA 2024) composed of PAP and GM-CSF is incubated in vitro with peripheral blood mononuclear cells, including DC precursors harvested from the patient.[77] GM-CSF is used for its ability to stimulate growth and maturation of macrophages and DCs.[78] Exposing the APCs to the antigen in vitro may offer the advantage of an augmented immune response by removing the cells from the immunotolerant environment of the patient.[79] Patients are then administered 3 doses of the vaccine over a 1-month period.[77] In two phase 3 double-blind, randomized, placebo-controlled trials in patients with advanced prostate cancer, men treated with sipuleucel-T showed a 33% reduction in the risk of death and 100% increase in 36-month survival compared with placebo.[80] The vaccine has a favorable side-effect profile. Most common side effects observed were chills, fever, headache, asthenia, dyspnea, and vomiting, and were usually transient and self-limited.[80] In the most recent and largest trial to date, Immunotherapy for Prostate Adenocarcinoma Treatment (IMPACT), sipuleucel-T was administered to men with metastatic castration-resistant prostate cancer (MCRPC). Patients in the sipuleucel-T group had a relative reduction in the risk of death of 22% compared with placebo.[76] Based on these trials, the FDA approved sipuleucel-T (Provenge) in April 2010 for the treatment of patients with asymptomatic or minimally symptomatic MCRPC.[78]

Prostvac-VF

Prostvac-VF is a vaccination system using recombinant poxviruses as vectors for prostate-specific antigen (PSA) and immunomodulatory molecules in a prime-boost strategy to enhance immunogenicity.[43] Prostvac-VF consists of a recombinant vaccinia vector vaccine and a fowlpox vector vaccine encoding the genes for PSA and the immunostimulator complex TRICOM, administered sequentially.[42] The vaccinia component is administered as a primary vaccination, followed by boosters using the fowlpox vaccine.[43] In a recent phase 2 trial in patients with MCRPC, the vaccine was associated with a 44% reduction in death rate and had an excellent safety profile.[81]

VACCINES IN AUTOIMMUNE DISEASES

Autoimmune diseases, such as systemic lupus erythematosus, rheumatoid arthritis and related connective tissue disorders, psoriasis, Crohn disease, and DM1, are a large group of entities of unknown etiology with a protracted and often fluctuating course, causing significant morbidity and mortality worldwide.[82] Although mechanisms are not exactly defined, most of their pathogenesis is mediated by loss of tolerance to self and attack by T cells and proinflammatory cytokines, and therefore subject to immunotherapy.[83] Since the advent of monoclonal antibodies 30 years ago, there has been increasing interest in anticytokine therapy, most notably directed against TNF-α, which has been clearly involved in the pathogenesis of multiple autoimmune conditions.[84] Active immunotherapy in autoimmune diseases, including anticytokine vaccines, is a relatively new development, but complements more established immunotherapies.[85] The authors now briefly discuss vaccine development in two autoimmune conditions: rheumatoid arthritis and multiple sclerosis.

Rheumatoid Arthritis

Rheumatoid arthritis is a relatively common autoimmune rheumatologic disease of unknown etiology characterized by synovial inflammation and significant nonarticular manifestations.[86] The proinflammatory cytokines TNF-α, IL-1β, IL-6 and, more recently, IL-17 have been shown to play an important role in the pathogenesis of rheumatoid arthritis. TNF-α and IL-1β produced by synovial macrophages stimulate the proliferation of synovial cells, which in turn produce collagenase that lyses cartilage, inhibits proteoglycan synthesis, and promotes bone resorption.[87] The inflamed synovium, infiltrated with inflammatory cells, causes irreversible destruction of the cartilage and bone components of the joint.[88] All 3 cytokines have been successfully targeted by passive anticytokine immunotherapy using soluble receptor antagonists, cell surface receptor antagonists, and monoclonal antibodies.[87] Although passive immunotherapy (particularly monoclonal antibodies targeting TNF-α) is highly effective in rheumatoid arthritis, it does not work for everyone, and has high cost and significant side effects, particularly opportunistic infections. These issues are a good reason for developing different anticytokine approaches, including active immunotherapy using various anticytokine vaccines.[85]

In an early experiment by Dalum and colleagues,[89] mice injected with recombinant murine TNF-α containing foreign T-helper epitopes to increase immunogenicity developed high titers of anti–TNF-α antibodies that were maintained by booster injections. Using a cachexia model obtained by injecting mice with murine TNF-α, the investigators were able to show that immunization with this vaccine before administration of TNF-α significantly reduced weight loss and mortality in the experimental animals. Also, in a murine model of rheumatoid arthritis, the vaccine significantly reduced the incidence of clinical symptoms and arthritis compared with controls. The investigators also noted that administration of anti–TNF-α monoclonal antibodies had no influence on the incidence of arthritis in this experimental model.[89]

More recently, a vaccine developed by coupling inactive human TNF-α with the career protein keyhole limpet hemocyanin (KLH) (TNF-kinoid) has been shown to be effective in a transgenic mouse model of rheumatoid arthritis in a series of experiments.[90–93]

Transgenic mice overexpressing human TNF-α genes spontaneously develop chronic inflammatory polyarthritis at 4 to 5 weeks of age. Development of arthritis is associated with increased TNF-α production, and administration of ant–TNF-α monoclonal antibodies at birth prevents it.[88] Using this animal model, Le Buanec and colleagues[91] showed induction of protective anti-TNF antibodies by the TNF-kinoid vaccine, demonstrated by prevention of TNF-induced shock and inflammatory polyarthritis. Subsequent experiments by Delavallee and colleagues[92,93] demonstrated early and long-term preventive and therapeutic effects of the TNF-kinoid vaccine in the transgenic mouse model of rheumatoid arthritis. Based on the promising responses thus far, several phase 1 and 2 trials involving the TNF-kinoid vaccine are being conducted by Neovacs in rheumatoid arthritis, Crohn disease, and lupus patients.[94] The ongoing rheumatoid arthritis phase 2 trial comprises patients who failed TNF-α antagonists or developed antidrug antibodies.[95] Other candidate anticytokine vaccines are targeting IL-1 and IL-17, two key mediators in the pathogenesis of joint and cartilage destruction in rheumatoid arthritis.[96–100] For a comprehensive list of targeted cytokines and candidate vaccines, the reader is referred to the excellent review by Delavallee and colleagues.[85]

Multiple Sclerosis

Multiple sclerosis is a chronic demyelinating disease with fluctuating course and heterogeneous characteristics. The animal model for multiple sclerosis is experimental autoimmune encephalomyelitis (EAE).[97,98] Although the etiology is unknown, there is increasing evidence that the principal pathogenic mechanism involves autoimmunity in the form of a Th1 inflammatory response.[99,100] More recently a subset of T cells producing IL-17, designated Th17, was also found to have an important role in pathogenesis of multiple sclerosis/EAE.[101] The inflammatory response is directed against self-antigens such as myelin basic protein (MBP), myelin oligodendrocyte glycoprotein, or proteolipid protein (PLP).[102] Approved therapies for multiple sclerosis include steroids, immunosuppressive agents, and immunomodulatory agents including IFN-β1b and glatiramer acetate.[103]

Several vaccine techniques are being considered for multiple sclerosis/EAE, including T-cell vaccines, T-cell receptor peptide vaccines, vaccines with altered peptide ligands (APL), DNA vaccines, and anticytokine vaccines. Similar to classic anti-infective vaccines, T-cell vaccines use attenuated T cells to induce a protective immune response against pathogenic T cells.[102] The T-cell receptors (TCR) on pathogenic Th1 cells that interact with autoantigens in multiple sclerosis use a limited number of variable-region elements (V regions) that are recognized by regulatory specific Th2 cells.[102,104] TCR candidate vaccines targeting peptides from the pathogenic Th1 cells receptors are being studied in EAE models and in clinical trials.[105] DNA vaccines using naked DNA or recombinant viral vectors are targeting genes encoding TCR peptides, MBP or other myelin antigens, and cytokines (TNF-α, IL-4, IL-10).[102] Recent clinical trials of DNA vaccines have improved magnetic resonance imaging findings in patients with multiple sclerosis.[40]

APL vaccines are an exciting new category for which self-antigen epitopes involved in the interaction with the TCR are changed by amino acid substitution, in an attempt to generate a new peptide that can induce a tolerant immune response to the original self-antigen.[102] In a phase 2 trial, an APL derived from immunodominant epitope of MBP (NBI 5788) was able to induce a shift from Th1 to Th2 response that may be protective in multiple sclerosis; however, the study was terminated early because of the high incidence of immediate-type hypersensitivity reactions (also Th2 mediated).[106]

Anticytokine vaccine candidates in multiple sclerosis target TNF-α and/or IL-17, and have also been studied in the EAE model.[85] A TNF-α naked DNA vaccine protected rats against EAE induced by injection of MBP combined with CFA.[107] In another study, immunization of rats with a naked DNA vaccine encoding genes for 4 chemokines from the C-C gene family conferred protection against EAE.[108] Cytokines from the C-C family are chemotactic for monocytes, macrophages, T cells, basophils, and eosinophils, and have been involved in the pathogenesis of EAE.[109] These cytokines include macrophage inflammatory protein 1a (MIP-1a), MIP-1b, monocyte-chemotactic protein-1 (MCP-1) and RANTES (CCL5).[108] An autologous anti–IL-17 vaccine protected mice against PLP-induced EAE in other experiments.[110] To further highlight the role of newly discovered IL-17 in multiple sclerosis and rheumatoid arthritis, a vaccine is using recombinant murine IL-17 covalently bound to a virus-like particle (VLP). VLPs are structures that have a similar antigenic pattern to that of actual viruses, without the viral genome.[110] VLPs are capable of inducing strong immune responses, similar with those induced by native viruses, and have found large applicability in the vaccine industry, both in established vaccines and in research. Examples of VLP-based vaccines are the two HBV and two HPV vaccines.[110,111]

VACCINES AS IMMUNOTHERAPY IN CARDIOVASCULAR DISEASES AND DIABETES MELLITUS

The renin-angiotensin system (RAS) plays an important role in the pathogenesis of hypertension. There is hope that immunization against components of RAS will eliminate the need for daily doses of antihypertensive drugs. PMD3117 is an angiotensin I peptide vaccine coupled with KLH and adsorbed on aluminum hydroxide to increase immunogenicity.[112] When administered to patients with essential hypertension in a clinical trial, it was able to stimulate production of angiotensin I antibodies, but did not reduce blood pressure significantly.[112] CYT006-AngQb is a VLP vaccine targeting angiotensin II. In a phase 2 trial, this vaccine was able to decrease the early-morning increase in blood pressure in patients with mild and moderate hypertension.[113] More research is needed before considering vaccines as serious alternatives to treat hypertension.[114]

Atherosclerosis is a multifactorial disease in which multiple risk factors converging on the endothelial cells produce a complex inflammatory cascade, leading to plaque formation.[115] Atherosclerosis remains the leading cause of cardiac disease, and current therapies targeting established risk factors have only a limited effect on its progression.[116] The idea of vaccine immunotherapy in atherosclerosis is based on the role of inflammation, immunity, and subendothelial neovascularization in the progression of atherosclerosis.[117] Candidate vaccines in atherosclerosis will be targeting proinflammatory cytokines such as IFN-γ and TNF-α, endothelial growth factor receptors, and protein component of low-density lipoprotein (apoB100).[115]

DM1 is an autoimmune disease in which the immune system attacks and progressively destroys pancreatic B cells responsible for insulin production.[118] DM1 has a strong genetic component: HLA genes, and especially the DQ locus on the short arm of chromosome 6, are the most important genetic determinant of DM1.[118,119] A large study in Finland, a country with a higher prevalence of DM1, showed that a small but significant proportion of children with the high-risk genotype would develop autoantibodies against islet cells and insulin well before clinical manifestations of DM.[119] In the NOD mouse model of spontaneous DM1, administration of intranasal insulin induces immune tolerance to insulin, results confirmed in humans in a pilot study.[120] Diabetes vaccines target specific autoantigens, such as insulin, glutamate decarboxylase, or heat-shock protein 60, and have been studied as primary prevention (to prevent autoantibodies in individual with high genetic susceptibility), secondary prevention (to prevent disease in patients with autoantibodies), or therapy for DM1 (to preserve remaining islet cells).[121] Although earlier prevention trials did not show a clear benefit for insulin administration in diabetes prevention, they demonstrated an excellent safety profile.[122,123] The pre-POINT trial is another ongoing phase 1 study to establish safety and feasibility of oral and intranasal insulin in primary prevention of DM1 in children at high genetic risk.[124]

Since the first attempts at vaccination in the seventh century, to the "golden" times of Jenner, Koch, and Pasteur, to modern vaccines of the twentieth and twenty-first centuries, vaccines have saved countless lives by preventing deadly infectious diseases for which no cure was available.[121] It is now only appropriate that they are being actively pursued as prevention and therapy in other incurable illnesses: cancer and autoimmune diseases. Despite the use of BCG vaccine in cancer immunotherapy for more than 30 years, use of vaccines as immunotherapeutic agents is still in its infancy. However, with the significant progress in recent years in immunology, molecular biology, and gene therapy, there is new impetus and great momentum in vaccine research and development, which likely in the next years will see new breakthroughs in the use of vaccines as immunotherapeutic agents.

REFERENCES

1. McGraw-Hill concise dictionary of modern medicine. The McGraw-Hill Companies, Inc; 2002.
2. Mandell: Mandell, Douglas, and Bennett's. Immunomodulators. Principles and practice of infectious diseases. 7th edition. 2009. p. 611–23. Chapter 42.
3. The American heritage dictionary of the English language. Houghton Mifflin Company; 2009.
4. Sylvester RJ. Bacillus Calmette-Guérin treatment of non-muscle invasive bladder cancer. Int J Urol 2011;18:113–20.

5. Balwit JM, Hwu P, Urba WJ, et al. The iSBTc/SITC primer on tumor immunology and biological therapy of cancer: a summary of the 2010 program. J Transl Med 2011;9(18):1–14.
6. Ochsenbein AF, Klenerman P, Karrer U, et al. Immune surveillance against a solid tumor fails because of immunological ignorance. Proc Natl Acad Sci U S A 1999;96(5):2233–8.
7. Plotkin S, Orenstein W, Offit P. Noninfectious disease vaccines. Vaccines: expert consult. 5th edition. 2008. p. 1275–81. Chapter 53.
8. Plotkin S, Orenstein W, Offit P. Immunologic adjuvants. Vaccines: expert consult. 5th edition. 2008. p. 59–71. Chapter 5.
9. Tagliabue A, Rappuoli R. Vaccine adjuvants: the dream becomes real. Landes Bioscience Journal. Hum Vaccin 2008;4(5):347–9.
10. HogenEsch H. Mechanisms of stimulation of the immune response by aluminum adjuvants. Vaccine 2002;31(20):S34–9.
11. Brunner R, Jensen-Jarolim E, Pali-Schöll I. The ABC of clinical and experimental adjuvants—a brief overview. Immunol Lett 2010;121(1):29–35.
12. Billiau A, Matthys P. Modes of action of Freund's adjuvants in experimental models of autoimmune diseases. J Leukoc Biol 2001;70:849–60.
13. Stills HF Jr. Adjuvants and antibody production: dispelling the myths associated with Freund's complete and other adjuvants. ILAR J 2005;46(3):280–93.
14. Rajput ZI, Hu S, Xiao C, et al. Adjuvants effects of saponins on animal immune responses. J Zhejiang Univ Sci B 2007;8(3):153–61.
15. Roitt IM, Delves PJ, Martin SJ, et al. Innate immunity. Roitt's essential immunology. 11th edition. 2006. p. 1–20. Chapter 1.
16. Wheeler AW, Marshall JS, Ulrich JT. A Th1-inducing adjuvant, MPL, enhances antibody profiles in experimental animals suggesting it has the potential to improve the efficacy of allergy vaccines. Int Arch Allergy Immunol 2001;126(2):135–9.
17. Dubensky TW Jr, Reed SG. Adjuvants for cancer vaccines. Semin Immunol 2010;22(3):155–61.
18. Baldridge JR, Crane RT. Monophosphoryl lipid A (MPL) formulations for the next generation of vaccines. Methods 1999;19(1):103–7.
19. Cluff CW. Monophosphoryl lipid A (MPL) as an adjuvant for anti-cancer vaccines: clinical results. Adv Exp Med Biol 2009;667:111–23.
20. Suntharalingam G, Perry MR, Ward S, et al. Cytokine storm in a phase 1 trial of the anti-CD28 monoclonal antibody TGN1412. N Engl J Med 2006;355(10): 1018–28.
21. Xu J, Kochanek KD, Murphy SL, et al. Deaths: final data for 2007. Natl Vital Stat Rep 2010;58(19):1–135.
22. Morales A, Eidinger D, Bruce AW. Intracavitary Bacillus Calmette-Guérin in the treatment of superficial bladder tumors. J Urol 1976;116(2):180–3.
23. Aldrich JF, Lowe DB, Shearer MH, et al. Vaccines and immunotherapeutics for the treatment of malignant disease. Clin Dev Immunol 2010;2010:697158, 1–12.
24. Plotkin S, Orenstein W, Offit P. Therapeutic cancer vaccines. Vaccines: expert consult. 5th edition. 2008. p. 1136–45. Chapter 41.
25. Cheever MA, Allison JP, Ferris AS, et al. The prioritization of cancer antigens: a National Cancer Institute Pilot Project for the Acceleration of Translational Research. Clin Cancer Res 2009;15(17):5323–37.
26. Bolhassani A, Safiyan S, Rafati S. Improvement of different vaccine delivery systems for cancer therapy. Mol Cancer 2011;10(3):1–20.
27. Steinman RM, Banchereau J. Taking dendritic cells into medicine. Nature 2007; 449:419–26.

28. Banchereau J, Briere F, Caux C, et al. Immunobiology of dendritic cells. Annu Rev Immunol 2000;18:767–811.
29. Palucka K, Ueno H, Banchereau J. Dendritic cells and immunity against cancer. J Intern Med 2011;269:64–73.
30. O'Neill DW, Adams S, Bhardwaj N. Manipulating dendritic cell biology for the active immunotherapy of cancer. Blood 2004;104:2235–46.
31. Boudreau JE, Bonehill A, Thielemans K, et al. Engineering dendritic cells to enhance cancer immunotherapy. Mol Ther 2011;19(5):841–53.
32. Antonia SJ, Nirza N, Frickie I, et al. Combination of p53 cancer vaccine with chemotherapy in patients with extensive stage small cell lung cancer. Clin Cancer Res 2006;12(3):878–87.
33. Ridolfi R, Petrini M, Fiammenghi L, et al. Improved overall survival in dendritic cell vaccination-induced immunoreactive subgroup of advanced melanoma patients. J Transl Med 2006;4(36):1–11.
34. Ridolfi L, Petrini M, Fiammenghi L, et al. Unexpected high response rate to traditional therapy after dendritic cell-based vaccine in advanced melanoma: update of clinical outcome and subgroup analysis. Clin Dev Immunol 2010;2010: 504979, 1–9.
35. Carballido E, Fishman M, Sipuleucel T. Prototype for development of anti-tumor vaccines. Curr Oncol Rep 2011;13:112–9.
36. Anderson RJ, Schneider J. Plasmid DNA and viral vector-based vaccines for the treatment of cancer. Vaccine 2007;25(Suppl 2):B24–34.
37. Hodi FS, O'Day SJ, McDermott DF, et al. Improved survival with ipilimumab in patients with metastatic melanoma. N Engl J Med 2010;363(8):711–23.
38. Fioretti D, Iurescia S, Fazio VM, et al. DNA vaccines: developing new strategies against cancer. J Biomed Biotechnol 2010;2010:174378, 1–16.
39. Webster RG, Robinson HL. DNA vaccines: a review of developments. BioDrugs 1997;8(4):273–92.
40. Fissolo N, Montalban X, Comabella M. DNA-based vaccines for multiple sclerosis: current status and future directions. Clin Immunol 2010. [Epub ahead of print].
41. Wildbaum G, Youssef S, Karin N. A targeted DNA vaccine augments the natural immune response to self TNF-α and suppresses ongoing adjuvant arthritis. J Immunol 2000;165:5860–6.
42. DiPaola RS, Plante M, Kaufman H, et al. A phase I trial of pox PSA vaccines (PROSTVAC-VF) with B7-1, ICAM-1, and LFA-3 co-stimulatory molecules (TRICOM) in patients with prostate cancer. J Transl Med 2006;4:1.
43. Madan RA, Arlen PM, Mohebtash M, et al. Prostvac-VF: a vector-based vaccine targeting PSA in prostate cancer. Expert Opin Investig Drugs 2009;18(7): 1001–11.
44. Franz SO, Downey SG, Klapper JA, et al. Treatment of metastatic melanoma using interleukin-2 alone or in conjunction with vaccines. Clin Cancer Res 2008;14(17):5610.
45. Hesseling AC, Behr MA. BCG: history, evolution, efficacy, and implications in the HIV era. Tuberculosis: a comprehensive clinical reference. Chapter 74. 2009.
46. Behr MA. BCG-different strains, different vaccines? Lancet Infect Dis 2002;2: 86–92.
47. Ritz N, Curtis N. Mapping the global use of different BCG vaccine strains. Tuberculosis 2009;89(4):248–51.
48. Brewer TF, Colditz GA. Relationship between bacille Calmette-Guérin (BCG) strains and the efficacy of BCG vaccine in the prevention of tuberculosis. Clin Infect Dis 1995;20(1):126–35.

49. CDC Division of Tuberculosis Elimination. BCG vaccine fact sheets. 2008. Available at: www.cdc.gov/tb. Accessed April 2011.
50. Comstock GW. Snippets from the past: 70 years ago in the Journal. Am J Epidemiol 1999;150(12):1263–5.
51. Zbar B, Bernstein ID, Rapp HJ. Suppression of tumor growth at the site of infection with living Bacillus Calmette-Guérin. J Natl Cancer Inst 1971;46(4):831–9.
52. Herr HW, Morales A. History of bacillus Calmette-Guérin and bladder cancer: an immunotherapy success story. J Urol 2008;179(1):53–6.
53. deKernion JB, Golub SH, Gupta RK, et al. Successful transurethral intralesional BCG therapy of a bladder melanoma. Cancer 1975;36(5):1662–7.
54. Bloomberg SD, Brosman SA, Hausman MS, et al. The effects of BCG on the dog bladder. Invest Urol 1975;12(6):423–7.
55. Lamm DL, Thor DE, Harris SC, et al. Bacillus Calmette-Guérin immunotherapy of superficial bladder cancer. J Urol 1980;124(1):38–40.
56. Pinsky CM, Camacho FJ, Kerr D, et al. Intravesical administration of bacillus Calmetter-Guérin in patients with recurrent superficial carcinoma of the urinary bladder: report of a prospective, randomized trial. Cancer Treat Rep 1985; 69(1):47–53.
57. Wittes RC. Immunology of bacille Calmette-Guérin and related topics. Clin Infect Dis 2000;31(Suppl 3):S59–63.
58. Kumar M, Behera K, Matsuse H, et al. A recombinant BCG vaccine generates a Th1-like response and inhibits IgE synthesis in BALB/c mice. Immunology 1999;97:515–21.
59. Kresowik TP, Griffith TS. Bacillus Calmette-Guérin immunotherapy for urothelial carcinoma of the bladder. Immunotherapy 2009;1(2):281–8.
60. Roitt IM, Delves PJ, Martin SJ, et al. The production of effectors. Roitt's essential immunology. 11th edition. 2006. p. 185–210. Chapter 9.
61. Wiley SR, Schooley K, Smolak PJ, et al. Identification and characterization of a new member of the TNF family that induces apoptosis. Immunity 1995;3(6): 673–82.
62. Ludwig AT, Morre JM, Luo Y, et al. Tumor necrosis factor-related apoptosis-inducing ligand: a novel mechanism for bacillus Calmette-Guérin-induced antitumor activity. Cancer Res 2004;64:3386–90.
63. Hall MC, Chang SS, Dalbagni G, et al. Guideline for the management of non-muscle invasive bladder cancer: (stages Ta, T1, and Tis): 2007 update. J Urol 2007;178(6):2314–30.
64. Böhle A, Jocham D, Bock PR. Intravesical bacillus Calmetter-Guérin versus mitomycin C for superficial bladder cancer: a formal meta-analysis of comparative studies on recurrence and toxicity. J Urol 2003;169(1):90–5.
65. Lamm DL, Blumenstein BA, Crissman JD, et al. Maintenance bacillus Calmette-Guérin immunotherapy for recurrent TA, T1 and carcinoma in situ transitional cell carcinoma of the bladder: a randomized Southwest Oncology Group Study. J Urol 2000;163(4):1124–9.
66. Shelley MD, Court JB, Kynaston H, et al. Intravesical bacillus Calmette-Guérin in Ta and T1 bladder cancer. Cochrane Database Syst Rev 2000;4:CD001986.
67. Lamm DL. Efficacy and safety of bacilli Calmette-Guérin immunotherapy in superficial bladder cancer. Clin Infect Dis 2000;31:S86–90.
68. Nepple KG, Lightfoot AJ, Rosevear HM, et al. Bacillus Calmetter-Guérin with or without interferon a-2b and megadose versus recommended daily allowance vitamins during introduction and maintenance intravesical treatment of non-muscle invasive bladder cancer. J Urol 2010;184(5):1915–9.

69. Joudi FN, Smith BJ, O'Donnell MA, et al. Final results from a national multicenter phase II trial of combination bacillus Calmette-Guérin plus interferon alpha-2B for reducing recurrence of superficial bladder cancer. Urol Oncol 2006;24(4): 344–8.

70. Morales A, Chin JL, Ramsey EW. Mycobacterial cell wall extract for treatment of carcinoma in situ of the bladder. J Urol 2001;166(5):1633–7.

71. Morales A. Evolution of intravesical immunotherapy for bladder cancer: mycobacterial cell wall preparation as a promising agent. Expert Opin Investig Drugs 2008;7(17):1067–73.

72. Bastos RG, Borsuk S, Seixas FK, et al. Recombinant *Mycobacterium bovis* BCG. Vaccine 2009;27:6495–503.

73. Murray PJ, Aldovini A, Young RA. Manipulation and potentiation of antimycobacterial immunity using recombinant bacilli Calmette-Guérin strains that secrete cytokines. Proc Natl Acad Sci U S A 1996;93:934–9.

74. Yuan S, Shi C, Liu L, et al. MUC1-based recombinant bacillus Calmette-Guérin vaccines as candidates for breast cancer immunotherapy. Expert Opin Biol Ther 2010;10(7):1037–48.

75. Yuan S, Shi C, Ling R, et al. Immunization with two recombinant bacillus Calmette-Guérin vaccines that combine the expression of multiple tandem repeats of mucin-1 and colony stimulating-factor suppress breast tumor growth in mice. J Cancer Res Clin Oncol 2010;136:1359–67.

76. Kantoff PW, Higano CS, Shore ND, et al. Sipuleucel-T immunotherapy for castration-resistant prostate cancer. N Engl J Med 2010;363(5):411–22.

77. Sipuleucel-T: APC 8015, APC-8015, prostate cancer vaccine—Denreon. Drugs R D 2006;7(3):197–201.

78. Cheever MA, Higano C. PROVENGE (Sipuleucel-T) in prostate cancer: the First FDA approved therapeutic cancer vaccine. Clin Cancer Res 2011;17(11): 3520–6.

79. Gabrilovich D. Mechanisms and functional significance of tumour-induced dendritic-cell defects. Nat Rev Immunol 2004;4(12):941–52.

80. Higano C, Schellhammer PF, Small EJ, et al. Integrated data from 2 randomized, double-blind, placebo-controlled, phase 3 trials of active cellular immunotherapy with sipuleucel-T in advanced prostate cancer. Cancer 2009;115(16): 3670–9.

81. Kantoff PW, Schuetz TJ, Blumenstein BA, et al. Overall survival analysis of a phase II randomized controlled trial of a Poxviral-based PSA-targeted immunotherapy in metastatic castration-resistant prostate cancer. J Clin Oncol 2010; 28(7):1099–105.

82. Kunz M, Ibrahim SM. Cytokines and cytokine profiles in human autoimmune diseases and animal models of autoimmunity. Mediators Inflamm 2009;2009: 979258.

83. Delavallee L, Assier E, Denys A, et al. Vaccination with cytokines in autoimmune diseases. Ann Med 2008;40(5):343–51.

84. Silva LC, Ortigosa LC, Benard G. Anti-TNF-α agents in the treatment of immune-mediated inflammatory diseases: mechanisms of action and pitfalls. Immunotherapy 2010;2(6):817–33.

85. Delavallee L, Duvallet E, Semerano L, et al. Anti-cytokine vaccination in autoimmune diseases. Swiss Med Wkly 2010;140:w13108.

86. Schur P. Overview of the systemic and nonarticular manifestations of rheumatoid arthritis. UpToDate 2011. Available at: www.uptodate.com. Accessed April 2011.

87. Stone JH. Overview of biological agents in the rheumatic diseases. UpToDate 2011. Available at: www.uptodate.com. Accessed April 2011.
88. Keffer J, Probert L, Cazlaris H, et al. Transgenic mice expressing human tumour necrosis factor: a predictive genetic model of arthritis. EMBO J 1991;10(13): 4025–31.
89. Dalum I, Butler DM, Jensen MR, et al. Therapeutic antibodies elicited by immunization against TNF-alpha. Nat Biotechnol 1999;17(7):666–9.
90. Bizzini B, Achour A. "Kinoids": the basis for anticytokine immunization and their use in HIV infection. Cell Mol Biol (Noisy-le-grand) 1995;41(3):351–6.
91. Le Buanec H, Delavallee L, Bessis N, et al. TNFalpha kinoid vaccination-induced neutralizing antibodies to TNFalpha protect mice from autologous TNFalpha-driven chronic and acute inflammation. Proc Natl Acad Sci U S A 2006;103(51):19442–7.
92. Delavallee L, Le Buanec H, Bessis N, et al. Early and long-lasting protection from arthritis in tumour necrosis factor alpha (TNFalpha) transgenic mice vaccinated against TNFalpha. Ann Rheum Dis 2008;67(9):1332–8.
93. Delavallee L, Semerano L, Assier E. Active immunization to tumor necrosis factor-alpha is effective in treating chronic established inflammatory disease: a long-term study in a transgenic model of arthritis. Arthritis Res Ther 2009; 11(6):R195.
94. Neovacs initiates a Phase II clinical study of its TNF-kinoid in Crohn's disease patients. Press release. Jan 2011. Available at: www.neovacs.com. Accessed April 2011.
95. Immunogenicity and safety of TNFa kinoid in rheumatoid arthritis with secondary resistance to TNFa antagonists and ADA. Ongoing Phase II trial. Available at: http://clinicaltrials.gov/ct2/show/NCT01040715. Accessed April 2011.
96. Spohn G, Keller I, Beck M, et al. Active immunization with IL-1 displayed on virus-like particles protects from autoimmune arthritis. Eur J Immunol 2008; 38(3):877–87.
97. Goldberg R, Zohar Y, Wildbaum G, et al. Suppression of ongoing experimental autoimmune encephalomyelitis by neutralizing the function of the p28 subunit of IL-27. J Immunol 2004;173(10):6465–71.
98. Bertin-Maghit SM, Capini CJ, Bessis N. Improvement of collagen-induced arthritis by active immunization against murine IL-1beta peptides designed by molecular modelling. Vaccine 2005;23(33):4228–35.
99. Weiner H. Multiple sclerosis is an inflammatory T-cell-mediated autoimmune disease. Arch Neurol 2004;61(10):1613–5.
100. Röhn TA, Jennings GT, Hernandez M. Vaccination against IL-17 suppresses autoimmune arthritis and encephalomyelitis. Eur J Immunol 2006;36(11): 2857–67.
101. Uyttenhove C, Van Snick J. Development of an anti-IL-17A auto-vaccine that prevents experimental auto-immune encephalomyelitis. Eur J Immunol 2006; 36(11):2868–74.
102. Correale J, Farez M, Gilmore W. Vaccines for multiple sclerosis: progress to date. CNS Drugs 2008;22(3):175–98.
103. Lublin F. History of modern multiple sclerosis therapy. J Neurol 2005;252(Suppl 3):iii3–9.
104. Vandenbark AA, Morgan E, Bartholomew R, et al. TCR peptide therapy in human autoimmune diseases. Neurochem Res 2001;26(6):713–30.
105. Vandenbark AA, Culbertson NE, Bartholomew RM, et al. Therapeutic vaccination with a trivalent T-cell receptor (TCR) peptide vaccine restores deficient

FoxP3 expression and TCR recognition in subjects with multiple sclerosis. Immunology 2008;123(1):66–78.

106. Kappos L, Comi G, Panitch H, et al. Induction of a non-encephalitogenic type 2 T helper-cell autoimmune response in multiple sclerosis after administration of an altered peptide ligand in a placebo-controlled, randomized phase II trial. Nat Med 2000;6(10):1176–82.

107. Wildbaum G, Karin N. Augmentation of natural immunity to a pro-inflammatory cytokine (TNF-alpha) by targeted DNA vaccine confers long-lasting resistance to experimental autoimmune encephalomyelitis. Gene Ther 1999;6(6): 1128–38.

108. Youssef S, Wildbaum G, Maor G, et al. Long-lasting protective immunity to experimental autoimmune encephalomyelitis following vaccination with naked DNA encoding C-C chemokines. J Immunol 1998;161(8):3870–9.

109. Karpus WJ, Lukacs NW, McRae BL. An important role for the chemokine macrophage inflammatory protein-1 alpha in the pathogenesis of the T cell-mediated autoimmune disease, experimental autoimmune encephalomyelitis. J Immunol 1995;155(10):5003–10.

110. Roldão A, Mellado MC, Castilho LR, et al. Virus-like particles in vaccine development. Expert Rev Vaccines 2010;9(10):1149–76.

111. Deschuyteneer M, Elouahabi A, Plainchamp D, et al. Molecular and structural characterization of the L1 virus-like particles that are used as vaccine antigens in Cervarix, the AS04-adjuvanted HPV-16 and -18 cervical cancer vaccine. Hum Vaccin 2010;6(5):407–19.

112. Brown MJ, Coltart J, Gunewardena K, et al. Randomized double-blind placebo-controlled study of an angiotensin immunotherapeutic vaccine (PMD3117) in hypertensive subjects. Clin Sci (Lond) 2004;107(2):167–73.

113. Tissot AC, Maurer P, Nussberger J, et al. Effect of immunisation against angiotensin II with CYT006-AngQb on ambulatory blood pressure: a double-blind, randomised, placebo-controlled phase IIa study. Lancet 2008;371(9615): 821–7.

114. Maurer P, Bachman MF. Immunization against angiotensins for the treatment of hypertension. Clin Immunol 2010;134(1):89–95.

115. Stoll G, Bendszus M. Inflammation and atherosclerosis. Novel insights into plaque formation and destabilization. Stroke 2006;37:1923–32.

116. Hauer AD, van Puijvelde GH, Peterse N, et al. Vaccination against VEGFR2 attenuates initiation and progression of atherosclerosis. Arterioscler Thromb Vasc Biol 2007;27(9):2050–7.

117. Petrovan R, Kaplan CD, Reisfeld RA, et al. DNA vaccination against VEGF receptor 2 reduces atherosclerosis in LDL receptor-deficient mice. Arterioscler Thromb Vasc Biol 2007;27(5):1095–100.

118. Harrison LC. The prospect of vaccination to prevent type I diabetes. Hum Vaccin 2005;1(4):143–50.

119. Kimpimäki T, Kupila A, Hämäläinen AM, et al. The first signs of beta-cell autoimmunity appear in infancy in genetically susceptible children from the general population: the Finnish Type 1 Diabetes Prediction and Prevention Study. J Clin Endocrinol Metab 2001;86(10):4782–8.

120. Harrison LC, Honeyman MC, Steele CE, et al. Pancreatic beta-cell function and immune responses to insulin after administration of intranasal insulin to humans at risk for type 1 diabetes. Diabetes Care 2004;27(10):2348–55.

121. Plotkin S, Orenstein W, Offit P. Immunologic adjuvants. vaccines: expert consult. Chapter 1. 5th edition. 2008. p. 1–16.

122. Skyler JS, Krischer JP, Wolfsdorf J, et al. Effects of oral insulin in relatives of patients with type 1 diabetes: the diabetes prevention trial—type 1. Diabetes Care 2005;28(5):1068–76.

123. Näntö-Salonen K, Kupila A, Simell S, et al. Nasal insulin to prevent type 1 diabetes in children with HLA genotypes and autoantibodies conferring increased risk of disease: a double-blind, randomised controlled trial. Lancet 2008; 372(9651):1746–55.

124. Rewers M, Gottlieb P. Immunotherapy for the prevention and treatment of type 1 diabetes: human trials and a look into the future. Diabetes Care 2009;32(10): 1769–82.

Polyclonal Immunoglobulins and Hyperimmune Globulins in Prevention and Management of Infectious Diseases

Jennifer L. Hsu, MD[a], Nasia Safdar, MD, PhD[b],*

KEYWORDS

• IVIG • Immunoglobulin • Sepsis • Toxic shock
• Cytomegalovirus • Viral hepatitis

Immunoglobulin replacement has long been used in the prevention and treatment of infectious diseases. In the late 1800s, scientists first recognized the protective effect of sera obtained from rabbits immunized with tetanus toxin. This finding led to an initial interest in curative sera, which were primarily antitoxins obtained from animals. Complications from serum sickness, however, limited the use of these products and prompted investigation of human convalescent sera. During World War I, there was widespread use of curative sera for treatment of tetanus, diphtheria, and pneumococcal disease. Immunoglobulin replacement therapy was greatly improved in the 1930s and 1940s when fractionation techniques were developed that allowed separation of plasma proteins into stable fractions with different biologic functions, including targeted treatment of poliomyelitis, measles, mumps, pertussis, and hepatitis A.[1] Although largely replaced by vaccines, this foundation for the production of polyclonal immunoglobulins remains in use today and has lead to the development of multiple applications of immunoglobulin therapy for infectious and noninfectious diseases.

The authors have nothing to disclose.
a Division of Infectious Disease, University of Wisconsin School of Medicine and Public Health, Room 5220 MFCB, 1685 Highland Avenue, Madison, WI 53705, USA
b Division of Infectious Disease, University of Wisconsin School of Medicine and Public Health, Room 5221 MFCB, 1685 Highland Avenue, Madison, WI 53705, USA
* Corresponding author.
E-mail address: ns2@medicine.wisc.edu

Intravenous immunoglobulin (IVIG) is a therapeutic preparation of pooled, normal, polyspecific immunoglobulin, which has activity against a broad spectrum of viral and bacterial pathogens.[2] Immunoglobulin products are used extensively for the replacement of antibody deficiencies in primary and secondary immunodeficiency states. However, the mechanisms of action are far more complicated than restoration of normal humoral immune function through increased antibody levels (**Box 1**). Data showing immunomodulatory and antiinflammatory effects have heightened interest in the use of IVIG for prophylaxis against infection and treatment of severe infections, including sepsis, toxic shock syndrome, *Clostridium difficile* infection (CDI), and cytomegalovirus (CMV) disease, among others.[3]

Despite the application of IVIG therapy in more than 150 noninfectious and infectious disease states, there are limited conditions for which this therapy is approved by the US Food and Drug Administration (FDA). These conditions include idiopathic thrombocytopenia purpura, Kawasaki disease, primary immunodeficiency, secondary hypogammaglobulinemia caused by B-cell chronic lymphocytic leukemia, prophylaxis in stem cell transplant recipients, and prophylaxis in pediatric HIV/AIDS.[4,5] The increased use of IVIG therapy in combination with its high cost, decreased reimbursement, and manufacturing limitations has placed new importance on determining the most efficacious and cost-effective applications of this treatment.[4,6] The following review focuses on infectious disease states for which immunoglobulin therapy has been applied in adult populations and for which there are data regarding efficacy. Infections for which the data are more limited are outlined in **Table 1**.

BACTERIAL INFECTIONS
Sepsis

Because of the high mortality associated with bacterial sepsis, there has long been interest in understanding and developing treatments adjunctive to antibiotics, such as IVIG. Mechanisms for a possible benefit of IVIG in sepsis include enhanced bactericidal activity through opsonizing immunoglobulin (Ig)G and IgM antibodies, stimulation of phagocytosis, and neutralization of bacterial toxins.[7,8] IVIG may also suppress the release of proinflammatory cytokines from endotoxin- or superantigen-activated blood cells.[7,8] Although multiple individual observational studies and randomized controlled trials have supported the use of IVIG in sepsis and septic shock, more

---

Box 1
Postulated mechanisms of immunoglobulin action in infection

Immunomodulatory Actions

    Neutralization of circulating superantigens

    Blockade of Fc receptor-mediated events

    Modulation of cytokines

    Regulation of T-cell production

Antiinflammatory Actions

    Reduction of complement-mediated damage

    Neutralization of microbial toxins

    Activation of leukocytes

Data from Durandy A, Kaveri SV, Kuijpers TW, et al. Intravenous immunoglobulins–understanding properties and mechanisms. Clin Exp Immunol 2009;158(Suppl 1):2–13.

Table 1 Infectious diseases with limited evidence for IVIG use	
Infection	**Rationale**
C jejuni	There was a single report of use in a patient with common variable immune deficiency with frequent recurrences; responded to treatment with oral Ig.[85]
Erythrovirus (Parvovirus B19)	Patients with congenital or acquired immunodeficiencies are at risk for chronic Erythrovirus infection, often manifested by pure red cell aplasia (PRCA). Case reports have shown success in treating erythrovirus-associated PRCA, and a single series showed success in treating dilated cardiomyopathy caused by Erythrovirus infection.[87,88]
Enteroviruses	Patients who are agammaglobulinemic are at risk for chronic enteroviral meningoencephalitis (CEM) with slowly progressive ataxia, loss of cognitive skills, and paresthesias. Twelve of 42 patients with CEM were treated with IVIG and intrathecal Ig and 6 were observed to have clinical improvement.[89]

recent meta-analyses have cast doubt on its benefit. In 2007, 3 systematic reviews were published showing a mortality benefit when IVIG was compared with placebo, with relative risk (RR) ratios of 0.74 and 0.79 in 2 of the reviews.[9–11] Similarly, Laupland, and colleagues[11] reported a significant reduction in mortality associated with IVIG treatment with a pooled odds ratio of 0.66 (95% confidence interval [CI] 0.53–0.83, $P<.0005$). However, these analyses were limited by considerable study heterogeneity and the result was not replicated when only high-quality trials were analyzed. Thus, the investigators emphasized the need for a well-designed, adequately powered, and transparently reported study.[11] This recommendation was confirmed by the most recent Cochrane review, which included 42 studies comparing IVIG (polyclonal and monoclonal) to placebo or no intervention in patients with bacterial sepsis or septic shock. There was a significant mortality benefit when IVIG was compared with placebo (RR 0.81; 95% CI 0.70–0.93). However, analysis of trials with a low risk of bias yielded no reduction in mortality (RR 0.97; 95% CI 0.81–1.15).[12]

Patients with postoperative sepsis have also been examined separately from mixed populations with sepsis. Rodriguez and colleagues[13] randomized patients with severe sepsis and septic shock of intra-abdominal origin to 2 treatment groups: antibiotics plus polyvalent IgM-enriched IVIG or antibiotics plus albumin (control). In this study, no specific benefit from the addition of IVIG was identified, and inappropriate antibiotic therapy was the only variable independently associated with death. Additionally, there has been interest in the use of IVIG in postcardiac surgery patients because of the high risk of postoperative sepsis in combination with postulated changes in immune function related to intraoperative extracorporeal membrane oxygenation.[14] Pilz and colleagues[15] showed a reduction in morbidity and severity of disease in patients treated with IVIG and IgM-enriched IVIG with an Acute Physiology and Chronic Health Evaluation II score greater than or equal to 24 on the first postoperative day following cardiac surgery with extracorporeal circulation. There are scant data, however, to draw any further conclusions regarding the benefit of IVIG in a general surgical population or specific subsets, such as cardiac surgery patients.

Overall, the small size of trials and heterogeneity, both in patient characteristics and treatment strategies, has limited the ability to draw conclusions regarding the use of IVIG in sepsis. Thus, IVIG is not routinely recommended for use in sepsis. High-quality randomized trials are needed to adequately answer this question.

Toxic Shock Syndrome

In 1992, IVIG was first reported as an adjunctive treatment in a previously healthy 32-year-old woman with refractory shock caused by toxin-producing *Streptococcus pyogenes*.[16] Based on the rapid clinical improvement reported in this patient, interest in IVIG as an adjunctive treatment of toxic shock syndrome (TSS) grew. Early observational work showed IVIG administration was associated with survival because of the postulated mechanisms of enhanced bacterial neutralization and reduced T-cell production.[17] IVIG also provides passive immunization against pyrogenic exotoxins.[18] In the first randomized, double-blind, placebo-controlled trial evaluating IVIG as an adjunctive therapy, a 3.6-fold higher mortality was identified in the placebo group, and a significant decrease in sepsis-related organ failure was seen in the IVIG group.[19] However, statistical significance in the primary end point of decreased mortality was not reached because the trial was terminated early because of slow patient recruitment.[19] Subsequent studies in mice have shown enhanced systemic clearance of bacteria and enhanced neutrophil infiltration into infected tissue, which would imply benefit. However, when penicillin and clindamycin were used concomitantly, IVIG did not confer additional benefit.[7] Similar results were seen in a pediatric population in which IVIG increased cost, but did not show an association with improved outcome.[20] The use of IVIG in sepsis is biologically plausible and, therefore, clinicians continue to use it in life-threatening disease, most commonly in a single dose of 400 mg/kg. The current data, however, do not support a recommendation for use in streptococcal TSS.

As with streptococcal TSS, staphylococcal TSS is linked to the bacterial production of superantigens, such as TSS toxin (TSST-1). However, the mortality is lower than streptococcal TSS, averaging 5%. Evidence evaluating IVIG for staphylococcal TSS is limited to in vitro studies showing neutralization of superantigens and case reports.[21] Thus, the level of evidence is weak, and IVIG is not recommended in staphylococcal TSS.

Clostridium Difficile Infection

Over the past decade, CDI has increased in incidence and severity, becoming the most common cause of health care–associated diarrhea in the United States, with an estimated cost of $1.1 billion per year. Additionally, there has been increasing concern for treatment failures with metronidazole, as well as failures among specific patient subsets, including elderly and immunocompromised patients.[22–24] Because of the inadequacy of the current treatments, attention has turned to alternative means of therapy. Previous studies of passive immunization in animal models have shown positive results, and human data have shown that patients with low serum antibody levels to *C difficile* toxin A are at risk for development of CDI.[25–28] Taken together, these observations provide a rationale for immunoglobulin therapy in CDI. Abougergi and Kwon[29] summarized the available case reports and series reporting the use of IVIG treatment in CDI. In studies evaluating protracted or relapsed CDI, 40 of 46 patients (87%) experienced resolution of diarrhea.[29] When severe CDI was examined separately, 32 of 51 patients (67%) survived their illness.[29] Similarly, O'Horo and Safdar[30] found an overall benefit in a small case series with the use of IVIG, but small sample sizes, publication bias, and lack of control groups did not allow for recommendation regarding the use of IVIG. Various dosages of IVIG, ranging from 1 dose of 150 mg/kg to 400 mg/kg weekly, have been used.[29,30] Additionally, there is variation in the level of *C difficile*–specific antibodies among various IVIG preparations, and this may lead to mixed study results.[31] This treatment strategy is biologically plausible and observational data are promising, but the level of evidence remains weak.

More recently, attention has turned to the treatment of CDI with human monoclonal antibodies directed against *C difficile* toxins A and B, which has the advantage of targeting therapy and avoiding the increased use of pooled IVIG. In a phase II trial, 200 patients receiving either metronidazole or vancomycin for CDI treatment were randomized to antibody and placebo. Among the antibody group, the rate of CDI recurrence was decreased compared with placebo (7% vs 25%; 95% CI 7–29; P<.001). No increase in adverse events was seen.[32] This strategy is promising and further study is underway.

Other Clostridial Infections

The treatment of tetanus is a 2-part approach: antibiotics to decrease bacterial burden and immunoglobulins to neutralize unbound toxin or tetanospasmin. Although unbound toxin is identified in a minority of patients at presentation, substantial decreases in mortality have been seen with immunoglobulin therapy.[33] Beginning in the late 1800s, equine antibodies, produced in response to vaccination with *Clostridium tetani*, were used for treatment of tetanus, resulting in a substantial decline in mortality rates in the United States. These rates further declined with the introduction of a tetanus vaccine in the 1940s and again, in 1960, with the introduction of human tetanus immunoglobulin (TIG).[34] Currently, the Centers for Disease Control (CDC) recommend 1 dose of 250 IU TIG (HyperTET S/D) given intramuscularly in unimmunized or inadequately immunized patients who sustain high-risk wounds, including deep punctures or contaminated wounds, in addition to vaccination with a tetanus toxoid-containing vaccine for development of long-term immunity.[33] Similar treatment is recommended for established tetanus infection; however, the recommended dose of TIG is 500 IU given in 1 dose.[35]

Unlike tetanus, equine antitoxin remains the treatment of choice for *Clostridium botulinum* infection, or botulism, because there is no human hyperimmune globulin available.[36] Heptavalent botulinum antitoxin is the only treatment available in the United States for the treatment of noninfant botulism, and it is available through a cosponsored CDC and FDA investigational new drug (IND) protocol.[37]

Diphtheria

The primary sequelae of *Corynebacterium diphtheriae* infection are related to a potent toxin causing respiratory, cardiac, and neurologic disease. Because of vaccination, the burden of diphtheria in the United States is low, with no cases reported since 2003.[38] However, travelers to endemic areas, such as sub-Saharan Africa, countries of the former Soviet Union, and much of Asia, are at risk.[39] At present, no human diphtheria immunoglobulin product is available in the United States. Treatment of *C diphtheriae* infection relies on an equine antitoxin, in conjunction with antimicrobial agents. Because of the risk of allergic reaction, postexposure prophylaxis with antitoxin is not recommended, but rather vaccination and antimicrobial therapy should be implemented. Currently, diphtheria antitoxin can only be obtained through the CDC as an IND, and the recommended dose is based on the site, duration, and severity of infection (range 20,000 IU –120,000 IU).[36] Skin sensitivity testing must be performed before use.[40]

VIRAL INFECTIONS
Cytomegalovirus Infection in Solid Organ Transplant

Neutralizing antibodies are thought to play a role in the immune response that controls CMV infection and, therefore, interest has risen in the use of immunoglobulins as a prophylaxis and adjunctive therapy for CMV in solid organ transplant (SOT) and hematopoietic stem cell transplant (HSCT) recipients. Both IVIG, containing a high titer of anti-CMV antibodies from healthy blood donors, and CMV hyperimmune globulin (CMV-Ig; CytoGam) have been used for the prevention of CMV disease, although supporting data are limited. IVIG and CMV-Ig use became widespread for SOT prophylaxis after the demonstration of benefit in reducing CMV disease in kidney and liver transplants.[41,42] A subsequent systematic review of 37 trials (2185 participants) evaluating IVIG and CMV-Ig for prophylaxis in SOT recipients showed decreased risk of mortality from CMV disease (**Fig. 1**).[43] However, there was no significant difference in the risk for CMV infection, CMV disease, or all-cause mortality when compared with placebo or antiviral therapy alone.[43] These data do not support routine use of prophylactic IVIG or CMV-Ig in SOT recipients.

The risks associated with established CMV disease are extensive in SOT recipients, including directly attributable mortality, late-onset malignancy, acute and chronic allograft injury, and chronic allograft vasculopathy.[44] Given these concerns, individual clinicians and transplant centers routinely elect to use immunoglobulin products in addition to first-line treatment with ganciclovir or valganciclovir. This practice is common in specific patient populations, such as lung transplants, in which as many as one-third of transplant centers use adjunctive immunoglobulins.[45] Currently, it is unclear if the addition of IVIG or CMV-Ig is beneficial in specific SOT populations, but it may be considered for patients with CMV pneumonitis and possibly other severe or treatment-refractory forms of disease.[44] Further research is needed to define appropriate use in SOT recipients with established CMV disease,

Review: Immunoglobulins, vaccines or interferon for preventing cytomegalovirus disease in solid organ transplant recipients
Comparison: 1IgG versus placebo/no treatment end (all patients)
Outcome: 3 All-cause mortality

Study or subgroup	IgG n/N	Placebo/no treatment n/N	Risk Ratio M - H,Random,95% CI	Risk Ratio M - H,Random,95% CI
1 CMV IgG				
Fassbinder 86-Kidney	0/42	0/34		0.0 [0.0, 0.0]
Greger 85a-Kidney	0/12	0/12		0.0 [0.0, 0.0]
Greger 85b-Kidney	0/12	0/12		0.0 [0.0, 0.0]
Grundmann 87-Kidney	0/50	0/50		0.0 [0.0, 0.0]
Kruger 03-Lung	2/22	4/22		0.50 [0.10, 2.45]
Snydman 87-Kidney	1/24	5/35		0.29 [0.04, 2.34]
Snydman 93-Liver	11/69	18/72		0.64 [0.33, 1.25]
Subtotal (95% CI)	**231**	**237**		**0.58 [0.32, 1.05]**
Total events: 14 (IgG), 27 (Placebo/no treatment)				
Heterogeneity: Tau² = 0.0; Chi² = 0.54, df = 2 (P = 0.76); I² =0.0%				
Test for overall effect: Z = 1.81 (P = 0.071)				
2 IgG				
Schechner 93-Kidney	0/14	1/20		0.47 [0.02, 10.69]
Subtotal (95% CI)	**14**	**20**		**0.47 [0.02, 10.69]**
Total events: 0 (IgG), 1 (Placebo/no treatment)				
Heterogeneity: not applicable				
Test for overall effect: Z = 0.48 (P = 0.63)				
Total (95% CI)	**245**	**257**		**0.57 [0.32, 1.03]**
Total events: 14 (IgG), 28 (Placebo/no treatment)				
Heterogeneity: Tau² = 0.0; Chi² = 0.56, df = 3 (P = 0.91); I² =0.0%				
Test for overall effect: Z = 1.86 (P = 0.063)				

0.01   0.1   1   10   100
IgG   Placebo/no treatment

Fig. 1. Comparison of IgG versus placebo/no treatment (all patients), all-cause mortality. Eight studies comparing IVIG versus placebo for prevention of CMV among HSCT recipients examined all-cause mortality as a primary endpoint. No significant difference in mortality was identified when IVIG was used compared with placebo. (*Reproduced From* Hodson EM, Jones CA, Strippoli GF, et al. Immunoglobulins, vaccines or interferon for preventing cytomegalovirus disease in solid organ transplant recipients. Cochrane Database Syst Rev 2007;2:CD005129. Copyright Cochrane Collaboration; with permission.)

especially lung and intestine recipients and hypogammaglobulinemic heart transplant recipients.[46,47]

Cytomegalovirus Infection in Hematopoietic Stem Cell Transplant

Similar to SOT recipients, hematopoietic stem cell transplant recipients are at a high risk from CMV infection and disease. Several trials published before 2000 prompted the National Institutes of Health to publish consensus guidelines endorsing the use of prophylactic IVIG after allogeneic bone marrow transplant (BMT).[48–51] However, with the increased use of prophylaxis, an increased risk of venoocclusive disease was seen without an associated survival benefit.[52] Thus, prophylaxis was examined further. In a recent meta-analysis, CMV infections were not significantly reduced with either polyvalent IVIG or CMG-Ig, and an increased risk of hepatic venoocclusive disease was seen with polyvalent IVIG.[50] Similarly, analysis of the newer studies examining interstitial pneumonitis showed no benefit with IVIG.[50] Based on these data, there seems to be no advantage for the use of IVIG or CMV-Ig in HSCT prophylaxis.

With the widespread use of ganciclovir and valganciclovir for CMV disease, the use of adjunctive IVIG or CMV-Ig has become less common in HSCT recipients. However, antiviral monotherapy failure rates often exceed 50%, which has prompted some clinicians and transplant centers to use combined CMV-Ig and ganciclovir. The benefit of CMV-Ig among HSCT recipients has been examined in several small studies.[47,53–55] In one study, 25 consecutive patients with CMV pneumonitis were treated with CMV-Ig and ganciclovir. Survival was enhanced in the combination therapy group (13/25, 52%) compared with antiviral monotherapy (13/89,15%) (P<.001).[54] Although this result was supported by other small studies, one trial found no benefit, with 4 out of 4 patients dying before hospital discharge.[53,56] Recently, retrospective analysis of 35 patients at a single center showed a mortality rate of 49% with combination therapy, comparable to other combination treatment studies but lower than in studies of antiviral monotherapy.[55] In summary, the available data limit drawing firm conclusions regarding the use of adjunctive immunoglobulin products in HSCT recipients with CMV disease. Given the high mortality of this disease and the tolerability of immunoglobulin products, further research should be pursued.

Hepatitis A

IVIG has been used for the prevention of hepatitis A (HAV) infection since the mid-1940s when it was found to end outbreaks in communal living situations, including children's camps, battlefields, and institutions for the mentally ill.[57,58] IVIG is 80% to 90% protective against the development of clinical hepatitis when administered as a postexposure prophylaxis within 2 weeks, and despite waning antibody levels in pooled IVIG, antibody levels in pooled IVIG seem to be sufficient for replacement.[58–61] The protection derived from IVIG results from the prevention of early clinical disease, whereas subclinical HAV viremia prompts the development of a longer-lived antibody response.[36]

In 1995, highly effective HAV vaccines were first licensed in the United States for preexposure prophylaxis, thus, limiting the use of IVIG. Preexposure IVIG is only recommended for high-risk persons who could not be vaccinated, including infants aged younger than 12 months, individuals with an allergy to vaccine components, or travelers declining vaccination.[60] More recently, HAV vaccination also became an acceptable option for postexposure prophylaxis based on data showing equivalent protection to IVIG when administered within 2 weeks of HAV exposure in persons aged 2 to 40 years.[62] The current Centers for Disease Control (CDC) guidelines recommend a single dose of IVIG 0.02 mL/kg for groups requiring postexposure prophylaxis in whom the vaccine has not been evaluated, including children aged younger than 12 months; immunocompromised individuals; individuals with chronic liver disease; and individuals for whom the vaccine is contraindicated.[59]

Hepatitis B

Hepatitis B immunoglobulin (HBIG; HepaGam B, HyperHEP B, Nabi-HB) is prepared from the plasma of donors with high concentrations of hepatitis B virus (HBV) surface antibody but no evidence of hepatitis B surface antigen (HBsAg). HBIG is most commonly used as part of passive-active immunization in postexposure settings, as well as in the prevention of maternal-child transmission. The combination of HBIG and vaccine are highly effective in preventing the transmission of HBV, with studies in health care workers and sexual contacts of HBV-infected persons showing 80% to 90% efficacy when treatment is completed within 7 days for needlesticks and 14 days for sexual contact.[63–65] Use of HBIG alone provides temporary protection (3–6 months) and is also efficacious.[66–68]

More recently, with an increase in liver transplantation for HBV infection, attention has turned to the use of HBIG for posttransplant treatment of HBV. Variation in antiviral regimens posttransplant, as well as dosing of HBIG, has limited conclusions regarding the efficacy of this therapy. A recent Cochrane review identified 4 randomized trials evaluating lamivudine or adefovir alone or combined with HBIG. The trials were underpowered and no statistically significant difference in all-cause mortality or recurrence of HBsAg was identified.[69] Chen and colleagues[70] completed a more recent systematic review on this subject. Examining 44 nonrandomized trials, they found that with long-term HBIG prophylaxis, hepatitis B recurrence ranged from 3.7% to 65.0% compared with lamivudine monotherapy, whereby recurrence ranged from 3.8% to 40.4%. The rate of recurrence was lowest with combination therapy, whereby recurrence decreased to less than 10%. These data are encouraging; however, larger, randomized, controlled trials are needed to best assess optimal HBV prevention after liver transplantation.

Varicella

In 1969, zoster immune globulin (ZIG), prepared from patients recovering from herpes zoster, was shown to prevent clinical varicella among children when administered within 72 hours after exposure and to lower disease rates in immunocompromised persons when given within 96 hours after exposure.[71,72] This effect was further demonstrated in patients receiving high-titer lots because they had a significantly lower rate of complications.[73] In 1978, varicella zoster immune globulin (VZIG), prepared from healthy volunteer blood donors with high varicella zoster virus antibody titers, became available. Serologic and clinical comparison of ZIG and VZIG showed equal efficacy.[74,75] As in other vaccine-preventable infections, use of immune globulin for varicella zoster infection has decreased since the varicella vaccine was implemented as part of a postexposure prophylaxis in healthy adults. VZIG as a prophylactic measure has not been evaluated in healthy or immunocompromised adults. However, VZIG can be considered in susceptible patients (no history of varicella disease or vaccination), if the exposure is likely to result in infection and the patient is at a greater risk for complications than the general population, including immunocompromised adults and pregnant women.[74] Because of the lack of data in adult prophylaxis, the appropriate dose of VZIG is unknown.[74] However, CDC guidelines state that 625 U should be sufficient to modify or prevent infection in healthy adults.[74] The appropriate dose for immunocompromised adults is unknown. Finally, administration of VZIG should take into account the high cost of this treatment ($400 for patients weighing more than 40 kg) in combination with the short-term nature of protection and limited production of VZIG.[74]

Rabies

Two human rabies immunoglobulin products (HRIG; HyperRab S/D, Imogam Rabies-HT) are derived from hyperimmunized donors and licensed for rabies postexposure prophylaxis in the United States. Two studies have demonstrated the role of HRIG administration in conjunction with vaccination as a postexposure prophylaxis, specifically in the development of a protective antibody response during the first 5 days after administration.[76,77] Simultaneous vaccination provides longer-term protection. Therefore, the CDC recommends the administration of HRIG 20 IU/kg body weight once at the beginning of rabies prophylaxis. If not begun at the time of initial vaccination, HRIG can be administered up to and including day 7 of the postexposure prophylaxis series.[78] If anatomically feasible, HRIG should be fully administered in and around the wound, and the first vaccine dose should be given at an anatomically distant location to prevent neutralization by HRIG.[79] If the entire dose cannot be infiltrated around the wound, the remaining volume should be administered intramuscularly at an anatomic site distant from that used for the active vaccine.

Respiratory Syncytial Virus Infection

There are limited data for the use of IVIG or hyperimmune globulin to treat adults with respiratory syncytial virus (RSV) infection because it is typically a self-limited infection. BMT recipients, however, are at risk for severe upper respiratory tract infection followed by pneumonia with an associated mortality rate of 60%.[80,81] Uncontrolled trials support the use of IVIG in combination with aerosolized ribavirin, especially in high-risk patients with an HSCT transplant in the pre-engraftment period.[81,82] No controlled trials examining aerosolized ribavirin and IVIG together have been performed. This treatment approach remains controversial because of the cost and logistical issues with the use of aerosolized ribavirin.

ADVERSE EFFECTS

Immunoglobulin therapy is complex and the incidence of adverse reactions is high. One previous study showed 440 of 1000 patients with primary immunodeficiency reported adverse effects that were not related to the rate of infusion.[5] These adverse effects are typically mild and nonanaphylactic, including back or abdominal pain, nausea, rhinitis, asthma, chills, fever, myalgia, or headache. Additionally, many of these reactions can be reversed by slowing the infusion or with the use of steroids and hydration. Up to 34% of reactions occur with the first infusion and the risk of adverse reaction declines with continued therapy.[5] However, given the potential for severe and life-threatening reactions, including anaphylaxis, hypotension, adult respiratory distress syndrome, thrombosis, and Stevens-Johnson syndrome, vigilance must be maintained with each infusion. In addition to the potential for immediate complications, patients must be counseled on the risk of infection transmission, such as prion diseases, HIV, and viral hepatitides, as well as the risk of nephrotoxicity, which has primarily been reported with the use of sucrose-containing products.[5,83] Lastly, complications related to venous access must also be considered when weighing the risks and benefits of Ig treatment.

Table 2
Infectious Diseases Society of America: US public health service grading system for ranking recommendations in clinical guidelines

Category, Grade	Definition
Strength of Recommendation	
A	Good evidence to support a recommendation for use
B	Moderate evidence to support a recommendation for use
C	Poor evidence to support a recommendation
D	Moderate evidence to support a recommendation against use
E	Good evidence to support a recommendation against use
Quality of evidence	
I	Evidence from ≥1 properly randomized controlled trial
II	Evidence from ≥1 well-designed clinical trial, without randomization; from cohort or case-controlled analytic studies (preferably from >1 center); from multiple time series; or from dramatic results from uncontrolled experiments
III	Evidence from opinions of respected authorities, based on clinical experience, descriptive studies, or reports of expert committees

Data from Nicolle LE, Bradley S, Colgan R, et al. Infectious Diseases Society of America guidelines for the diagnosis and treatment of asymptomatic bacteriuria in adults. Clin Infect Dis 2005; 40(5):643–54.

ROUTE OF ADMINISTRATION

Outside of the specific examination of oral Ig therapy in gastrointestinal infections with rotavirus, *Campylobacter jejuni*, and *C difficile*, intravenous Ig has been the primary route of administration.[84,85] More recently, subcutaneous infusion of Ig has been investigated as an alternative given the improved side-effect profile and enhanced

Table 3
Summary of evidence for use of IVIG in infectious diseases

Indication	Level of Evidence	Plain Language
Sepsis	IIC	May be beneficial
Streptococcal TSS	IIC	May be beneficial
Staphylococcal TSS	IIIC	May be beneficial
C difficile	IIIC	May be beneficial
C tetani	IIIB	Standard of care
C botulinum	IIIB	Standard of care
C diphtheriae	IIIB	Likely beneficial
CMV prophylaxis in SOT	IID	Likely not beneficial
CMV prophylaxis in HSCT	IIE	Not beneficial
CMV treatment in SOT	IIIC	May be beneficial
CMV treatment in HSCT	IIE	Not beneficial
Hepatitis A	IIB	Beneficial
Hepatitis B	IIB	Beneficial
Varicella	IIIC	Beneficial
Rabies	IIIB	Beneficial
RSV	IIB	May be beneficial

levels of IgG in the blood.[86] However, data exist for use in primary immunodeficiency only at this point. It is unclear if there is equivalent activity between intravenous and subcutaneous in conditions, such as infection, that may benefit primarily from immunomodulatory effects seen at high-peak IgG levels.

SUMMARY

The spectrum of IVIG use in the prevention and treatment of infectious disease is broad and particularly focuses on areas where disease is life threatening and effective treatment options are limited. The evidence for common uses of IVIG in infectious disease is summarized in **Tables 2** and **3**. In summary, limited data are available to guide therapy in the most infectious diseases. Although a great need for additional research exists, particularly focusing on randomized and controlled trials, these may be difficult to undertake in the United States for conditions that are becoming increasingly rare (eg, diphtheria) and for which the use of IVIG is firmly entrenched as the standard of care. For new or emerging pathogens that continue to pose a significant problem, such as C difficile, CMV, and sepsis, examination of the efficacy of IVIG is essential.

REFERENCES

1. Eibl MM. History of immunoglobulin replacement. Immunol Allergy Clin North Am 2008;28(4):737–64, viii.
2. Krause I, Wu R, Sherer Y, et al. In vitro antiviral and antibacterial activity of commercial intravenous immunoglobulin preparations–a potential role for adjuvant intravenous immunoglobulin therapy in infectious diseases. Transfus Med 2002;12(2):133–9.
3. Durandy A, Kaveri SV, Kuijpers TW, et al. Intravenous immunoglobulins–understanding properties and mechanisms. Clin Exp Immunol 2009;158(Suppl 1): 2–13.
4. Leong H, Stachnik J, Bonk ME, et al. Unlabeled uses of intravenous immune globulin. Am J Health Syst Pharm 2008;65(19):1815–24.
5. Orange JS, Hossny EM, Weiler CR, et al. Use of intravenous immunoglobulin in human disease: a review of evidence by members of the Primary Immunodeficiency Committee of the American Academy of Allergy, Asthma and Immunology. J Allergy Clin Immunol 2006;117(Suppl 4):S525–53.
6. Darabi K, Abdel-Wahab O, Dzik WH. Current usage of intravenous immune globulin and the rationale behind it: the Massachusetts General Hospital data and a review of the literature. Transfusion 2006;46(5):741–53.
7. Sriskandan S, Ferguson M, Elliot V, et al. Human intravenous immunoglobulin for experimental streptococcal toxic shock: bacterial clearance and modulation of inflammation. J Antimicrob Chemother 2006;58(1):117–24.
8. Werdan K. Pathophysiology of septic shock and multiple organ dysfunction syndrome and various therapeutic approaches with special emphasis on immunoglobulins. Ther Apher 2001;5(2):115–22.
9. Kreymann KG, de Heer G, Nierhaus A, et al. Use of polyclonal immunoglobulins as adjunctive therapy for sepsis or septic shock. Crit Care Med 2007;35(12): 2677–85.
10. Turgeon AF, Hutton B, Fergusson DA, et al. Meta-analysis: intravenous immunoglobulin in critically ill adult patients with sepsis. Ann Intern Med 2007;146(3): 193–203.

11. Laupland KB, Kirkpatrick AW, Delaney A. Polyclonal intravenous immunoglobulin for the treatment of severe sepsis and septic shock in critically ill adults: a systematic review and meta-analysis. Crit Care Med 2007;35(12):2686–92.
12. Alejandria MM, Lansang MA, Dans LF, et al. Intravenous immunoglobulin for treating sepsis and septic shock. Cochrane Database Syst Rev 2002;1:CD001090.
13. Rodriguez A, Rello J, Neira J, et al. Effects of high-dose of intravenous immunoglobulin and antibiotics on survival for severe sepsis undergoing surgery. Shock 2005;23(4):298–304.
14. Sablotzki A, Muhling J, Dehne MG, et al. Treatment of sepsis in cardiac surgery: role of immunoglobulins. Perfusion 2001;16(2):113–20.
15. Pilz G, Kreuzer E, Kaab S, et al. Early sepsis treatment with immunoglobulins after cardiac surgery in score-identified high-risk patients. Chest 1994;105(1):76–82.
16. Barry W, Hudgins L, Donta ST, et al. Intravenous immunoglobulin therapy for toxic shock syndrome. JAMA 1992;267(24):3315–6.
17. Kaul R, McGeer A, Norrby-Teglund A, et al. Intravenous immunoglobulin therapy for streptococcal toxic shock syndrome–a comparative observational study. The Canadian Streptococcal Study Group. Clin Infect Dis 1999;28(4):800–7.
18. Stevens DL. Rationale for the use of intravenous gamma globulin in the treatment of streptococcal toxic shock syndrome. Clin Infect Dis 1998;26(3):639–41.
19. Darenberg J, Ihendyane N, Sjolin J, et al. Intravenous immunoglobulin G therapy in streptococcal toxic shock syndrome: a European randomized, double-blind, placebo-controlled trial. Clin Infect Dis 2003;37(3):333–40.
20. Shah SS, Hall M, Srivastava R, et al. Intravenous immunoglobulin in children with streptococcal toxic shock syndrome. Clin Infect Dis 2009;49(9):1369–76.
21. Darenberg J, Soderquist B, Normark BH, et al. Differences in potency of intravenous polyspecific immunoglobulin G against streptococcal and staphylococcal superantigens: implications for therapy of toxic shock syndrome. Clin Infect Dis 2004;38(6):836–42.
22. Archibald LK, Banerjee SN, Jarvis WR. Secular trends in hospital-acquired Clostridium difficile disease in the United States, 1987-2001. J Infect Dis 2004;189(9): 1585–9.
23. Fernandez A, Anand G, Friedenberg F. Factors associated with failure of metronidazole in Clostridium difficile-associated disease. J Clin Gastroenterol 2004; 38(5):414–8.
24. Kyne L, Hamel MB, Polavaram R, et al. Health care costs and mortality associated with nosocomial diarrhea due to Clostridium difficile. Clin Infect Dis 2002; 34(3):346–53.
25. Kim PH, Iaconis JP, Rolfe RD. Immunization of adult hamsters against Clostridium difficile-associated ileocecitis and transfer of protection to infant hamsters. Infect Immun 1987;55(12):2984–92.
26. Lyerly DM, Bostwick EF, Binion SB, et al. Passive immunization of hamsters against disease caused by Clostridium difficile by use of bovine immunoglobulin G concentrate. Infect Immun 1991;59(6):2215–8.
27. Gerding DN, Johnson S. Management of Clostridium difficile infection: thinking inside and outside the box. Clin Infect Dis 2010;51(11):1306–13.
28. Kyne L, Warny M, Qamar A, et al. Asymptomatic carriage of Clostridium difficile and serum levels of IgG antibody against toxin A. N Engl J Med 2000;342(6): 390–7.
29. Abougergi MS, Kwon JH. Intravenous immunoglobulin for the treatment of Clostridium difficile infection: a review. Dig Dis Sci 2011;56(1):19–26.

30. O'Horo J, Safdar N. The role of immunoglobulin for the treatment of Clostridium difficile infection: a systematic review. Int J Infect Dis 2009;13(6):663–7.
31. Salcedo J, Keates S, Pothoulakis C, et al. Intravenous immunoglobulin therapy for severe Clostridium difficile colitis. Gut 1997;41(3):366–70.
32. Lowy I, Molrine DC, Leav BA, et al. Treatment with monoclonal antibodies against Clostridium difficile toxins. N Engl J Med 2010;362(3):197–205.
33. Kretsinger K, Broder KR, Cortese MM, et al. Preventing tetanus, diphtheria, and pertussis among adults: use of tetanus toxoid, reduced diphtheria toxoid and acellular pertussis vaccine recommendations of the Advisory Committee on Immunization Practices (ACIP) and recommendation of ACIP, supported by the Healthcare Infection Control Practices Advisory Committee (HICPAC), for use of Tdap among health-care personnel. MMWR Recomm Rep 2006;55(RR-17): 1–37.
34. Centers for Disease Control and Prevention (CDC). Tetanus surveillance—United States, 2001–2008. MMWR Morb Mortal Wkly Rep 2011;60(12):365–9.
35. Afshar M, Raju M, Ansell D, et al. Narrative review: tetanus–a health threat after natural disasters in developing countries. Ann Intern Med 2011;154(5):329–35.
36. Keller MA, Stiehm ER. Passive immunity in prevention and treatment of infectious diseases. Clin Microbiol Rev 2000;13(4):602–14.
37. Investigational heptavalent botulinum antitoxin (HBAT) to replace licensed botulinum antitoxin AB and investigational botulinum antitoxin E. MMWR Morb Mortal Wkly Rep 2010;59(10):299.
38. Organization WH. WHO vaccine-preventable diseases monitoring system: 2010 global summary, vol. 2. Geneva (Switzerland): World Health Organization; 2010. p. R-234.
39. Centers for Disease Control and Prevention. CDC health information for international travel 2010. Atlanta (GA): U.S. Department of Health and Human Services PHS; 2009.
40. Centers for Disease Control and Prevention (CDC). Availability of diphtheria antitoxin through an investigational new drug protocol. MMWR Morb Mortal Wkly Rep 1997;46(17):380.
41. Snydman DR, Werner BG, Heinze-Lacey B, et al. Use of cytomegalovirus immune globulin to prevent cytomegalovirus disease in renal-transplant recipients. N Engl J Med 1987;317(17):1049–54.
42. Snydman DR, Werner BG, Dougherty NN, et al. Cytomegalovirus immune globulin prophylaxis in liver transplantation. A randomized, double-blind, placebo-controlled trial. Ann Intern Med 1993;119(10):984–91.
43. Hodson EM, Jones CA, Strippoli GF, et al. Immunoglobulins, vaccines or interferon for preventing cytomegalovirus disease in solid organ transplant recipients. Cochrane Database Syst Rev 2007;2:CD005129.
44. Humar A, Snydman D. Cytomegalovirus in solid organ transplant recipients. Am J Transplant 2009;9(Suppl 4):S78–86.
45. Zuk DM, Humar A, Weinkauf JG, et al. An international survey of cytomegalovirus management practices in lung transplantation. Transplantation 2010;90(6):672–6.
46. Carbone J, Sarmiento E, Palomo J, et al. The potential impact of substitutive therapy with intravenous immunoglobulin on the outcome of heart transplant recipients with infections. Transplant Proc 2007;39(7):2385–8.
47. Kotton CN, Kumar D, Caliendo AM, et al. International consensus guidelines on the management of cytomegalovirus in solid organ transplantation. Transplantation 2010;89(7):779–95.

48. Bowden RA, Sayers M, Flournoy N, et al. Cytomegalovirus immune globulin and seronegative blood products to prevent primary cytomegalovirus infection after marrow transplantation. N Engl J Med 1986;314(16):1006–10.

49. Condie RM, O'Reilly RJ. Prevention of cytomegalovirus infection by prophylaxis with an intravenous, hyperimmune, native, unmodified cytomegalovirus globulin. Randomized trial in bone marrow transplant recipients. Am J Med 1984;76(3A): 134–41.

50. Raanani P, Gafter-Gvili A, Paul M, et al. Immunoglobulin prophylaxis in hematopoietic stem cell transplantation: systematic review and meta-analysis. J Clin Oncol 2009;27(5):770–81.

51. Winston DJ, Ho WG, Lin CH, et al. Intravenous immune globulin for prevention of cytomegalovirus infection and interstitial pneumonia after bone marrow transplantation. Ann Intern Med 1987;106(1):12–8.

52. Cordonnier C, Chevret S, Legrand M, et al. Should immunoglobulin therapy be used in allogeneic stem-cell transplantation? A randomized, double-blind, dose effect, placebo-controlled, multicenter trial. Ann Intern Med 2003;139(1):8–18.

53. Verdonck LF, de Gast GC, Dekker AW, et al. Treatment of cytomegalovirus pneumonia after bone marrow transplantation with cytomegalovirus immunoglobulin combined with ganciclovir. Bone Marrow Transplant 1989;4(2):187–9.

54. Reed EC, Bowden RA, Dandliker PS, et al. Treatment of cytomegalovirus pneumonia with ganciclovir and intravenous cytomegalovirus immunoglobulin in patients with bone marrow transplants. Ann Intern Med 1988;109(10):783–8.

55. Alexander BT, Hladnik LM, Augustin KM, et al. Use of cytomegalovirus intravenous immune globulin for the adjunctive treatment of cytomegalovirus in hematopoietic stem cell transplant recipients. Pharmacotherapy 2010;30(6):554–61.

56. Emanuel D, Cunningham I, Jules-Elysee K, et al. Cytomegalovirus pneumonia after bone marrow transplantation successfully treated with the combination of ganciclovir and high-dose intravenous immune globulin. Ann Intern Med 1988; 109(10):777–82.

57. Havens WP Jr. The etiology of infectious hepatitis. J Am Med Assoc 1947;134(8): 653–5 [discussion: 676–9].

58. Ashley A. Use of gamma globulin for control of infectious hepatitis in an institution for the mentally retarded. N Engl J Med 1955;252(3):88–91.

59. Advisory Committee on Immunization Practices (ACIP) Centers for Disease Control and Prevention (CDC). Update: prevention of hepatitis A after exposure to hepatitis A virus and in international travelers. Updated recommendations of the Advisory Committee on Immunization Practices (ACIP). MMWR Morb Mortal Wkly Rep 2007;56(41):1080–4.

60. Fiore AE, Wasley A, Bell BP. Prevention of hepatitis A through active or passive immunization: recommendations of the Advisory Committee on Immunization Practices (ACIP). MMWR Recomm Rep 2006;55(RR-7):1–23.

61. Liu JP, Nikolova D, Fei Y. Immunoglobulins for preventing hepatitis A. Cochrane Database Syst Rev 2009;2:CD004181.

62. Victor JC, Monto AS, Surdina TY, et al. Hepatitis A vaccine versus immune globulin for postexposure prophylaxis. N Engl J Med 2007;357(17):1685–94.

63. Mast EE, Weinbaum CM, Fiore AE, et al. A comprehensive immunization strategy to eliminate transmission of hepatitis B virus infection in the United States: recommendations of the Advisory Committee on Immunization Practices (ACIP) Part II: immunization of adults. MMWR Recomm Rep 2006;55(RR-16):1–33 [quiz: CE31–4].

64. Mitsui T, Iwano K, Suzuki S, et al. Combined hepatitis B immune globulin and vaccine for postexposure prophylaxis of accidental hepatitis B virus infection in hemodialysis staff members: comparison with immune globulin without vaccine in historical controls. Hepatology 1989;10(3):324–7.

65. Roumeliotou-Karayannis A, Papaevangelou G, Tassopoulos N, et al. Post-exposure active immunoprophylaxis of spouses of acute viral hepatitis B patients. Vaccine 1985;3(1):31–4.

66. Grady GF, Lee VA, Prince AM, et al. Hepatitis B immune globulin for accidental exposures among medical personnel: final report of a multicenter controlled trial. J Infect Dis 1978;138(5):625–38.

67. Redeker AG, Mosley JW, Gocke DJ, et al. Hepatitis B immune globulin as a prophylactic measure for spouses exposed to acute type B hepatitis. N Engl J Med 1975;293(21):1055–9.

68. Seeff LB, Wright EC, Zimmerman HJ, et al. Type B hepatitis after needle-stick exposure: prevention with hepatitis B immune globulin. Final report of the Veterans Administration Cooperative Study. Ann Intern Med 1978;88(3):285–93.

69. Katz LH, Tur-Kaspa R, Guy DG, et al. Lamivudine or adefovir dipivoxil alone or combined with immunoglobulin for preventing hepatitis B recurrence after liver transplantation. Cochrane Database Syst Rev 2010;7:CD006005.

70. Chen J, Yi L, Jia JD, et al. Hepatitis B immunoglobulins and/or lamivudine for preventing hepatitis B recurrence after liver transplantation: a systematic review. J Gastroenterol Hepatol 2010;25(5):872–9.

71. Gershon AA, Piomelli S, Karpatkin M, et al. Antibody to varicella-zoster virus after passive immunization against chickenpox. J Clin Microbiol 1978;8(6):733–5.

72. Hanngren K, Falksveden L, Grandien M, et al. Zoster immunoglobulin in varicella prophylaxis. A study among high-risk patients. Scand J Infect Dis 1983;15(4):327–34.

73. Prevention of varicella: recommendations of the Advisory Committee on Immunization Practices (ACIP). Centers for Disease Control and Prevention. MMWR Recomm Rep 1996;45(RR-11):1–36.

74. Marin M, Guris D, Chaves SS, et al. Prevention of varicella: recommendations of the Advisory Committee on Immunization Practices (ACIP). MMWR Recomm Rep 2007;56(RR-4):1–40.

75. Paryani SG, Arvin AM, Koropchak CM, et al. Varicella zoster antibody titers after the administration of intravenous immune serum globulin or varicella zoster immune globulin. Am J Med 1984;76(3A):124–7.

76. Habel K, Koprowski H. Laboratory data supporting the clinical trial of anti-rabies serum in persons bitten by a rabid wolf. Bull World Health Organ 1955;13(5):773–9.

77. Lin FT, Chen SB, Wang YZ, et al. Use of serum and vaccine in combination for prophylaxis following exposure to rabies. Rev Infect Dis 1988;10(Suppl 4):S766–70.

78. Khawplod P, Wilde H, Chomchey P, et al. What is an acceptable delay in rabies immune globulin administration when vaccine alone had been given previously? Vaccine 1996;14(5):389–91.

79. Manning SE, Rupprecht CE, Fishbein D, et al. Human rabies prevention–United States, 2008: recommendations of the Advisory Committee on Immunization Practices. MMWR Recomm Rep 2008;57(RR-3):1–28.

80. Harrington RD, Hooton TM, Hackman RC, et al. An outbreak of respiratory syncytial virus in a bone marrow transplant center. J Infect Dis 1992;165(6):987–93.

81. Whimbey E, Champlin RE, Englund JA, et al. Combination therapy with aerosolized ribavirin and intravenous immunoglobulin for respiratory syncytial virus disease in adult bone marrow transplant recipients. Bone Marrow Transplant 1995;16(3):393–9.
82. Ghosh S, Champlin RE, Englund J, et al. Respiratory syncytial virus upper respiratory tract illnesses in adult blood and marrow transplant recipients: combination therapy with aerosolized ribavirin and intravenous immunoglobulin. Bone Marrow Transplant 2000;25(7):751–5.
83. Nydegger UE, Sturzenegger M. Adverse effects of intravenous immunoglobulin therapy. Drug Saf 1999;21(3):171–85.
84. Guarino A, Guandalini S, Albano F, et al. Enteral immunoglobulins for treatment of protracted rotaviral diarrhea. Pediatr Infect Dis J 1991;10(8):612–4.
85. Hammarstrom V, Smith CI, Hammarstrom L. Oral immunoglobulin treatment in Campylobacter jejuni enteritis. Lancet 1993;341(8851):1036.
86. Gaspar J, Gerritsen B, Jones A. Immunoglobulin replacement treatment by rapid subcutaneous infusion. Arch Dis Child 1998;79(1):48–51.
87. Dennert R, Velthuis S, Schalla S, et al. Intravenous immunoglobulin therapy for patients with idiopathic cardiomyopathy and endomyocardial biopsy-proven high PVB19 viral load. Antivir Ther 2010;15(2):193–201.
88. Mouthon L, Guillevin L, Tellier Z. Intravenous immunoglobulins in autoimmune- or parvovirus B19-mediated pure red-cell aplasia. Autoimmun Rev 2005;4(5):264–9.
89. McKinney RE Jr, Katz SL, Wilfert CM. Chronic enteroviral meningoencephalitis in agammaglobulinemic patients. Rev Infect Dis 1987;9(2):334–56.

Monoclonal Antibodies in Infectious Diseases: Clinical Pipeline in 2011

Jan ter Meulen, MD, DTM&H

KEYWORDS

• Monoclonal antibodies • Infectious diseases • Pipeline

Based on an impressive body of preclinical work, anti-infectious disease antibodies are considered to have great potential to address the unmet medical needs associated with viral and bacterial infections, particularly nosocomial infections. For example, the recent discovery of human monoclonal antibodies (mAbs) that broadly neutralize different clades and strains of influenza virus has generated considerable interest in the field and raised the possibility that universal anti-influenza mAbs could enhance pandemic preparedness.[1] However, despite progress in the field and many candidates in clinical development, which have been summarized in several comprehensive reviews,[2–5] it seems that anti-infectious disease (anti-ID) mAbs may not change medical practice within the optimistic time frames that have been projected. Actual progress has been slow; several high-profile anti-ID mAbs have not performed as well as anticipated in clinical trials, and, to date, there is still only 1 anti-ID mAb approved for clinical use (palivizumab [Synagis]). This review briefly summarizes the current clinical pipeline of anti-ID mAbs that are actively being developed, based on publicly accessible information, and highlights conceptual problems in the discovery and development of these biological drugs, which may contribute to the slower-than-expected progress in this field. Development of mAbs by research institutions or manufacturers located in emerging markets is not covered in this article.

THE SCIENTIFIC AND TECHNOLOGICAL BASIS FOR THE GENERATION OF ANTI-ID mAbs

Because the antibody response of a naive individual takes 1 to 2 weeks to fully develop, the innate immune response as the first-line defense is pivotal in determining

Disclosure: The author is a full-time employee of Merck & Co.
Vaccine Research, Merck Research Laboratories, 16-100, 770 Sumneytown Pike, West Point, PA 19486, USA
E-mail address: jan.ter.meulen@merck.com

Infect Dis Clin N Am 25 (2011) 789–802
doi:10.1016/j.idc.2011.07.006
0891-5520/11/$ – see front matter © 2011 Elsevier Inc. All rights reserved.

id.theclinics.com

the outcome of an infection. The surfaces of many infectious agents contain conserved motifs that react with evolutionarily conserved pattern recognition receptors of the host, such as toll-like receptors. This interaction initiates a powerful innate immune response, which forms the basis of a strong and durable adaptive immune response. Because of the pronounced antigenic difference between infectious agents and the mammalian host, the components of the infectious agent that come into contact with B-cell receptors (membrane-bound IgM/IgD), usually surface proteins (eg, viral structural proteins) and carbohydrates (eg, bacterial capsular polysaccharides), often induce potent antibody responses. Antibodies that block important receptor functions are clearly associated with protection against many viruses and toxins, both in natural infection and after immunization, and complement-fixing antibodies opsonize and kill bacteria. Specific antibody titers have been identified as correlates or surrogates of protection against several toxins, viruses, or encapsulated bacteria (eg, neutralizing antibody titer against poliovirus, serum bactericidal titer against *Meningococcus*[6]). However, for some viral and most bacterial infections, no correlates of protection have been established, and the significance of antibody titers other than indicating past exposure is not clear (eg, *Staphylococcus*).

Immune avoidance mechanisms may help explain why total antibody titers are not always correlates of protection. For example, the constantly mutating surface proteins and glycan-shielded epitopes of many infectious organisms, including influenza virus, human immunodeficiency virus (HIV), malaria-causing organisms, and *Streptococcus pneumoniae*, subvert the humoral immune response by diverting the antibody response away from functionally important epitopes in favor of highly immunogenic, highly variable, and functionally irrelevant epitopes. In addition, some pathogens, such as *Pseudomonas*, *Staphylococcus*, and *Streptococcus*, directly disable antibodies by binding the Fc receptor (eg, staphylococcal protein A, streptococcal proteins G and H) or secreting proteases that cleave the Fc portion from the antigen-binding site. Therefore, the ability to effectively eliminate pathogens depends not only on the magnitude of the antibody response but also on the ability to target functionally important antigens. Likewise, in the development of candidate therapeutic mAbs, selection for functionality as well as high affinity seems critical, as evidenced by the discovery of potent and broadly neutralizing anti-HIV mAbs that do not bind the monomeric recombinant gp120 or gp41 envelope proteins that are commonly used as screening antigens.[7]

Although the use of antibacterial sera was only common in the preantibiotic era, antiviral immunoglobulins are still in clinical use today, notably antirabies immunoglobulin. Historically, polyclonal sera have been most effective against viruses with long incubation periods, such as hepatitis A virus, and bacterial toxins, such as diphtheria toxin and tetanus toxin. Rather than relying on polyclonal sera as a source of therapeutic antibodies, modern technology enables the efficient generation of mAbs from the antibody repertoires of animals or humans. In one approach, B cells or plasma cells of naturally infected or immunized human donors are enriched for specific antigen binding and taken into short-term culture or immortalized. The antibody genes are cloned out of single cells and used to express full-length IgG molecules of different subclasses in a recombinant mammalian expression system. The mAbs cloned directly from humans have the obvious advantage of low intrinsic immunogenicity compared with mAbs cloned from animals and then humanized. In addition, the kinetics of human B cells and plasma cells after infection and vaccination are well studied, making it possible to precisely harvest plasma cells producing a large variety of affinity-matured antibodies when they leave the lymph node and migrate to the bone marrow.[8] This study also allows the characterization of the entire human antibody repertoire directed against a given antigen and identification of dominant epitopes.

Another common approach to producing mAbs is antibody phage display, in which the genes for the variable regions of the heavy and light chains of the entire antibody repertoire are cloned separately. The heavy and light chain genes are then randomly combined and expressed as single-chain antibodies on the coat of a bacteriophage. Thus, one drawback of phage display is the possibility that the random unnatural pairing of variable region of heavy chain and variable region of light chain genes may increase the immunogenicity of some of these antibodies. In addition, antibodies derived from phage libraries typically have lower affinities than those derived from plasma cells, so they are affinity matured in the laboratory by rationally mutating their antigen-binding regions. However, there are several advantages to this approach. Phage display produces an antibody library with a vast repertoire of specificities, which is readily available for panning with any antigen and includes antibodies against antigens that are weakly immunogenic or too toxic to use for immunizations. Thus, technological advances have made it possible to generate anti-ID mAbs with a broad repertoire of specificities and to harness the power of the adaptive immune system for anti-ID therapies.

ANTIVIRAL mAbs IN CLINICAL DEVELOPMENT

The only approved anti-ID mAb, palivizumab (Synagis), is the basis for second- and third-generation mAbs under development by AstraZeneca/MedImmune for prevention of respiratory syncytial virus (RSV) infection in infants. The third-generation mAb, a YTE mutant of the second-generation mAb motavizumab, has an extended half-life and is currently in phase 2 trials (MEDI-557). Motavizumab (Numax) was derived from palivizumab by affinity maturation (13 amino acids difference) and showed promise in early trials, with a 70-fold increase in in vitro affinity to the F protein of RSV and a neutralizing potency increased by 18-fold in in vitro and increased up to 100-fold in the cotton rat model.[9] In published clinical efficacy data for 3 phase 3 trials, one of which involved 300 study locations and 6600 preterm infants with or without chronic lung disease, motavizumab was shown to be noninferior to palivizumab for the prevention of serious lower respiratory tract disease caused by RSV. In 2010, the Food and Drug Administration's Antiviral Drugs Advisory Committee declined to endorse MedImmune's request for licensure of motavizumab in children at high risk for RSV disease, citing concerns about safety, allergic reactions (3-fold increase in nonfatal hypersensitivity adverse reactions, including urticaria, compared with palivizumab[10]), and the study design to prove noninferiority as opposed to superiority. This example demonstrates that antibody engineering to increase affinity and potency does not necessarily translate into improved clinical efficacy and may come at the risk of increased side effects because of increased immunogenicity.

Four mAbs against hepatitis C virus (HCV) are in phase 1 or 2 development, either for therapy for chronic infection or prophylaxis for liver reinfection after transplantation. A phase 2 trial was initiated in 2010 for the MBL-HCV1 mAb (MassBiologics), the only of these 4 mAbs to neutralize the virus by binding to a viral protein.[11] The other anti-HCV mAbs target cellular proteins. Bavituximab (Peregrine) is directed against phosphatidylserine, an anionic phospholipid that is found on the inner surface of the cellular membranes of normal cells but is on the exterior surface of enveloped viruses and tumor-associated vascular endothelium.[12] In preclinical models, bavituximab demonstrated neutralizing activity against a wide range of enveloped viruses and inhibited the growth of various solid tumors by inhibiting angiogenesis. Antiviral activity (decline of $\geq 0.5\ \log_{10}$ in HCV RNA level) was observed in phase 1a and phase 1b repeat-dose trials at all doses. At a dose of 3 mg/kg, 83% of patients demonstrated a maximum peak reduction in HCV RNA levels of at least 75% (0.6 log), and these patients showed an average peak reduction of 84% (0.8 log). Bavituximab is in phase 2 clinical development for HCV infection and in phase 1 trial for HCV/HIV coinfection. Two other mAbs (CT-011, CureTech; BMS-936558, Bristol-Myers Squibb) exert anti-HCV activity by modulating the immune response to HCV. The immunoinhibitory receptor programmed death 1 (PD-1) is upregulated on dysfunctional virus-specific $CD8^+$ T cells during chronic HCV infection. CT-011 and BMS-936558 block PD-1 signaling, thus restoring the function of anti-HCV $CD8^+$ T cells.[13] MDX1106 is also in phase 2 clinical trials for a variety of tumors. These examples highlight the potential value of anti-ID mAbs that target host-derived proteins.

HIV therapy with mAbs such as 2G12, 2F5, and 4E10, which are directed against the HIV envelope glycoprotein, has been complicated by escape variants that produce a rebound of viral load. HIV entry into $CD4^+$ T cells requires the presence of a coreceptor, either CCR5 or CXCR4, on the target cell. Therefore, it has been proposed that blocking the interaction of the virus with its conserved cellular coreceptors could prevent viral entry and thereby increase the breadth of protection while reducing or eliminating the development of escape variants. Two mAbs, ibalizumab (Tanox), directed against CD4, and PRO 140 (Progenics), directed against the coreceptor CCR5, are being developed based on this hypothesis.[14,15] At nanomolar concentrations, ibalizumab demonstrated potent in vitro neutralization against almost all 116 HIV envelope–pseudotyped viruses tested and exhibited extremely broad in vitro neutralization irrespective of envelope diversity by geography, clade, tropism, and stage of infection. In phase 1b and phase 2a clinical trials, multiple doses of ibalizumab given intravenously decreased viral load by approximately 1 log in HIV-infected volunteers, and no evidence of adverse effects on CD4 T cells was noted. A return toward baseline viral loads by week 9 was associated with reduced susceptibility to ibalizumab (increase in IC50) and a loss of asparagine-linked glycosylation sites in variable region 5 of HIV type 1 envelope protein.[16] Ibalizumab is currently in a phase 2b trial and is being developed by the Ibalizumab Development Consortium under the guidance of Dr David Ho (http://www.cavd.org/grantees/Pages/HoIDC.aspx).

PRO 140 is a humanized monoclonal CCR5 antibody that binds CCR5 and inhibits R5-tropic HIV. In a phase 2 study, 44 patients were randomized to receive subcutaneous infusions either of PRO 140 in 3 weekly doses of 162 mg or 324 mg (days 1, 8 and 15) or 2 biweekly doses of 324 mg (days 1 and 15) or placebo. With 3 weekly doses of 324-mg PRO 140, the mean maximum viral load reduction was 1.77 $\log_{10}$, and 100% of the patients in this group achieved a maximum reduction in viral load of greater than 1.0 $\log_{10}$. In both the 324-mg weekly and biweekly dose groups, a mean reduction in viral load of greater than 1.0 $\log_{10}$ was maintained for 2 weeks after the last dose. Thus, this study demonstrated potent and prolonged antiviral activity of PRO 140 at a 324-mg weekly or biweekly dose given subcutaneously. Subcutaneous PRO 140 was generally well tolerated compared with placebo, with mild and transient local reactions at the site of infusion occurring in a minority of individuals. There were no drug-related serious adverse events and no study discontinuations.[17] Virologic failure was seen in some individuals as a result of the outgrowth of virus with dual/mixed tropism. Decreased susceptibility of R5-tropic virus to PRO 140 was not seen despite the slow washout of the drug, suggesting a high barrier to resistance. Although mAbs against neutralizing epitopes on the viral envelope have disappointed because of rapid generation of escape mutants, there is cautious optimism that targeting the conserved cellular receptors of the virus may open new avenues for a viable antibody therapy for HIV infection.

Rabies postexposure prophylaxis (PEP) is performed by concomitant administration of killed rabies vaccine and rabies immunoglobulin prepared from immunized human donors (HRIG) or horses. Because of a shortage of vaccine and rabies immunoglobulins and logistic problems with PEP, more than 50,000 people die of rabies annually, mostly in Asia. Crucell/Sanofi are developing foravirumab, a cocktail of 2 potent noncompeting rabies virus neutralizing mAbs (CL184) directed against highly conserved epitopes on the viral glycoprotein G, to replace HRIG in PEP. In a phase 2 trial in 140 healthy volunteers, the antibody product was tested in association with Sanofi Pasteur human diploid cell rabies vaccine. The study compared foravirumab with a currently marketed HRIG or placebo, in association with the rabies vaccine in a simulated rabies postexposure setting. Individuals were randomized to receive foravirumab (N = 80), HRIG (N = 40), or placebo (N = 20). All individuals completed the study. By day 14, in all individuals administered foravirumab together with the rabies vaccine, the level of neutralizing antibody activity in serum reached 0.5 IU/mL, which is associated with protection. Of note, the development of the active immune response to the rabies vaccine was comparable in the foravirumab and HRIG treatment groups.[18]

MGAWN1 is a humanized mAb that is being developed by MacroGenics for therapy for West Nile virus (WNV) infections. This mAb neutralizes the virus by binding to the domain III of the envelope glycoprotein.[19] Since 1999, there have been more than 29,000 cases of confirmed symptomatic WNV infection in the United States, which include more than 12,000 neurologic cases and more than 1100 deaths. In 2009, 722 cases of WNV infection were reported to the Centers for Disease Control and Prevention for the year, with 33 of these cases resulting in death. MGAWN1 is being tested in a randomized, double-blind, multicenter, placebo-controlled phase 2 clinical study that is designed to evaluate the safety and efficacy in patients older than 18 years with signs and symptoms of acute West Nile neuroinvasive disease as well as in those with WNV fever with laboratory evidence of infection with the virus.

ANTIBACTERIAL AND ANTITOXIN mAbs IN CLINICAL DEVELOPMENT

The past years have seen several failures in the development of polyclonal (Altastaph, Veronate) and monoclonal (Aurograb) antibody products against Staphylococcus aureus infections, which underlines the difficulty to treat with passive immunotherapy a complex organism expressing a multitude of pathogenicity factors that are involved in a variety of different clinical manifestations. A comprehensive review of staphylococcal vaccines and immunotherapies was recently published.[20]

Biosynexus is developing pagibaximab (PMAB), a chimeric mAb directed against lipoteichoic acid (LTA), a highly conserved glycolipid component of the staphylococcal cell walls. In a phase 2 study, 2- to 5-day-old 700- to 1300-g neonates were randomized to receive 3 doses 7 days apart of either PMAB or placebo. A total of 88 newborns, with a mean birth weight of 992 g and mean gestation of 28 weeks received at least 1 dose of study drug at 60 mg/kg (N = 20), 90 mg/kg (N = 22), or placebo (N = 46). There were no significant demographic, mortality, or morbidity differences between study groups. All serious adverse events seemed unrelated or probably not related to PMAB. PMAB was nonimmunogenic and demonstrated linear pharmacokinetics. Mean sustained PMAB levels of more than 500 µg/mL were seen for 3 weeks after the second infusion of 90 mg/kg. There was a trend for those treated with this dose to have fewer positive blood culture results due to any organism than other groups (18% vs 40% and 30% in the 60 mg/kg and placebo groups, respectively; $P<.3$). No individual in the 90 mg/kg group had confirmed staphylococcal sepsis compared with 20% and 13% in the 60 mg/kg and placebo groups, respectively ($P<.11$). Estimated or observed PMAB levels were less than 500 µg/mL at the time of staphylococcal sepsis in all cases except one.[21] A phase 2b/3 trial is underway in the United States in 1550 very-low–birth weight neonates to determine whether the antibody can prevent staphylococcal sepsis. Based on a pharmacokinetic study performed in this patient population, a dosing regimen of 100 mg/kg daily for 3 days and then weekly for 3 weeks maintains serum levels at or greater than 500 µg/ml.[22]

Sanofi/Alopexx are developing SAR279356 (mAb F598), a human mAb directed against a carbohydrate found on the surface of staphylococci, polysaccharide poly-N-acetylated glucosamine (PNAG). F598 bound the best to nonacetylated or backbone epitopes on PNAG and had superior complement deposition and opsonophagocytic activity compared with 2 mAbs that bound optimally to PNAG that was expressed with a native level (>90%) of N-acetyl groups (mAbs F628 and F630). Protection of mice against lethality due to S aureus strains Mn8 and Reynolds further showed that the backbone-specific mAb had optimal protective efficacy compared with the acetate-specific MAbs. These results provide evidence for the importance of epitope specificity in inducing the optimal protective antibody response to PNAG and indicate that MAbs to the deacetylated form of PNAG could be immunotherapeutic agents for preventing or treating staphylococcal infections.[23]

Bacterial toxins are highly sensitive to antibody neutralization, as illustrated by the impressive efficacy of preexposure and postexposure passive mAb treatment of highly lethal inhalational anthrax in animal models. Three mAbs for prophylaxis of pulmonary anthrax infection are in clinical development; all are directed against the protective antigen (PA). Bacillus anthracis produces a tripartite A-B toxin that is an essential virulence factor for the development of anthrax disease. The toxin is composed of 2 alternative A subunits, lethal factor (LF) and edema factor (EF), and a single receptor-binding B subunit, designated as PA. PA combines with LF to form lethal toxin and with EF to form edema toxin. Toxin entry into cells involves PA receptor binding and proteolytic activation to generate an oligomeric prepore and binding EF and/or LF and internalization of the toxin-receptor complexes by cellular endocytosis. Recommended prophylaxis of inhalational anthrax after exposure to B anthracis spores includes 60 days of ciprofloxacin. Of concern is that ciprofloxacin may be contraindicated, the complete dosing schedule not complied with or infection might be caused by mutant B anthracis strains made intentionally resistant to the antibiotic.

Valortim (PharmAthene), ThravixaTM (Emergent BioSolutions), and AnthimTM (Elusys) are human mAbs in phase 1 of clinical development. ABThrax (raxibacumab, Human Genome Sciences) is a human mAb in phase 3. In preclinical studies, a single dose of raxibacumab, administered without the use of antibiotics, improved survival rates of nonhuman primates by up to 64%, even when administered after animals were already showing clinical symptoms as a result of anthrax spore inhalation exposure to 100 to 200 times the dose required to kill 50% of untreated animals.[24] Human safety studies were conducted in 438 individuals, 333 receiving raxibacumab at a dose of 40 mg/kg of bodyweight (the recommended dose for licensure) and 105 receiving placebo. Adverse events recorded for individuals receiving raxibacumab alone or with ciprofloxacin did not differ significantly from the placebo groups and were transient and mild to moderate in severity. More than 20,000 doses of raxibacumab have been delivered to the US Strategic National Stockpile.

Merck & Co. is developing MK3415A, a cocktail of 2 human mAbs (CDA-1 and CDB-1) directed against toxins A and B of *Clostridium difficile*, for therapy for *C difficile*–associated disease. In a randomized, double-blind, placebo-controlled study involving 200 patients with symptomatic *C difficile* infection who were receiving either metronidazole or vancomycin, MK3415A was administered intravenously at a dose of 10 mg/kg. The rate of laboratory-documented recurrence of infection during the 84 days after the administration of MK3415A or placebo was lower among patients treated with mAbs (7% vs 25%; 95% confidence interval, 7–29; $P<.001$). The recurrence rates among patients with the epidemic BI/NAP1/027 strain were 8% for the antibody group and 32% for the placebo group ($P = .06$); among patients with more than one previous episode of *C difficile* infection, recurrence rates were 7% and 38%, respectively ($P = .006$). The mean duration of the initial hospitalization for inpatients did not differ significantly between the antibody and placebo groups (9.5 and 9.4 days, respectively). This study demonstrates that the addition of MK3415A to standard of care significantly reduced the recurrence of *C difficile* infection.[25]

Shigamabs, a cocktail of 2 chimeric mAbs (caStx1, caStx2) neutralizing Shiga toxins 1 and 2, is being developed by Thallion for treatment of Shiga toxin–producing *Escherichia coli* (STEC) infections, causing bloody diarrhea and hemolytic uremic syndrome. In animal models of STEC, each antibody has independently demonstrated a protective effect at low doses, and animal rescue was demonstrated possible even when administration of cαStx2 was initiated up to 72 hours postinfection.[26] The safety and pharmacokinetic properties of cαStx1 and cαStx2 have been evaluated in 4 phase 1 clinical trials. Overall, 50 healthy volunteers have been exposed to one or both antibodies. A total of 40 healthy volunteers have received a single infusion of Stx1 (n = 15) or Stx2 (n = 25), and an additional 10 have received a single concomitant infusion of Stx1 and Stx2. It was concluded that the antibodies were safe and well tolerated at a dose of up to 10 mg/kg of each antitoxin (for a final dose of 20 mg/kg when administered concomitantly), which exceeds the maximal intended dose of 3 mg/kg for the target pediatric population. No serious adverse events were reported in any of the studies. Minimal immunogenicity to the antibodies was observed. Of the 49 volunteers tested for human antichimeric antibody (HACA), 5 (10%) tested positive for low HACA concentrations approximately 8 weeks after administration of the antibodies. At the targeted pediatric therapeutic dose of 3 mg/kg, the elimination half-life of each antibody is approximately 9 days, suggesting that a single infusion of Shigamabs is sufficient for treating patients diagnosed with STEC infection. A randomized, double-blind, placebo-controlled trial is underway to enroll 42 patients, aged 6 months to 18 years testing positive for STEC infection, distributed in 2 cohorts, comparing standard of care combined with a low (1 mg/kg) or high (3 mg/kg) dose of Shigamabs with standard of care with placebo. Primary end points for the phase 2 trial are safety and tolerability; secondary endpoints include pharmacokinetics and efficacy of STEC-associated disease.

Pseudomonas aeruginosa infection remains a very important nosocomial problem, especially for patients requiring mechanical ventilation and for burn patients. Kenta Biotech developed panobacumab, a human IgM-mAb directed against lipopolysaccharide of the O11 serotype of *P aeruginosa*. In a murine pulmonary infection model, panobacumab was able to reach the bronchoalveolar space and reduce the pulmonary bacterial load as well as lung inflammation in a dose-dependent manner. Furthermore, panobacumab treatment lead to enhanced neutrophil recruitment in bronchoalveolar lavage fluid while reducing the host-derived production of proinflammatory mediators and lung injury.[27] Results from a phase 2a trial in patients with ventilator-associated pneumonia (N = 12) or hospital-acquired pneumonia

(N = 1) caused by *P aeruginosa* serotype O11 showed that all patients who received the full treatment cycle of panobacumab survived, despite a predicted mortality of 24% according to the severity of disease classification (Acute Physiology and Chronic Health Evaluation II). In the study, patients received 3 single intravenous infusions of panobacumab, 1.2 mg/kg, on days 1, 4, and 7, administered in addition to standard antibacterial therapy. A total of 18 patients were treated; 13 patients received 3 doses, and 5 patients received 1 dose. The 28-day mortality rate in this trial was 7%.[28]

Sanofi-Pasteur/KaloBios developed KB001, a humanized pegylated Fab fragment directed against the type 3 secretion system (TTSS) PcrV of *P aeruginosa*. The instillation of a single dose of Fab into the lungs of mice provided protection against lethal pulmonary challenge of *P aeruginosa* and led to a substantial reduction of viable bacterial counts in the lungs. These results demonstrate that blocking of the TTSS by a Fab lacking antibody Fc-mediated effector functions can be sufficient for the effective clearance of pulmonary *P aeruginosa* infection.[29] Trends toward improved clinical outcomes were observed in KB001-treated patients in a pilot clinical study of the candidate in the prevention of serious *P aeruginosa* pneumonia in mechanically ventilated patients confirmed to be colonized with the bacterium. The double-blind 4-week study randomized patients to either a single intravenous infusion of KB001 at 3 or 10 mg/kg or placebo. More than 90% of patients in all cohorts received antibacterials within 14 days of study entry, with the majority on mechanical ventilation for at least 7 days. Of the 35 evaluable patients, 46% of those treated with high-dose KB001 were alive at day 28 without *P aeruginosa* infection compared with only 20% of placebo recipients. The proportion of patients with *P aeruginosa* pneumonia was lower in KB001-treated patients (33% and 31% for low and high doses, respectively) compared with placebo recipients (60%).

SUMMARY AND CONSIDERATIONS

The surge in antibiotic-resistant nosocomial infections highlights a serious unmet medical need in anti-infective drugs. However, in 2011, the pipeline for anti-ID mAbs consists primarily of antibodies directed against viruses and toxins, and all but 2 of these are in phase 1 or 2 programs (**Table 1**). In recent years, 3 late-stage mAb products (Aurograb and Mycograb, both single-chain antibodies, and Numax) as well as polyclonal products (Veronate) have failed, and their development has been discontinued. In addition, the development of some polyclonal and monoclonal products has been placed on hold, in some cases for several years. Considering recent technical progress in antibody engineering and manufacturing, it is surprising that there is still only 1 licensed product in the market (Synagis). The possible reasons because of which mAbs seem to not have delivered on their promise as "magical bullets" against infectious diseases are discussed in the following paragraphs.

One likely explanation is that the development path to a viable mAb product becomes unclear with increasing biological complexity of the target because the mechanisms by which antibodies neutralize complex targets are intricate and often poorly understood. For many years, rudimentary passive immunotherapy has been successful against simple targets such as toxins and viruses, and immune sera are still in clinical use against these targets. Bacterial toxins are the simplest targets of passive immunotherapy because neutralization of toxins requires only high-affinity binding of the antibody to inhibit receptor interactions, and Fc receptor functions are not involved. It is therefore fairly straightforward to develop antitoxin mAbs, provided the neutralizing epitopes are known.

Similar to toxins, virus neutralization requires usually only antibody binding, although complement fixation may enhance neutralization. In some cases, mAbs to viruses are being developed as alternatives to immune sera (eg, cytomegalovirus, hepatitis B virus, rabies virus). Several strategies are also being used to increase the affinity and neutralizing potency of existing antiviral mAbs. However, the results of the motavizumab trials show that these changes do not necessarily translate into increased clinical efficacy. The development of new antiviral antibody products has been complicated by antigenic variability, especially for RNA viruses. Effective targeting of such viruses may require a combination of mAbs to increase the breadth of protection and prevent the selection of immune escape variants in the patient. Indeed, in several examples, the combination of antibodies exerts an additive or even synergist effect on neutralization, which may allow for a lower concentration of final product and lower cost of goods.[30,31] For viruses that are difficult to neutralize and especially prone to variability, antibody therapies may be ineffective or may be effective only in combination with other therapies, such as antiviral drugs or immunomodulators that stimulate T-cell responses.

Just as antibody titer is a correlation of protection against some viruses, serum bactericidal activity and opsonic activity of antibodies are known correlates of protection for some bacterial infections. However, passive immunotherapy has been much less successful against bacteria. Paradoxically, the current paradigm that anti-ID mAbs should have maximum affinity and be narrowly focused on their targets may have hindered efforts to develop antibacterial antibodies. Natural IgM antibodies have low affinity for their targets, are broadly cross-reactive, and fix complement well, which makes them an important first line of defense against invading encapsulated bacteria.[32] In addition, most antibacterial mAbs work by engaging other components of the immune system, such as neutrophils, through the Fc receptor, but antibacterial mAbs are used primarily in patient populations that are predisposed to nosocomial infections because of immature or compromised immune systems. Furthermore, it is increasingly clear that innate immunity plays an essential role in preventing invasive infection with bacteria that colonize mucosal membranes, for example, methicillin-resistant S aureus, and that T cells are also critical for protective immunity against extracellular bacteria. For example, neutrophils are critical for host defense against both Staphylococcus and Candida, killing the organisms by phagocytosis and reactive oxygen burst. Neutrophil proliferation and recruitment are facilitated by interleukin (IL) 17, and individuals who lack IL-17–secreting CD4$^+$ T cells suffer from recurrent staphylococcal infection.[33] Therefore, most antibacterial mAbs are effective only in patients with some level of immunocompetence, and immune function should be assessed in patient populations selected for clinical trials.

mAbs have been described as a panacea for infectious diseases, but that view is changing. The success of mAbs as therapeutic tools will require a further paradigm shift and new approaches to mAbs development. Although elaborate technologies make it possible to clone even very rare antibody specificities from the human repertoire, the procedures to screen for leads are still fairly simple and rely mostly on high-affinity binding. The development of high-throughput screening technologies that access the complex functionality of antibodies, their synergy with each other, and their synergy with small-molecule anti-ID drugs or immunomodulators will be particularly important for the success of mAbs against complex and highly variable targets. Conceptually, anti-ID mAb therapy needs to become more polyclonal and polyfunctional to be efficient against complex biological pathogens.

Table 1
Anti-infective mAbs in clinical development in 2011

Target	Compound	Company	Structure	Mechanism	Indication	Status	Refs
RSV	Palivizumab	AZ/Medimmune	humanized mAb	Virus neutralisation (anti-glycoprotein F)	Treatment and prevention of RSV pneumonia in at-risk infants. Treatment of RSV pneumonia in stem-cell transplant patients.	Approved	34
	Motavizumab (Numax)	AZ/Medimmune	humanized mAb	as above, increased potency	2nd generation anti-RSV mAb	Phase III, discontinued[a]	35
	MEDI 557	AZ/Medimmune	Motavizumab, YTE mutation	as above, plus extended halflife	3rd generation anti-RSV mAb	Phase I	
HCV	Bavituximab	Peregrine	chimeric mAb	Virus neutralisation (anti-phosphatidyl serine). Also antitumor activity	Therpy of chronic HCV infection. Co-adminstered with Ribavirin	Phase II	11
	CT-011	CureTech	humanized mAb	anti-PD1 (immunomodulation)	Therapy of chronic HCV infection	Phase I/II	
	BMS 936558 (MDX1106)	Bristol-Myers Squibb/ Medarex	human mAb	anti-PD-1 (immunomodulation)	Therapy of chronic HCV infection	Phase I	
	MBL-HCV1	MassBiologics	human mAb	Virus neutralisation (anti-E2)	Prevention of liver reinfection wit HCV after transplantation	Phase II	10
Rabies	Foravirumab (CL184)	J&J/Crucell	Two human mAbs (cocktail)	Virus neutralization (anti-Glycoprotein G)	Postexposure prophylaxis of rabies in conjunction with rabies vaccine	Phase II	17
HIV	Ibalizumab	TaiMed Biologics/ Tanox	humanized mAb	Viral entry blocking (anti-CD4 receptor)	Therapy of HIV infection	Phase II	13,15
	Pro-140	Progenics/PDL	humanized mAb	Viral entry blocking (anti-CCR5 receptor)	Therapy of HIV infection	Phase IIb	14,16

Disease	Compound	Company	mAb type	Target	Indication	Phase	Ref.
West Nile	MGAWN1	MacroGenics	humanized mAb	Virus neutralization (anit-E)	Therapy of WNV infections	Phase II	18
Staphylococcus	Pagibaximab	Biosynexus	chimeric mAb	Anti-lipoteichoic acid	Prevention of Staph infections in neonates	Phase IIb/III	20,21
	SAR279356 (F598)	Sanofi-Aventis/Alopexx	human mAb	Anti-poly-N-acetylglucosamine (PNAG)	Therapy of Staph and other bacterial infections	Phase I	22
Bacillus anthracis	ETI-204 (Anthim)	Elusys	human mAb	Toxin neutralisation (PA)	Prevention and treatment of pulmonary anthrax	Phase II	23
	Raxibacumab (ABThrax)	Human Genome Sciences	human mAb	Toxin neutralisation (PA)	as above	Phase III	37
	Valortim (MDX-1303)	PharmAthene	human mAb	Toxin neutralisation (PA)	as above	Phase I	36
	AVP 21D9 (Thravixa)	Emergent BioSolutions/Avanir	human mAb	Toxin neutralisation (PA)	as above	Phase I	
E coli (STEC)	Shigamabs (caStx1, caStx2)	Thallion/LFB Biotechnologies	Two chimeric mAbs (cocktail)	Toxin neutralization (Stx1, Stx2)	Treatment of shiga toxin producing E coli infections	Phase II	25
C difficile	MK3415A (CDA-1 and CDB-1)	Merck	Two humanized mAbs (cocktail)	anti-toxin A and B	Therapy of C. difficile associated disease	Phase II	24
P aeruginosa	Panobacumab (KBPA 101)	Kenta Biotech	human mAb (IgM)	anti-LPS (O11)	P aeruginosa infection	Phase II	26,27
	KB 001	Sanofi-Pasteur/KaloBios	Humanized, PEGylated Fab fragment	anti-type 3 secretion system (PcrV)	P aeruginosa infection	Phase II	28

a Data were collected from the Adis R&D Insight database, homepages of listed companies in May 2011, and selected scientific publications.

ACKNOWLEDGMENTS

I thank Donald Capra for helpful discussions and Kalpit Vora for critical reading of the manuscript.

REFERENCES

1. Wang TT, Palese P. Universal epitopes of influenza virus hemagglutinins? Nat Struct Mol Biol 2009;16(3):233–4.
2. Saylor C, Dadachova E, Casadevall A. Monoclonal antibody-based therapies for microbial diseases. Vaccine 2009;275:G38–46.
3. Nagy E, Giefing C, von Gabain A. Anti-infective antibodies: a novel tool to prevent and treat nosocomial diseases. Exper Rev Anti Infect Therapy 2008;6(1):21–30.
4. Bebbington C, Geoffrey Y. Antibodies for the treatment of bacterial infections: current experience and future prospects. Curr Opin Biotechnol 2008;19:613–9.
5. ter Meulen J. Monoclonal antibodies for prophylaxis and therapy of infectious diseases. Expert Opin Emerg Drugs 2007;12(4):525–40.
6. Plotkin SA. Correlates of protection induced by vaccination. Clin Vaccine Immunol 2010;17(7):1055–65.
7. Walker LM, Phogat SK, Chan-Hui PY, et al. Broad and potent neutralizing antibodies from an African donor reveal a new HIV-1 vaccine target. Science 2009; 326(5950):285–9.
8. Smith K, Garman L, Wrammert J, et al. Rapid generation of fully human monoclonal antibodies specific to a vaccinating antigen. Nat Protoc 2009;4(3):372–84.
9. Cingoz O. Motavizumab. mAbs 2009;1(5):439–42.
10. Available at: http://www.fda.gov/downloads/AdvisoryCommittees/Committees MeetingMaterials/ Drugs/AntiviralDrugsAdvisoryCommittee/UCM224182.pdf. Accessed July 28, 2011.
11. Broering TJ, Garrity KA, Boatright NK, et al. Identification and characterization of broadly neutralizing human monoclonal antibodies directed against the E2 envelope glycoprotein of hepatitis C virus. J Virol 2009;83(23):12473–82.
12. Soares MM, King SW, Thorpe PE. Targeting inside-out phosphatidylserine as a therapeutic strategy for viral diseases. Nat Med 2008;14(12):1357–62, 3.
13. Nakamoto N, Kaplan DE, Coleclough J, et al. Functional restoration of HCV-specific CD8 T cells by PD-1 blockade is defined by PD-1 expression and compartmentalization. Gastroenterology 2008;134(7):1927–37.
14. Bruno CJ, Jacobson JM. Ibalizumab: an anti-CD4 monoclonal antibody for the treatment of HIV-1 infection. J Antimicrob Chemother 2010;65(9):1839–41.
15. Li L, Sun T, Yang K, et al. Monoclonal CCR5 antibody for treatment of people with HIV infection [review]. Cochrane Database Syst Rev 2010;8(12):CD008439.
16. Toma J, Weinheimer SP, Stawiski E, et al. Loss of asparagine-linked glycosylation sites in variable region 5 of human immunodeficiency virus type 1 envelope is associated with resistance to CD4 antibody ibalizumab. J Virol 2011;85(8):3872–80.
17. Tenorio AR. The monoclonal CCR5 antibody PRO-140: the promise of once-weekly HIV therapy. Curr HIV/AIDS Rep 2011;8(1):1–3.
18. Quiambao B, Bakker A, Bermal NN, et al. Evaluation of the safety and neutralizing activity of CL184, a monoclonal antibody cocktail against rabies, in a phase II study in healthy adolescents and children. Quebec (Canada): RITA XX, Rabies in the Americas; 2009.
19. Beigel JH, Nordstrom JL, Pillemer SR, et al. Safety and pharmacokinetics of single intravenous dose of MGAWN1, a novel monoclonal antibody to West Nile virus. Antimicrob Agents Chemother 2010;54(6):2431–6.

20. Schaffer AC, Lee JC. Staphylococcal vaccines and immunotherapies. Infect Dis Clin North Am 2009;23:153–71.
21. Weisman LE, Thackray HM, Garcia-Prats JA, et al. Phase 1/2 double-blind, placebo-controlled, dose escalation, safety, and pharmacokinetic study of pagibaximab (BSYX-A110), an antistaphylococcal monoclonal antibody for the prevention of staphylococcal bloodstream infections, in very-low-birth-weight neonates. Antimicrob Agents Chemotherapy 2009;53(7):2879–86.
22. Mould DR, Weisman LE, Bloom B, et al. Predicted and measured pagibaximab serum levels in high-risk neonates. Pediatric Academic Societies and European Society for Pediatric Infectious Diseases Meeting; 2010. Available at: http://www.biosynexus.com/phase2b-3.html.
23. Kelly-Quintos C, Cavacini LA, Posner MR, et al. Characterization of the opsonic and protective activity against Staphylococcus aureus of fully human monoclonal antibodies specific for the bacterial surface polysaccharide poly-N-acetylglucosamine. Infect Immun 2006;74(5):2742–50.
24. Migone T, Subramanian GM, Bolmer SD, et al. Raxibacumab for the treatment of inhalational anthrax. N Engl J Med 2009;361(2):135–44.
25. Lowy I, Molrine DC, Leav BA, et al. Treatment with monoclonal antibodies against Clostridium difficile toxins. N Engl J Med 2010;362(3):197–205.
26. López EL, Contrlni MM, Glatstein E, et al. Safety and pharmacokinetics of urtoxazumab, a humanized monoclonal antibody, against Shiga-like toxin 2 in healthy adults and in pediatric patients infected with Shiga-like toxin-producing Escherichia coli. Antimicrob Agents Chemother 2010;54(1):239–43.
27. Secher T, Fauconnier L, Szade A, et al. Anti-Pseudomonas aeruginosa serotype O11 LPS immunoglobulin M monoclonal antibody panobacumab (KBPA101) confers protection in a murine model of acute lung infection. J Antimicrob Chemother 2011;66(5):1100–9.
28. Lu Q, Rouby JJ, Laterre PF, et al. Pharmacokinetics and safety of panobacumab: specific adjunctive immunotherapy in critical patients with nosocomial Pseudomonas aeruginosa O11 pneumonia. J Antimicrob Chemother 2011; 66(5):1110–6.
29. Baer M, Sawa T, Flynn P, et al. An engineered human antibody Fab fragment specific for Pseudomonas aeruginosa PcrV antigen has potent anti-bacterial activity. Infect Immun 2009;77(3):1083–90.
30. ter Meulen J, van den Brink EN, Poon LL, et al. Human monoclonal antibody combination against SARS coronavirus: synergy and coverage of escape mutants. PLoS Med 2006;3(7):e237.
31. Bakker AB, Marissen WE, Kramer RA, et al. Novel human monoclonal antibody combination effectively neutralizing natural rabies virus variants and individual in vitro escape mutants. J Virol 2005;79(14):9062–8.
32. Kruetzmann S, Rosado MM, Weber H, et al. Human immunoglobulin M memory B cells controlling Streptococcus pneumoniae infections are generated in the spleen. J Exp Med 2003;197(7):939–45.
33. Milner JD, Sandler NG, Douek DC. Th17 cells, Job's syndrome and HIV: opportunities for bacterial and fungal infections. Curr Opin HIV AIDS 2010;5(2):179–83.
34. Krilov LR. Respiratory syncytial virus disease: update on treatment and prevention. Expert Rev Anti Infect Ther 2011;9(1):27–32.
35. Feltes TF, Sondheimer HM, Tulloh RM, et al. A randomized controlled trial of motavizumab versus palivizumab for the prophylaxis of serious respiratory syncytial virus disease in children with hemodynamically significant congenital heart disease. Pediatr Res 2011;70(2):186–91.

36. Wang F, Ruther P, Jiang I, et al. Human monoclonal antibodies that neutralize anthrax toxin by inhibiting heptamer assembly. Hum Antibodies 2004;13(4): 105–10.

37. Mohamed N, Clagett ML, Li J, et al. A high affinity monoclonal antibody to anthrax protective antigen passively protects rabbits pre and post aerosolized bacillus anthracis spore challenge. Infect Immun 2005;73(2):795–802.

Colony-Stimulating Factors in the Prevention and Management of Infectious Diseases

Andrea V. Page, MD[a], W. Conrad Liles, MD, PhD[b],*

KEYWORDS

- Granulocyte colony-stimulating factor
- Granulocyte macrophage colony-stimulating factor
- Macrophage colony-stimulating factor • Neutropenia • Cancer
- Sepsis • Pneumonia • Diabetic foot infection

Colony-stimulating factors (CSFs) are attractive adjunctive anti-infective therapies from a variety of perspectives. CSFs are well-tolerated and widely available in recombinant form, and have a long history of clinical use.[1] Administered with the goal of enhancing innate host defenses against microbial pathogens, the myeloid CSFs—granulocyte CSF (G-CSF), granulocyte-macrophage CSF (GM-CSF), and macrophage CSF (M-CSF)—increase absolute numbers of circulating innate immune effector cells by accelerating bone marrow production and maturation, or augment the function of those cells through diverse effects on chemotaxis, phagocytosis, and microbicidal functions, including oxidative (respiratory) burst activity. Despite a solid rationale for their use and promising results in preclinical studies, CSFs have not been shown to improve outcomes obtained with conventional antimicrobial therapy

Financial Support. This work was supported by the University of Toronto Department of Medicine Clinician-Scientist Training Program (Dr Page), the McLaughlin Centre for Molecular Medicine (Dr Liles), and the Canadian Institutes of Health Research Canada Research Chair program (Dr Liles).

Potential conflicts of interest. The authors have no relevant conflicts of interest to disclose.

[a] Division of Infectious Diseases, Department of Medicine and SA Rotman Laboratories, McLaughlin-Rotman Centre for Global Health, Toronto General Hospital, University Health Network, University of Toronto, 13 Eaton North, Room 208, 200 Elizabeth Street, Toronto, Ontario M5G 2C4, Canada

[b] Division of Infectious Diseases, Department of Medicine and SA Rotman Laboratories, McLaughlin-Rotman Centre for Global Health, Toronto General Hospital, University Health Network, University of Toronto, 13 Eaton North, Room 220, 200 Elizabeth Street, Toronto, Ontario M5G 2C4, Canada

* Corresponding author.

E-mail address: conrad.liles@uhn.on.ca

Infect Dis Clin N Am 25 (2011) 803–817
doi:10.1016/j.idc.2011.07.007
0891-5520/11/$ – see front matter © 2011 Elsevier Inc. All rights reserved.

id.theclinics.com

in all clinical settings. This article summarizes the evidence supporting the accepted clinical uses of the myeloid CSFs in patients with congenital or chemotherapy-induced neutropenia, and presents an overview of proposed and emerging uses of the CSFs for the prevention and treatment of infectious diseases in other immunosuppressed and immunocompetent patient populations.

G-CSF

Among the myeloid CSFs, G-CSF has been the most widely studied in clinical investigations and the most frequently used in clinical practice. Endogenous G-CSF is produced by monocytes/macrophages, fibroblasts, and endothelial cells and acts primarily on neutrophils (polymorphonuclear leukocytes [PMNs]) and their precursors to regulate both steady-state and responsive or emergency granulopoiesis.[1] G-CSF–deficient (G-CSF−/−; G-CSF "knock-out") mice have a reduced number of both circulating neutrophils in the peripheral blood and granulopoietic precursors in the bone marrow, and display an impaired ability to mobilize additional peripheral blood neutrophils in response to infection.[2] The absence of G-CSF also impairs immune function in a qualitative manner, with diminished inducible oxidative burst activity despite exposure to *Listeria monocytogenes*.[3] The combined quantitative and qualitative immune defects translate into more severe bacterial infections in G-CSF–deficient mice. As predicted, these defects are normalized through administration of exogenous G-CSF.[2] Similarly, exposure of human neutrophils to exogenous or endogenous G-CSFs leads to reduced apoptosis and enhanced oxidative burst and microbicidal activity when neutrophils are studied ex vivo.[4–6]

Primary Prophylaxis in Patients With Neutropenia and Malignancy

Given its potential to enhance the absolute number and function of circulating neutrophils, recombinant human G-CSF has been studied in patients at risk for chemotherapy-induced neutropenia. Although the risk of neutropenia varies with the type of malignancy and chemotherapeutic regimen, when it does occur it is often associated with infection, increased use of health care resources, and significant morbidity and mortality.[7] In one recent study of 3638 patients from across the United States who were beginning a new chemotherapeutic regimen, 24% of those not receiving a CSF experienced severe (absolute neutrophil count [ANC] $<0.5 \times 10^3/mm^3$) or febrile neutropenia during their first cycle of chemotherapy.[8] Furthermore, the in-hospital mortality rate during an episode of febrile neutropenia has been shown to be approximately 10%.[9] Thus, a pressing need exists for therapeutic agents that can prevent or shorten neutropenia, and thereby reduce the risk of infection, in patients undergoing chemotherapy for solid organ and hematologic malignancies.

Although G-CSF has been studied extensively in the setting of cancer chemotherapy-associated neutropenia, individual randomized controlled trials have often lacked sufficient power to show a significant reduction in clinically important outcomes, such as infection-related mortality. Accordingly, much of the strongest recent evidence supporting the use of G-CSF has been derived from meta-analyses. In one such study of 17 randomized controlled trials published through December 2006, a total of 3493 patients with a solid tumor or malignant lymphoma received either a G-CSF within 1 to 3 days of completing their first cycle of chemotherapy or placebo/no treatment.[10] Febrile neutropenia occurred in 39.5% of control patients and 22.4% of those receiving G-CSF. The latter group also had a significantly lower risk of infection-related and all-cause mortality during the chemotherapy period, making this one of the rare studies to show a mortality benefit.

A meta-analysis of 13 randomized controlled trials that had enrolled a total of 2607 patients who were receiving chemotherapy for malignant lymphoma and who were randomized to either prophylactic G-CSF/GM-CSF or placebo/no treatment showed a reduction in episodes of febrile neutropenia and documented infection, but no reduction in infection-related mortality, mortality during the chemotherapy period (whether related to infection or not), or overall survival.[11] Similarly, a meta-analysis designed to explore the potential usefulness of prophylactic CSFs before neutrophil engraftment during autologous or allogeneic hematopoietic stem cell transplantation that included 34 studies published to January 2006, with 2669 participants randomized to receive a CSF (20 studies used G-CSF, 13 used GM-CSF, and 1 used both agents) or placebo/no treatment found an 8% reduction in documented infection with CSF use (resulting in a number needed to treat of 13 to prevent one infection) but no change in infection-related mortality.[12] However, G-CSF use in allogeneic bone marrow transplantation has been associated with acute and chronic graft-versus-host disease, and its use remains controversial in this patient population.[13,14]

Finally, a large meta-analysis of 148 studies that included 16,839 adults and children who were undergoing chemotherapy for solid tumors or hematologic malignancies or who were receiving conditioning regimens before hematopoietic stem cell transplantation and were randomized to receive either G-CSF/GM-CSF or placebo/no treatment before the onset of neutropenia showed an overall reduction in febrile neutropenia and documented infections but no difference in infection-related or all-cause mortality.[15] In this analysis, the median rate of febrile neutropenia in patients not receiving CSF support was 44.2%. CSF administration had the same effect regardless of whether the baseline febrile neutropenia rate was greater or less than 20% (the risk cut-off most commonly used to guide prophylactic CSF use). This study has also been one of the few meta-analyses to specifically examine the effect of CSFs in leukemia, reporting a reduction in febrile neutropenia and documented infection in this subgroup of patients. The number of patients with leukemia included in this meta-analysis (N = 5322) far exceeds those in individual studies, for which results have varied depending on the type of leukemia and the age of study participants.[16]

A meta-analysis exploring the use of G-CSF or GM-CSF in children with acute lymphoblastic leukemia (ALL) found a statistically significant reduction in the number of episodes of febrile neutropenia; however, there was significant heterogeneity among the included studies.[17] Although two small meta-analyses of studies comparing G-CSF with placebo/no treatment in adult patients with acute myelogenous leukemia (AML) reached opposite conclusions regarding the benefit of G-CSF, a larger systematic review of G-CSF/GM-CSF in patients with AML showed that primary prophylaxis with a CSF shortened the time to neutrophil recovery and the duration of hospitalization, yet had no impact on the incidence of documented infections or on overall survival.[18–20]

Taken together, these meta-analyses show that the use of CSFs as primary prophylaxis is effective in reducing the incidence of febrile neutropenia and documented infection in patients receiving chemotherapy as treatment for solid organ tumors or malignant lymphoma, or for conditioning before hematopoietic stem cell transplantation. Many of these studies also reported a concomitant reduction in the use of health care resources related to infection.[12,15] Improved survival has not been consistently shown.

In contrast, a large meta-analysis of studies comparing primary antibiotic prophylaxis with placebo/no treatment in patients with afebrile neutropenia undergoing chemotherapy for solid tumors or hematologic malignancies, and before hematopoietic stem cell transplantation found a reduction in documented infection, infection-related mortality, and all-cause mortality with any antibiotic prophylaxis, and with fluoroquinolone prophylaxis in particular.[21] Few studies, however, have found a significant difference between the strategies when directly compared for the prevention of either infection or mortality. An attempted meta-analysis of G-CSF/GM-CSF versus antimicrobial therapy for primary prophylaxis in patients with afebrile neutropenia reported only two small studies of sufficient quality for inclusion, both conducted in patients with solid organ tumors and neither reporting enough similar outcome measures to allow data to be analyzed in aggregate.[22] Although some authors have documented fewer episodes of febrile neutropenia with the use of both strategies simultaneously, this finding has not been universal.[23,24] Larger randomized controlled trials of primary prophylaxis are needed to compare CSFs with antimicrobial therapy in afebrile patients at risk of neutropenia, and to explore the possible superiority of one strategy over the other.

Guidelines from both the American Society of Clinical Oncology (ASCO) and the European Organisation for Research and Treatment of Cancer (EORTC) recommend the use of G-CSF as primary prophylaxis for patients receiving chemotherapy regimens associated with a 20% or greater risk of febrile neutropenia, or for those whose individual characteristics increase their risk.[25,26] Details of specific treatment regimens and the associated risk of febrile neutropenia are provided in the guidelines and are not repeated here. The ASCO guidelines also make specific recommendations for the use of G-CSFs as primary prophylaxis in patients with AML after consolidation chemotherapy and perhaps after induction chemotherapy; in those with ALL after initial induction or first postremission chemotherapy; and after autologous, but not allogeneic, stem cell transplantation.[25] Indications for use that are approved by the U.S. Food and Drug Administration are listed in **Table 1**.

Although neither guideline recommends one G-CSF formulation over another, emerging literature suggests important differences may exist. G-CSF is available for clinical use in three recombinant forms: filgrastim, a nonglycosylated protein; pegfilgrastim, a pegylated formulation with a long half-life; and lenograstim, a glycosylated form produced in mammalian cells and bearing the greatest similarity to the naturally occurring human cytokine.[27] Neutrophils stimulated with lenograstim in vivo have been shown to have the least perturbation of normal phenotype and function when

Table 1
Indications for myeloid CSFs approved by the U.S. Food and Drug Administration for the prevention and treatment of infectious diseases

CSF	Indication
G-CSF (filgrastim, pegfilgrastim)	After myelosuppressive chemotherapy for nonmyeloid malignancy[a]
	After induction or consolidation chemotherapy for AML in adults
	Myeloid reconstitution after hematopoietic stem cell transplantation for nonmyeloid malignances
	Symptomatic patients with congenital, cyclic, or idiopathic neutropenia
GM-CSF (sargramostim)	After induction chemotherapy for AML in patients older than 55 years
	After autologous bone marrow transplantation in patients with Hodgkin's disease, non-Hodgkin's lymphoma, or ALL
	After allogeneic bone marrow transplantation from a human leukocyte antigen–matched donor
	After bone marrow transplantation failure or engraftment delay
M-CSF	No approved indications

[a] Sole approved indication for pegfilgrastim.

studied ex vivo.[27] However, evidence is now accumulating showing superiority of peg-filgrastim in clinical use. Pegylation of filgrastim extends its duration of biologic activity, often reducing the regimen to a single dose for primary prophylaxis of chemotherapy-induced neutropenia, compared with unpegylated filgrastim, which must be administered daily. Although peak neutrophil count is achieved in less than 12 hours after administration of filgrastim to healthy volunteers, followed by a slow decline over approximately 48 hours, the peak neutrophil count is reached instead in 48 hours after administration of pegfilgrastim to healthy volunteers, followed by a slow decline in the peripheral blood neutrophil count over approximately 10 days.[28,29]

A meta-analysis of five randomized controlled trials comparing once-daily filgrastim to single-dose pegfilgrastim for the prevention of chemotherapy-induced neutropenia in a mixed population of patients with solid organ and hematologic malignancies concluded that prophylaxis with pegfilgrastim resulted in significantly fewer episodes of febrile neutropenia across all cycles of chemotherapy compared with prophylaxis with filgrastim.[30] Since the publication of the meta-analysis, individual studies have also reported a reduction in neutropenia-related hospitalization with pegfilgrastim.[31,32] However, not all studies have documented improved outcomes with pegfilgrastim, and in the absence of large prospective studies, no definitive conclusions can be drawn.[33] Ensuring an adequate duration of CSF support, whether using once-per-cycle pegfilgrastim or daily-dose filgrastim/lenograstim, is likely the most significant factor in the successful primary prophylaxis of febrile neutropenia.

Secondary Prophylaxis in Patients With Neutropenia and Malignancy

Secondary prophylaxis applies to individuals who experienced a neutropenic compli-cation, most commonly an episode of febrile neutropenia, during a prior cycle of chemotherapy. The risk of a subsequent episode of febrile neutropenia is estimated to be greater than 50% without CSF support.[23] A retrospective cohort study of elderly patients with non-Hodgkin's lymphoma registered in a Medicare database showed that administration of G-CSF as secondary prophylaxis during at least four subse-quent cycles of chemotherapy reduced mortality compared with no secondary CSF prophylaxis.[34] The 2010 update of the EORTC guidelines clearly states that patients should receive prophylactic G-CSF for all subsequent courses of chemotherapy after an episode of febrile neutropenia, even if the chemotherapeutic regimen falls below the 20% risk threshold, with the goal of preventing further episodes.[26] The older ASCO guidelines differ slightly in that dose reduction or delay of chemotherapy is considered equally acceptable to G-CSF prophylaxis in this situation, provided that this alteration of the chemotherapeutic regimen is not expected to compromise disease-free survival or treatment outcomes.[25]

Treatment for Febrile Neutropenia in Patients With Malignancy

When combined with antibiotics, G-CSF has been studied for the treatment of estab-lished febrile neutropenia. In a meta-analysis of 13 randomized controlled trials comparing G-CSF or GM-CSF and antibiotics with antimicrobial therapy alone for the treatment of febrile neutropenia in adults and children after chemotherapy for a solid organ or hematologic malignancy, the addition of G-CSF shortened the dura-tion of neutropenia and the length of hospitalization but did not change overall mortality.[35] The authors reported a statistically significant reduction in infection-related mortality with the use of G-CSF, but a large proportion of the patients included in this analysis were drawn from a single positive study. Therefore, both the ASCO and EORTC guidelines recommend that adjunctive G-CSF be reserved for patients at high risk of infection-related complications or who are not experiencing response to standard antimicrobial therapy.[25,26]

Prevention of Infection in Patients With Nonmalignant Neutropenia

Individuals with primary (congenital) neutropenic disorders, including severe congenital neutropenia, cyclic neutropenia, and idiopathic neutropenia, in which the ANC may remain less than $0.5 \times 10^3/mm^3$ for months or years, are also at increased risk of frequent, recurrent, and severe bacterial and fungal infections. In this patient population, routine prophylactic administration of G-CSF significantly increases the ANC, accompanied by a concomitant decrease in infection, antibiotic use, and hospitalization.[36] As a result, long-term G-CSF administration is now considered standard care for this patient population.[37]

Given its proven benefits in chemotherapy-induced and primary congenital neutropenia, G-CSF has also been investigated for preventing infection in patients with neutropenia and a variety of other underlying illnesses. Neutropenia occurs frequently in the setting of HIV, as a direct result of HIV infection on neutrophil production or function, or secondary to medications and opportunistic infections. HIV-related neutropenia has been associated with an increased risk of bacterial infection and increased mortality after bacterial or fungal bloodstream infection.[38,39] Early studies reported that G-CSF could reverse the accelerated neutrophil apoptosis seen in patients with HIV whose CD4 count was less than 200 cells/μL, and that the use of G-CSF for treatment of HIV-related neutropenia reduced the incidence of bacteremia and increased survival in patients with advanced HIV.[40,41] However, G-CSF use has not been rigorously studied in the era of modern antiretroviral regimens. An assessment of 1729 patients in the Women's Interagency HIV Study found that neutropenia, although frequent, was not independently associated with mortality, and was instead a reflection of more advanced disease.[42] Therefore, the critical intervention in this patient population is likely to be the initiation of combination antiretroviral therapy rather than supplementary G-CSF.

In contrast, interferon-induced neutropenia in patients with hepatitis C infection, with or without HIV coinfection, has not been associated with an increased risk of bacterial infection.[43,44] However, interferon is known to suppress endogenous G-CSF production, and therefore G-CSF has been studied as adjunctive therapy to avoid reductions in the dose of interferon as a result of neutropenia.[45] Some preliminary reports suggest that more patients can experience a sustained virologic response when full-dose interferon therapy is continued with G-CSF support; however, rigorous randomized controlled studies are needed before routine use of G-CSF can be recommended in this setting.[46,47]

Neutropenia caused by immunosuppressive medications, cytomegalovirus infection, antiviral therapy, or a combination thereof may also occur in patients who receive solid organ transplants. Neutropenia has been documented in 28% of renal transplant recipients in the first year posttransplant.[48] A small retrospective study reported fewer bacterial infections in association with the use of G-CSF in neutropenic renal transplant recipients.[49] G-CSF has also been used to avoid dose reduction of antiviral therapy for cytomegalovirus infection in this population.[50] Although G-CSF is effective in increasing the ANC in solid organ transplant recipients, recommendations for routine use in this population cannot be made in the absence of large, prospective studies. Existing studies did not find an association between G-CSF use and allograft rejection.

Finally, CSF therapy may have a supportive role in the care of neutropenic preterm neonates. Administration of G-CSF or GM-CSF to neutropenic neonates with sepsis reduced 14-day mortality compared with a control group of infants with sepsis who did not receive a CSF.[51] Furthermore, when administered prophylactically as a 3-day course of therapy to neutropenic premature infants before the onset of sepsis, G-CSF significantly improved infection-free survival at 2 but not 4 weeks after treatment.[52]

Prevention and Treatment of Infection in Nonneutropenic Patients

The rationale for G-CSF use in neutropenic patients is clear. In nonneutropenic patients, G-CSF has been proposed as adjunctive therapy to enhance the function of existing neutrophils. In patients with severe community-acquired pneumonia, treatment with a single dose of G-CSF reduced apoptosis and increased cell surface marker expression and antiinflammatory cytokine release when neutrophils were studied ex vivo.[53] Despite these promising results, a systematic review of six randomized controlled trials with a total enrollment of 2018 adult patients with pneumonia concluded that the addition of G-CSF to standard antimicrobial therapy had no impact on 28-day mortality.[54] Consequently, G-CSF is not included in current guidelines for the treatment of community-acquired pneumonia.[55]

Similarly, promising ex vivo results in the setting of critical illness have not translated into clinically meaningful outcomes in vivo. Administration of G-CSF to nonneutropenic patients with poor wound healing in a surgical intensive care unit resulted in enhanced oxidative burst activity and phagocytosis when neutrophils were studied ex vivo and compared with neutrophils from healthy controls.[56] However, administration of G-CSFs to patients with the systemic inflammatory response syndrome (SIRS) did not enhance neutrophil function compared with a control group of patients with SIRS who had not received G-CSF.[57] Furthermore, clinical studies have shown no consistent benefit in the use of G-CSF as adjunctive therapy for sepsis in nonneutropenic adults or neonates.[51,58,59] A recent meta-analysis included 12 randomized controlled trials published to October 2010 involving 2380 nonneutropenic patients with sepsis who were randomized to receive either G-CSF/GM-CSF or placebo. Compared with placebo, receipt of a CSF was associated with increased resolution of infection but no change in in-hospital or 28-day mortality.[60]

Although G-CSF has been shown to significantly reduce the need for surgical interventions in nonneutropenic patients with diabetic foot infections, and to lead to a shorter duration of hospitalization when compared with standard therapy, it did not shorten either the time to resolution of infection or the duration of antibiotic therapy.[61] A separate systematic review focusing only on patients with diabetic foot infections complicated by osteomyelitis concluded that evidence was insufficient to recommend the routine use of G-CSFs.[62] Updated guidelines from the Infectious Diseases Society of America (IDSA) on the management of diabetic foot infections are expected in late 2011; however, the quality of the current evidence is not sufficiently high to recommend the routine use of G-CSFs in this patient population.

Finally, although G-CSF reverses transplantation-induced impairment of the neutrophil oxidative burst in vitro, perioperative administration of G-CSF failed to reduce the incidence of infection in liver transplant recipients.[63,64] Similarly, perioperative G-CSF had no impact on postoperative infection rates in patients undergoing esophagectomy for esophageal cancer.[65]

GM-CSF

GM-CSF is produced in vivo by a variety of stromal cells. Although it can stimulate production of neutrophils, monocytes, and eosinophils, unlike G-CSF, it does not seem to be crucial for normal steady-state hematopoiesis.[66] Rather, the primary role of endogenous GM-CSF is to enhance or support the function of mature hemato-poietic cells. GM-CSF–deficient (GM-CSF −/−; GM-CSF "knock-out") mice have normal numbers of peripheral blood cells and bone marrow progenitors, yet develop alveolar proteinosis as a result of impaired macrophage clearance of surfactant.[66] GM-CSF −/− mice also have a higher rate of bacterial and fungal pneumonia when compared with GM-CSF +/+ mice.[67]

Recombinant GM-CSF has been studied in various forms that differ according to mode of production, amino acid structure, and degree of glycosylation, and include sargramostim (produced in yeast), molgramostim (produced in Escherichia coli), and regramostim (produced in mammalian cells), but it is approved for use in the United States, Canada, and Europe only as sargramostim. When administered to healthy volunteers, GM-CSF produces a gradual rise in the absolute neutrophil count to a peak of 3.5 times baseline levels through the increased release of mature cells from the bone marrow.[68] GM-CSF also enhances the induced neutrophil oxidative burst in vitro and results in eosinophilia in vivo.

GM-CSF has been studied primarily as an alternative to G-CSF to prevent or limit neutropenia, and therefore reduce infectious risk, in patients undergoing myelosup-pressive chemotherapy. However, individual studies have shown mixed results. Many of the largest meta-analyses in this area have combined studies using either G-CSF or GM-CSF and were discussed earlier. Among the studies that present results stratified by the type of CSF used, the effect of GM-CSF has been similarly variable.

In the meta-analysis by Sung and colleagues,[15] GM-CSF was less effective than G-CSF in reducing the incidence of febrile neutropenia and documented infection in patients with hematologic or solid organ malignancies. Among patients with malignant lymphoma, GM-CSF did not reduce the incidence of neutropenia or documented infection (unlike G-CSF); however, far fewer studies used GM-CSF.[11] In patients who had undergone hematopoietic stem cell transplantation, use of GM-CSF resulted in a significant reduction in the incidence of documented infection, whereas G-CSF resulted only in a trend toward the same; however, neither agent reduced infection-related or overall mortality.[12]

Two recent studies have attempted to clarify the existence of a meaningful differ-ence between the efficacy of GM-CSF and G-CSF; however, divergent results were reported. In a retrospective matched (by age and gender) cohort study, sargramostim prophylaxis was found to result in lower infection-related hospitalization rates, but not febrile neutropenia hospitalization rates, compared with either filgrastim or pegfilgras-tim prophylaxis[69] although the number of hospitalizations in each group was low. In contrast, a retrospective, nonmatched cohort study that analyzed almost 80 000 cycles of chemotherapy in which prophylactic CSFs were administered according to two United States health care claims databases found that hospitalization for neu-tropenic complications (neutropenia, fever, or infection) was higher with sargramostim and filgrastim than with pegfilgrastim.[70] The apparent increased risk with sargramos-tim occurred even in patients who received an optimal duration of therapy.

Trials of GM-CSF for the treatment of febrile neutropenia have also failed to show a survival benefit.[71] As a result, the ASCO guidelines from 2005 state that no conclu-sion can be drawn regarding the relative efficacy of the two agents, whereas the EORTC guidelines limit the recommendations to G-CSF alone.[25,26] Furthermore, GM-CSF has limited approved indications for use in the United States: to shorten the time to neutrophil recovery and reduce the incidence of infection in older patients after induction chemotherapy for AML; to aid in myeloid recovery after autologous bone marrow transplantation in patients with Hodgkin's disease, non-Hodgkin's lymphoma, and ALL; after allogeneic bone marrow transplantation from a human leukocyte antigen (HLA)–matched donor; and in the setting of bone marrow transplant failure or engraftment delay (see **Table 1**).

Like G-CSF, GM-CSF has also been studied as an immunostimulatory agent for the treatment of serious infections in nonneutropenic patients. GM-CSF treatment of monocytes from patients with septic shock produced enhanced oxidative burst activity in response to Gram-positive and Gram-negative stimuli ex vivo compared with unprimed cells from the same patients.[72] A murine model of systemic zygomycosis showed greater reduction in fungal burden when GM-CSF was combined with liposomal amphotericin B and compared with liposomal amphotericin B alone, and published reports have shown the successful use of GM-CSF and interferon-γ as adjunctive therapy for refractory invasive fungal infections in neutropenic and nonneutropenic patients.[73–75] In a randomized, double-blind, placebo-controlled trial of 38 patients with severe sepsis or septic shock and sepsis-induced immunosuppression (characterized by monocytes with reduced HLA class II cell surface expression), administration of GM-CSF was associated with increased cell surface expression of HLA markers and enhanced proinflammatory cytokine production, a shorter duration of mechanical ventilation, and improved Acute Physiology and Chronic Health Evaluation II (APACHE II) scores immediately after the course of GM-CSF.[76] Although interesting, larger studies that focus on clinically relevant outcomes are needed, particularly because previous studies have shown a GM-CSF–induced improvement in ex vivo immune function without a corresponding improvement in morbidity or mortality.[77,78] In low-birthweight preterm neonates, only 20% of whom were neutropenic, prophylactic GM-CSF raised the neutrophil count but did not affect sepsis-free survival at 14 days.[79]

Unique among the CSFs, GM-CSF has been used as a vaccine adjuvant. When given concomitantly with the hepatitis B (HBV) vaccine, GM-CSF has been found to produce higher postvaccination HBV surface antibody titres in patients with chronic renal failure and those with HIV, although this effect was not seen when the HBV vaccine was administered on an accelerated schedule to individuals with HIV.[80–82] Furthermore, GM-CSF did not improve the response to the 23-valent polysaccharide pneumococcal vaccine in patients with chronic lymphocytic leukemia nor to a peptide anti-HIV vaccine in healthy volunteers, indicating that its usefulness as an adjuvant is not universal.[83,84]

M-CSF

M-CSF is produced by monocytes/macrophages, fibroblasts, and endothelial cells and enhances the microbicidal activity of cells in the monocyte/macrophage lineage.[1] Found to improve natural killer cell numbers and function, and neutrophil oxidative burst when administered to patients after chemotherapy for ovarian cancer, M-CSF was also found to reduce the incidence and duration of febrile neutropenia in AML.[85,86] Nonetheless, M-CSF has been supplanted by the other more neutrophil-specific CSFs in postchemotherapeutic supportive care regimens.

SUMMARY

The advent of recombinant forms of the myeloid CSFs was met with enthusiasm, and all three—G-CSF, GM-CSF, and M-CSF—have been studied in diverse patient populations. However, the initial promise of the myeloid CSFs as immunomodulatory agents has been tempered by the recurrent failure of impressive in vitro and ex vivo stimulatory effects on phagocyte function to translate into clinically relevant outcomes for nonneutropenic patients. Instead, G-CSF has found an established role in the primary prophylaxis of neutropenia among high-risk patients undergoing myelosuppressive chemotherapy, and among those with primary or congenital neutropenia, in whom its use is considered standard care. Use of the myeloid CSFs for other indications will depend on the results of the large, prospective trials needed to confirm potential benefits shown in preliminary studies.

REFERENCES

1. Hubel K, Dale DC, Liles WC. Therapeutic use of cytokines to modulate phagocyte function for the treatment of infectious diseases: current status of granulocyte colony-stimulating factor, granulocyte-macrophage colony-stimulating factor, macrophage colony-stimulating factor, and interferon-γ. J Infect Dis 2002;185: 1490–501.
2. Lieschke GJ, Grail D, Hodgson G, et al. Mice lacking granulocyte colony-stimulating factor have chronic neutropenia, granulocyte and macrophage progenitor cell deficiency, and impaired neutrophil mobilization. Blood 1994;84: 1737–46.
3. Zhan Y, Basu S, Lieschke GJ, et al. Functional deficiencies of peritoneal cells from gene-targeted mice lacking G-CSF or GM-CSF. J Leukoc Biol 1999;65: 256–64.
4. Leavey PJ, Sellins KS, Thurman G, et al. In vivo treatment with granulocyte colony-stimulating factor results in divergent effects on neutrophils functions measured in vitro. Blood 1998;11:4366–74.
5. Barth E, Fischer G, Schneider EM, et al. Peaks of endogenous G-CSF serum concentrations are followed by an increase in respiratory burst activity of granulocytes in patients with septic shock. Cytokine 2002;17:275–84.
6. Lejeune M, Sariban E, Cantinieaux B, et al. Defective polymorphonuclear leukocyte functions in children receiving chemotherapy for cancer are partially restored by recombinant human granulocyte colony-stimulating factor in vitro. J Infect Dis 1996;174:800–5.
7. Crawford J, Dale DC, Lyman GH. Chemotherapy-induced neutropenia. Risks, consequences, and new directions for its management. Cancer 2004;100: 228–37.
8. Lyman GH, Kuderer NM, Crawford J, et al. Predicting individual risk of neutropenic complications in patients receiving cancer chemotherapy. Cancer 2011; 117:1917–27.
9. Kuderer NM, Dale DC, Crawford J, et al. Mortality, morbidity, and cost associated with febrile neutropenia in adult cancer patients. Cancer 2006;106:2258–66.
10. Kuderer NM, Dale DC, Crawford J, et al. Impact of primary prophylaxis with granulocyte colony-stimulating factor on febrile neutropenia and mortality in adult cancer patients receiving chemotherapy: a systematic review. J Clin Oncol 2007;25:3158–67.
11. Bohlius J, Herbst C, Reiser M, et al. Granulopoiesis-stimulating factors to prevent adverse effects in the treatment of malignant lymphoma. Cochrane Database Syst Rev 2008;4:CD003189.
12. Dekker A, Bulley S, Beyene J, et al. Meta-analysis of randomized controlled trials of prophylactic granulocyte colony-stimulating factor and granulocyte-macrophage colony-stimulating factor after autologous and allogeneic stem cell transplantation. J Clin Oncol 2006;24:5207–15.

13. Ringden O, Hassan Z, Karlsson H, et al. Granulocyte colony-stimulating factor induced acute and chronic graft-versus-host disease. Transplantation 2010;90: 1022–9.
14. Trivedi M, Martinez S, Corringham S, et al. Optimal use of G-CSF administration after hematopoietic SCT. Bone Marrow Transplant 2009;43:895–908.
15. Sung L, Nathan PC, Alibhai SM, et al. Meta-analysis: effect of prophylactic hematopoietic colony-stimulating factors on mortality and outcomes of infection. Ann Intern Med 2007;147:400–11.
16. Wheatley K, Goldstone AH, Littlewood T, et al. Randomized placebo-controlled trial of granulocyte colony stimulating factor (G-CSF) as supportive care after induction chemotherapy in adult patients with acute myeloid leukaemia: a study of the United Kingdom Medical Research Council Adult Leukaemia Working Party. Br J Haematol 2009;146:54–63.
17. Sasse EC, Sasse AD, Brandalise SR, et al. Colony-stimulating factors for prevention of myelosuppressive therapy-induced febrile neutropenia in children with acute lymphoblastic leukaemia. Cochrane Database Syst Rev 2005;3:CD004139.
18. Wang J, Zhan P, Ouyang J, et al. Prophylactic use of granulocyte colony-stimulating factor after induction chemotherapy in patients with newly diagnosed acute myeloid leukemia may increase the complete remission rate: a meta-analysis of five randomized controlled trials. Leuk Lymphoma 2009;50:457–9.
19. Wang J, An L, Ouyang J, et al. Prophylactic use of granulocyte colony-stimulating factor after chemotherapy does not affect survival rate in acute myeloid leukemia: a meta-analysis. Acta Haematol 2009;121:223–6.
20. Heuser M, Zapf A, Morgan M, et al. Myeloid growth factors in acute myeloid leukemia: a systematic review of randomized controlled trials. Ann Hematol 2011;90:273–81.
21. Gafter-Gvili A, Fraser A, Paul M, et al. Meta-analysis: antibiotic prophylaxis reduces mortality in neutropenic patients. Ann Intern Med 2005;142:979–95.
22. Herbst C, Naumann F, Kruse EB, et al. Prophylactic antibiotics or G-CSF for the prevention of infections and improvement of survival in cancer patients undergoing chemotherapy. Cochrane Database Syst Rev 2009;1:CD007107.
23. Timmer-Bonte JN, de Boo TM, Smit HJ, et al. Prevention of chemotherapy-induced febrile neutropenia by prophylactic antibiotics plus or minus granulocyte colony-stimulating factor in small-cell lung cancer: a Dutch randomized phase III study. J Clin Oncol 2005;23:7974–84.
24. Lalami Y, Paesmans A, Aoun M, et al. A prospective randomized evaluation of G-CSF or G-CSF plus oral antibiotics in chemotherapy-treated patients at high risk of developing febrile neutropenia. Support Care Cancer 2004;12:725–30.
25. Smith TJ, Khatcheressian J, Lyman GH, et al. 2006 Update of recommendations for the use of white blood cell growth factors: an evidence-based clinical practice guideline. J Clin Oncol 2006;24:3187–205.
26. Aapro MS, Bohlius J, Cameron DA, et al. 2010 update of EORTC guidelines for the use of granulocyte-colony stimulating factor to reduce the incidence of chemotherapy-induced febrile neutropenia in adult patients with lymphoproliferative disorders and solid tumors. Eur J Cancer 2011;47:8–32.
27. Ribeiro D, Veldwijk MR, Benner A, et al. Differences in functional activity and antigen expression of granulocytes primed in vivo with filgrastim, lenograstim, or pegfilgrastim. Transfusion 2007;47:969–80.
28. Wang B, Ludden TM, Cheung EN, et al. Population pharmacokinetic-pharmacodynamic modeling of filgrastim (r-metHuG-CSF) in healthy volunteers. J Pharmacokinet Pharmacodyn 2001;28:321–42.

29. Roskos LK, Lum P, Lockbaum P, et al. Pharmacokinetic/pharmacodynamic modeling of pegfilgrastim in healthy subjects. J Clin Pharmacol 2006;46:747–57.
30. Pinto L, Liu Z, Doan Q, et al. Comparison of pegfilgrastim with filgrastim on febrile neutropenia, grade IV neutropenia and bone pain: a meta-analysis of randomized controlled trials. Curr Med Res Opin 2007;23:2283–95.
31. Tan H, Tomic K, Hurley D, et al. Comparative effectiveness of colony-stimulating factors for febrile neutropenia: a retrospective study. Curr Med Res Opin 2011;27: 79–86.
32. Weycker D, Malin J, Kim J, et al. Risk of hospitalization for neutropenic complications of chemotherapy in patients with primary solid tumors receiving pegfilgrastim or filgrastim prophylaxis: a retrospective cohort study. Clin Ther 2009;31: 1069–81.
33. Skarlos DV, Timotheadou E, Galani E, et al. Pegfilgrastim administered on the same day with dose-dense adjuvant chemotherapy for breast cancer is associated with a higher incidence of febrile neutropenia as compared to conventional growth factor support: matched case-control study of the Hellenic Cooperative Oncology Group. Oncology 2009;77:107–12.
34. Gruschkus SK, Lairson D, Dunn JK, et al. Comparative effectiveness of white blood cell growth factors on neutropenia, infection, and survival in older people with non-Hodgkin's lymphoma treated with chemotherapy. J Am Geriatr Soc 2010;58:1885–95.
35. Clark OA, Lyman G, Castro AA, et al. Colony stimulating factors for chemotherapy induced febrile neutropenia. Cochrane Database Syst Rev 2000;4:CD003039.
36. Dale DC, Bonilla MA, Davis MW, et al. A randomized controlled phase III trial of recombinant human granulocyte colony-stimulating factor (filgrastim) for treatment of severe chronic neutropenia. Blood 1993;81:2496–502.
37. Dale DC, Bolyard AA, Schwinzer BG, et al. The severe chronic neutropenia international registry: 10-year follow-up report. Support Cancer Ther 2006;3:223–34.
38. Moore RD, Keruly JC, Chaisson RE. Neutropenia and bacterial infection in acquired immunodeficiency syndrome. Arch Intern Med 1995;155:1965–70.
39. Ortega M, Almela M, Soriano A, et al. Bloodstream infections among human immunodeficiency virus-infected adult patients: epidemiology and risk factors for mortality. Eur J Clin Microbiol Infect Dis 2008;27:969–76.
40. Pitrak DL, Sutton SH, Tsai HC, et al. Reversal of accelerated neutrophil apoptosis and restoration of respiratory burst activity with r-metHuG-CSF (Filgrastim) therapy in patients with AIDS. AIDS 1999;13:427–9.
41. Keiser P, Rademacher S, Smith JW, et al. Granulocyte colony-stimulating factor use is associated with decreased bacteremia and increased survival in neutropenic HIV-infected patients. Am J Med 1998;104:48–55.
42. Levine AM, Karim R, Mack W, et al. Neutropenia in Human Immunodeficiency Virus Infection. Data from the Women's Interagency HIV Study. Arch Intern Med 2006;166:4405–10.
43. Cooper CL, Al-Bedwawi S, Lee C, et al. Rate of infectious complications during interferon-based therapy for hepatitis C is not related to neutropenia. Clin Infect Dis 2006;42:1674–8.
44. Cooper CL, Bedwawi S. Infection rates in HIV-HCV patients treated with interferon are similar to those in HCV mono-infection and not related to neutropenia. HIV Clin Trials 2006;7:251–4.
45. Tajuddin T, Ryan EJ, Norris S, et al. Interferon-alpha suppressed granulocyte colony stimulating factor production is reversed by CL097, a TLR 7/8 agonist. J Gastroenterol Hepatol 2010;25:1883–90.

46. Koskinas J, Zacharakis G, Sidiropoulos J, et al. Granulocyte colony stimulating factor in HCV genotype-1 patients who develop Peg-IFN-alpha2b related severe neutropenia: a preliminary report on treatment, safety and efficacy. J Med Virol 2009;81:848–52.
47. Koirala J, Gandotra SD, Rao S, et al. Granulocyte colony-stimulating factor dosing in pegylated interferon alpha-induced neutropenia and its impact on outcome of anti-HCV therapy. J Viral Hepat 2007;14:782–7.
48. Zafrani L, Truffaut L, Kreis H, et al. Incidence, risk factors and clinical consequences of neutropenia following kidney transplantation: a retrospective study. Am J Transplant 2009;9:1816–25.
49. Schmaldienst S, Bekesi G, Deicher R, et al. Recombinant human granulocyte colony-stimulating factor after kidney transplantation: a retrospective analysis to evaluate the benefit or risk of immunostimulation. Transplantation 2000;69: 527–31.
50. Turgeon N, Hovingh GK, Fishman JA, et al. Safety and efficacy of granulocyte colony-stimulating factor in kidney and liver transplant recipients. Transpl Infect Dis 2000;2:15–21.
51. Carr R, Modi N, Dore C. G-CSF and GM-CSF for treating or preventing neonatal infections. Cochrane Database Syst Rev 2003;3:CD003066.
52. Kuhn P, Messer J, Paupe A, et al. A multicentre, randomized, placebo-controlled trial of prophylactic recombinant granulocyte-colony stimulating factor in preterm neonates with neutropenia. J Pediatr 2009;155:324–30.
53. Droemann D, Hansen F, Aries SP, et al. Neutrophil apoptosis, activation and anti-inflammatory cytokine response in granulocyte colony-stimulating factor-treated patients with community-acquired pneumonia. Respiration 2006;73:340–6.
54. Cheng AC, Stephens DP, Currie BJ. Granulocyte-colony stimulating factor (G-CSF) as an adjunct to antibiotics in the treatment of pneumonia in adults. Cochrane Database Syst Rev 2007;2:CD004400.
55. Mandell LA, Wunderink RG, Anzueto A, et al. Infectious Diseases Society of America/American Thoracic Society consensus guidelines on the management of community-acquired pneumonia in adults. Clin Infect Dis 2007;44:S27–72.
56. Gerber A, Struy H, Weiss G, et al. Effect of granulocyte colony-stimulating factor treatment on ex vivo neutrophil functions in nonneutropenic surgical intensive care patients. J Interferon Cytokine Res 2000;20:1083–90.
57. Weiss M, Voglic S, Harms-Schirra B, et al. Effects of exogenous recombinant human granulocyte colony-stimulating factor (filgrastim, rhG-CSF) on neutrophils of critically ill patients with systemic inflammatory response syndrome depend on endogenous G-CSF plasma concentrations on admission. Intensive Care Med 2003;29:904–14.
58. Cheng AC, Limmathurotsakul D, Chierakul W, et al. A randomized controlled trial of granulocyte colony-stimulating factor for the treatment of severe sepsis due to melioidosis in Thailand. Clin Infect Dis 2007;45:308–14.
59. Stephens DP, Thomas JH, Dip G, et al. Randomized, double-blind, placebo-controlled trial of granulocyte colony-stimulating factor in patients with septic shock. Crit Care Med 2008;36:448–54.
60. Bo L, Wang F, Zhu J, et al. Granulocyte-colony stimulating factor (G-CSF) and granulocyte-macrophage colony stimulating factor (GM-CSF) for sepsis: a meta-analysis. Crit Care 2011;15:R58.
61. Cruciani M, Lipsky BA, Mengoli C, et al. Granulocyte-colony stimulating factors as adjunctive therapy for diabetic foot infections. Cochrane Database Syst Rev 2009;3:CD006810.

62. Berendt AR, Peters EJ, Bakker K, et al. Diabetic foot osteomyelitis: a progress report on diagnosis and a systematic review of treatment. Diabetes Metab Res Rev 2008;24:S145–61.

63. Pursell K, Verral S, Daraiesh F, et al. Impaired phagocyte respiratory burst responses to opportunistic fungal pathogens in transplant recipients: *in vitro* effect of r-metHuG-CSF (Filgrastim). Transpl Infect Dis 2003;5:29–37.

64. Winston DJ, Foster PF, Somberg KA, et al. Randomized, placebo-controlled, double-blind, multicenter trial of efficacy and safety of granulocyte colony-stimulating factor in liver transplant recipients. Transplantation 1999;68:1298–304.

65. Schaefer H, Engert A, Grass G, et al. Perioperative granulocyte colony-stimulating factor does not prevent severe infections in patients undergoing esophagectomy for esophageal cancer. A randomized placebo-controlled clinical trial. Ann Surg 2004;240:68–75.

66. Dranoff G, Crawford AD, Sadelain M, et al. Involvement of granulocyte-macrophage colony-stimulating factor in pulmonary hemostasis. Science 1994; 264:713–6.

67. Stanley E, Lieschke GJ, Grail D, et al. Granulocyte/macrophage colony-stimulating factor-deficient mice show no major perturbation of hematopoiesis but develop a characteristic pulmonary pathology. Proc Natl Acad Sci U S A 1994;91:5592–6.

68. Dale DC, Liles WC, Llewellyn C, et al. Effects of granulocyte-macrophage colony-stimulating factor (GM-CSF) on neutrophils kinetics and function in normal human volunteers. Am J Hematol 1998;57:7–15.

69. Heaney ML, Toy EL, Vekeman F, et al. Comparison of hospitalization risk and associated costs among patients receiving sargramostim, filgrastim, and pegfilgrastim for chemotherapy-induced neutropenia. Cancer 2009;115:4839–48.

70. Weycker D, Malin J, Barron R, et al. Comparative effectiveness of filgrastim, pegfilgrastim, and sargramostim as prophylaxis against hospitalization for neutropenic complications in patients with cancer receiving chemotherapy. Am J Clin Oncol 2011. [Epub ahead of print].

71. Anaissie EJ, Vartivarian S, Bodey GP, et al. Randomized comparison between antibiotics alone and antibiotics plus granulocyte-macrophage colony-stimulating factor (*Escherichia coli*-derived) in cancer patients with fever and neutropenia. Am J Med 1996;100:17–23.

72. Williams MA, White SA, Miller JJ, et al. Granulocyte-macrophage colony-stimulating factor induces activation and restores respiratory burst activity in monocytes from septic patients. J Infect Dis 1998;177:107–15.

73. Rodriguez MM, Calvo E, Marine M, et al. Efficacy of liposomal amphotericin B combined with gamma interferon or granulocyte-macrophage colony-stimulating factor for treatment of systemic zygomycosis in mice. Antimicrob Agents Chemother 2009;53:3569–71.

74. Bandera A, Trabattoni D, Ferrario G, et al. Interferon-γ and granulocyte-macrophage colony stimulating factor therapy in three patients with pulmonary aspergillosis. Infection 2008;36:368–73.

75. Lewis R, Hogan H, Howell A, et al. Progressive fusariosis: unpredictable posaconazole bioavailability, and feasibility of recombinant interferon-gamma plus granulocyte macrophage-colony stimulating factor for refractory disseminated infection. Leuk Lymphoma 2008;49:163–5.

76. Meisel C, Schefold JC, Pschowski R, et al. Granulocyte-macrophage colony-stimulating factor to reverse sepsis-associated immunosuppression. Am J Respir Crit Care Med 2009;180:640–8.

77. Rosenbloom AJ, Linden PK, Dorrance A, et al. Effect of granulocyte-monocyte colony-stimulating factor therapy on leukocyte function and clearance of serious infection in nonneutropenic patients. Chest 2005;127:2139–50.

78. Presneill JJ, Harris T, Stewart AG, et al. A randomized phase II trial of granulocyte-macrophage colony-stimulating factor therapy in severe sepsis with respiratory dysfunction. Am J Respir Crit Care Med 2002;166:138–43.

79. Carr R, Brocklehurst P, Dore CJ, et al. Granulocyte-macrophage colony stimulating factor administered as prophylaxis for reduction of sepsis in extremely preterm, small for gestational age neonates (the PROGRAMS trial): a single-blind, multicentre, randomized controlled trial. Lancet 2009;373:226–33.

80. Cruciani M, Mengoli C, Serpelloni G, et al. Granulocyte macrophage colony-stimulating factor as an adjuvant for hepatitis B vaccination: a meta-analysis. Vaccine 2007;25:709–18.

81. Sasaki MG, Foccacia R, de Messias-Reason IJ. Efficacy of granulocyte-macrophage colony-stimulating factor (GM-CSF) as a vaccine adjuvant for hepatitis B virus in patients with HIV infection. Vaccine 2003;21:4545–9.

82. Overton ET, Kang M, Peters MG, et al. Immune response to hepatitis B vaccine in HIV-infected subjects using granulocyte-macrophage colony-stimulating factor (GM-CSF) as a vaccine adjuvant: ACTG study 5220. Vaccine 2010;28:5597–604.

83. Safdar A, Rodriguez GH, Rueda AM, et al. Multiple-dose granulocyte-macrophage-colony-stimulating factor plus 23-valent polysaccharide pneumococcal vaccine in patients with chronic lymphocytic leukemia. A prospective, randomized trial of safety and immunogenicity. Cancer 2008;113:383–7.

84. Spearman P, Kalams S, Elizaga M, et al. Safety and immunogenicity of a CTL multiepitope peptide vaccine for HIV with or without GM-CSF in a phase 1 trial. Vaccine 2009;27:243–9.

85. Hidaka T, Akada S, Teranishi A, et al. Mirimostim (macrophage colony-stimulating factor; M-CSF) improves chemotherapy-induced impaired natural killer cell activity, Th1/Th2 balance, and granulocyte function. Cancer Sci 2003;94:812–20.

86. Ohno R, Miyawaki S, Hatake K, et al. Human urinary macrophage colony-stimulating factor reduces the incidence and duration of febrile neutropenia and shortens the period required to finish three courses of intensive consolidation therapy in acute myeloid leukemia: a double-blind controlled study. J Clin Oncol 1997;15:2954–65.

Interferons as Therapeutic Agents for Infectious Diseases

Scott J. Bergman, PharmD, BCPS[a,b,*],
McKenzie C. Ferguson, PharmD, BCPS[a], Cathy Santanello, PhD[c]

KEYWORDS

- Interferon-α • Viral hepatitis • Respiratory tract infection viruses
- Common cold • Human papillomavirus • Genital warts
- Vaccine • Adjuvant

Interferons (IFNs) are attractive biological response modifiers for use as therapeutic agents in infectious diseases, because they have both antiviral and immunomodulatory activity. Their name even comes from the fact that they can "interfere" with viral replication.[1] IFN-α ("leukocyte interferon") and IFN-β ("fibroblast interferon") are released by human cells infected with certain viruses, whereas IFN-γ ("immune interferon") is produced by natural killer (NK) cells (T-cell lymphocytes) in response to antigen exposure. These cytokines then act on uninfected host tissue cells to induce a state of relative resistance to viral infections.[2] The agents bind to specific cell-surface receptors that initiate a series of intracellular events: induction of certain enzymes, inhibition of cell proliferation, and enhancement of immune activities, including increased phagocytosis by macrophages and augmentation of specific cytotoxicity by T lymphocytes.[3] Further details on endogenous IFN action and an explanation of their activity as biological response modifiers, including in bacterial infections, can be found elsewhere in this issue.[4]

Even though IFNs' role against viruses is most prominent, they can also be induced by, and active against, rickettsia, mycobacteria, and several protozoa.[1] Therapeutically, however, their use has generally been limited to treatment or prevention of viral infections. Although their potent antiviral activity is promising—inhibiting viral

The authors have nothing to disclose.
[a] Department of Pharmacy Practice, Southern Illinois University Edwardsville (SIUE) School of Pharmacy, 220 University Park Drive, Box 2000, Edwardsville, IL 62026, USA
[b] Division of Infectious Diseases, SIU School of Medicine, 701 North 1st Street, Box 19636, Springfield, IL 62794, USA
[c] Department of Pharmaceutical Sciences, SIUE School of Pharmacy, 220 University Park Drive, Box 2000, Edwardsville, IL 62026, USA
* Corresponding author. Division of Infectious Diseases, SIU School of Medicine, 701 North 1st Street, Box 19636, Springfield, IL 62794.
E-mail address: scbergm@siue.edu

Infect Dis Clin N Am 25 (2011) 819–834
doi:10.1016/j.idc.2011.07.008
0891-5520/11/$ – see front matter
id.theclinics.com

replication in vitro at concentrations as low as pg/mL—the development of IFNs as clinically useful drugs has been largely disappointing. This fact can be attributed partly to their short half-life in vivo and their extensive side effects. In fact, many symptoms of viral infections such as influenza can be blamed on endogenous IFN release. The adverse effects prevalent at therapeutic doses include fever, myalgia, and headache, dubbed "flulike symptoms," along with bone marrow suppression leading to leukocytopenia and thrombocytopenia, plus central nervous system manifestations including depression.[1]

IFNs have been studied for the treatment or prevention of herpes zoster, herpes simplex, and cytomegalovirus infections, but the successful development of acyclovir and ganciclovir gave clinicians safer and more effective alternatives for dealing with these viruses.[5,6] IFNs can also be used in the treatment of multiple sclerosis and certain cancers, but this article reviews the therapeutic applications of IFNs for infectious diseases, focusing on viral infections.

INTERFERONS AND INTERFERON INDUCERS AVAILABLE COMMERCIALLY

IFNs are not absorbed orally because of their large amino acid sequence, which is susceptible to the proteolytic enzymes in the digestive tract. However, IFN-α is readily absorbed after both intramuscular and subcutaneous injection.[7] This rapid absorption combined with a short half-life means that frequent injections are needed to maintain adequate concentrations in the body. Both commercially available IFN-α products in the United States have now been chemically attached to polyethylene glycol (PEG) to enhance their half-life and make once-weekly dosing possible. This coupling not only makes administration easier, but also reduces side effects by having a predictably lower peak concentration of the exogenous cytokine.

Both pegylated INF-α2a (Pegasys) and IFN-α2b (Peg-Intron) are obtained from *Escherichia coli* by recombinant methods. These agents consist of naturally occurring small proteins with molecular weights of 15,000 to 27,600 Da.[3] Each is considered a first-line option for the treatment of chronic hepatitis C virus (HCV) infection in combination with ribavirin. More details on this use and others are described later in this article. Along with the list of additional indications approved by the Food and Drug Administration shown in **Table 1**, IFN-α was shown to be an effective treatment for the symptoms of an aggressive case of chronic active Epstein-Barr virus, but did not eliminate infection entirely.[8] Therefore, additional studies would need to be performed before recommendation for this use.

Human leukocyte derived IFN-αn3 (Alferon N) injection contains a spectrum of α IFNs, and is only approved for the treatment of refractory or recurring condylomata acuminata in adult patients. A low-dose oral version is in development for use in the treatment and prevention of influenza.[9] Both versions have been studied against human immunodeficiency virus (HIV)-1 infection, but with little success.[10,11] IFN alfacon-1 (Infergen) is considered the synthetic "consensus interferon" because it contains a nonnatural sequence of IFN-α amino acids all chosen for the highest activity against viral hepatitis. To date, no pegylated formulation of this product has been brought to market. All the α IFNs include a black-box warning in their prescribing information about how their use

...may cause or aggravate fatal or life-threatening neuropsychiatric, autoimmune, ischemic and infectious disorders. Patients should be monitored closely with periodic clinical and laboratory evaluations. Therapy should be withdrawn in patients with persistently severe or worsening signs and symptoms related to side effects. In many, but not all cases, these resolve after stopping therapy.[12,13]

Table 1
Commercially available interferon products

Product	Brand Name	FDA-Approved Indications	Usual Doses in Adults for Treatment of Indicated Infections
Interferon-α2a & Peginterferon-α2a injection	Roferon-A Pegasys	Chronic HCV, hairy cell leukemia and AIDS-related Kaposi sarcoma Chronic HBV, HCV	3 million units SC 3 times/wk 180 μg SC every wk × 24 or 48 wk
Interferon-α2b & Peginterferon-α2b injection	Intron A Peg-Intron, Sylatron	Chronic HBV, chronic HCV, condylomata acuminuta, hairy cell leukemia, follicular lymphoma, ard AIDS-related Kaposi sarcoma Chronic HCV, melanoma	3 million units SC 3 times/wk 1.5 μg/kg SC every wk × 24 or 48 wk
Interferon alfacon injection	Infergen	Chronic HCV	15 μg SC daily with ribavirin for retreatment of IFN refractory disease
Interferon-αn3 injection	Alferon N	Refractory or recurring external condylomata acuminata	Intralesional injection of 250,000 IU (0.05 mL) per wart twice weekly for up to 8 wk
Interferon-β1a injection	Avonex Rebif	Relapsing multiple sclerosis	Not indicated for infection
Interferon-β1b injection	Betaseron	Relapsing multiple sclerosis	Not indicated for infection
Interferon-γ1b injection	ACTIMMUNE	Reduction in the frequency and severity of serious infections associated with CGD or treatmert of severe, malignant osteopetrosis	50 μg/m^2 (1 million IU/m^2) for patients whose BSA is greater than 0.5 m^2 SC 3 times/wk
Imiquimod 5% topical cream	Aldara	Actinic keratoses of the face or scalp, superficial basal cell carcinoma, external genital and perianal warts/condyloma acuminata	Apply topically 3 times/wk until total clearance of warts or a maximum of 16 wk
Imiquimod 3.75% cream	Zyclara	Actinic keratoses of the full face or balding scalp, external genital and perianal warts/condyloma acuminata	Apply once daily to the warts until total clearance or up to 8 wk

Abbreviations: AIDS, acquired immunodeficiency syndrome; BSA, body surface area; CGD, chronic granulomatous disease; HBV, hepatitis B virus infection; HCV, hepatitis C virus infection; IU, international units; SC, subcutaneously.

IFN-β1a (Avonex or Rebif) and IFN-β1b (Betaseron) are recombinant proteins with 166 and 165 amino acids, respectively. These β IFNs have antiviral and immunomodulatory properties too, but their use at this time is limited to treatment of multiple sclerosis, not infections. IFN-γ1b (ACTIMMUNE) injection is used regularly for the prevention of infections in patients with chronic granulomatous disease along with antibacterials and antifungals.[14] Its mechanism of action for this purpose is not entirely known, but long-term studies show a definite benefit.[15] IFN-γ can also be used as a salvage therapy for mycobacterial infections, but is not routinely used for treatment of this or other infections.[16]

Topical imiquimod 5% (Aldara) and 3.75% (Zyclara) creams do not have inherent antiviral activity alone, but instead induce IFN-α, IFN-β, and IFN-γ plus tumor necrosis factor (TNF)-α through Toll-like receptors (TLRs). Local application to external genital and perianal warts results in an immunomodulatory response that stimulates cytokines, which have antiviral action and cause a reduction in both viral load and wart size.[3]

USE OF INTERFERONS FOR HEPATITIS VIRUSES

Chronic infection with hepatitis B virus (HBV) and HCV affects over 400 million people worldwide.[17–19] Chronic viral hepatitis is a leading cause of cirrhosis, liver transplantation, and hepatocellular carcinoma. With the development of a vaccination series for hepatitis B in the mid-1980s, along with increased public education and awareness, acute infection rates of both HBV and HCV in the United States have declined steadily.[19]

HBV is a double-stranded DNA virus whereas HCV is a single-stranded RNA virus, both of which are capable of significant morbidity and mortality in chronic infection. The exact mechanisms of hepatic injury from HBV and HCV infection are not completely understood. Because asymptomatic carriers with normal liver transaminases exist, it is likely multiple immune-mediated mechanisms result in hepatocyte damage as opposed to the virus itself being directly cytotoxic.

Following acute viral infection, the innate immune response initiates formation of NK cells, followed by virus-specific CD4$^+$ T cells and CD8$^+$ cytotoxic T lymphocytes. NK cells stimulate production of IFN-α/β and promote cellular clearance of viral proteins through disruption of the replication process. Following successful clearance, either spontaneously or by treatment with IFN, peripheral cytotoxic T lymphocytes and CD4$^+$ T-cell response persists.[20] Chronic infection is likely a result of failed innate and adaptive immunity. Specifically, chronic infection with HCV has been associated with impaired T-cell and NK-cell response.[21–24] Genetic factors also likely influence progression of disease and predisposition to adverse effects.[25] Although an abundance of research has investigated the immune response in relation to chronic viral hepatitis, many areas of uncertainty still exist.

Standard IFN-α, the first approved IFN for viral hepatitis, lacked several desirable pharmacokinetic properties. The addition of PEG created an IFN that has a slower rate of absorption, reduced elimination, and a longer half-life, necessitating less frequent dosing and fewer adverse effects. Furthermore, the PEG moiety results in reduced immunogenicity and sterically hinders the antigenic binding site.[26,27] Although pegylated IFN has replaced standard IFN-α in treatment of chronic HBV and HCV, as many as 40% to 50% of patients still fail to respond to treatment. Successful response depends on many factors including but not limited to viral genotype, viral load, and degree of liver fibrosis.[25]

Chronic hepatitis B and C are treated similarly with peginterferon (pegIFN); however, only pegIFN-α2a is FDA-approved in the United States for treatment of HBV. Both pegIFN products are administered as subcutaneous injections once weekly for durations up to 48 weeks, dependent on viral genotype and early viral response for treatment of HCV. PegIFN-α2b is dosed based on body weight (1.5 μg/kg once weekly) whereas pegIFN-α2a is a fixed dose (180 μg/wk). Ribavirin is used in combination with pegIFN for treatment of HCV. The exact mechanism of action of ribavirin as an adjunctive antiviral agent in HCV is not completely understood.[12,13] Some studies have proposed ribavirin to act as an IFN-stimulated gene inducer to improve second-phase viral decline.[28] Protease inhibitors (boceprevir and telaprevir) are recently approved adjunctive oral agents for the treatment of chronic HCV with pegIFN and ribavirin. To date, all studies of protease inhibitors have been conducted in patients with HCV genotype 1, and have shown an increase in sustained virologic response (SVR) rates particularly for patients previously unresponsive to IFN therapy.[29–35]

The use of IFN for the treatment of chronic HBV and HCV has represented a mainstay of treatment for several decades. The specific mechanisms behind the antiviral effects of IFN for hepatitis are complex. IFN-stimulated genes are induced by IFN and disrupt viral replication. Hundreds of IFN-stimulated genes are thought to exist. Viperin, ISG20 and protein kinase R (PKR) are just a few of the most commonly cited. It is also highly possible that IFN-stimulated genes work synergistically to produce antiviral activities.[36,37] A lack of PKR can lead to an environment conducive to HCV replication, though it may not be a good predictor of exogenous IFN response. The study of IFN-stimulated genes and their role in determining who responds to IFN therapy has been evaluated in several studies.[25,36,38] Additional studies of IFN-stimulated gene expression are needed to clarify which are directly involved in successful viral response, in what capacity they affect response, and whether pharmacotherapy directed at induction of IFN-stimulated genes can help improve treatment response.

Hepatitis B

Chronic HBV infection can be successfully treated with IFN monotherapy.[39] Loss of viral DNA and antibody formation are successful outcomes associated with IFN treatment. The mechanism of IFN antiviral activity varies depending on hepatitis Be antigen (HBeAg)-positive or HBeAg-negative disease. In HBeAg-positive patients, an immune response is stimulated by IFN whereas in HBeAg-negative disease, IFN acts directly as an antiviral.[5] HBeAg-negative disease tends to be more difficult to treat, and is associated with a longer duration of disease and a higher likelihood of complications such as cirrhosis.[20] Several oral nonnucleoside reverse transcriptase inhibitors are also available for treatment of HBV (entecavir, tenofovir, adefovir, lamivudine, and telbivudine). Although IFN is still considered a first-line alternative and provides the advantage of defined treatment duration rather than potentially lifelong administration, these oral agents are often used in therapy because of their ease of use and reduced number of side effects associated with treatment.

Hepatitis C

The ability of HCV to evade the host immune response has produced a complex RNA virus capable of lingering infection, ultimately resulting in opportunities for increased risk of transmission and complications from advanced liver disease. Much of the research regarding the use of IFN for chronic viral hepatitis has focused on use in HCV. Following treatment with IFN, a decline in HCV RNA occurs over several phases. A rapid inhibition of RNA production within the first 1 to 2 days of treatment is followed by a second, slower phase associated with clearance of infected cells.[23,40,41] The immune response to endogenous IFN produced by innate immunity and that administered exogenously can differ in terms of antiviral activities based on the phase of viral decline.

Studies have shown that response to IFN-based treatment for HCV may be affected by differences in IFN signaling and induction. It is likely that HCV has mechanisms to avoid recognition by the innate immune response, and as such inhibits the ability of HCV-infected cells to generate IFN.[25,38,42] Early studies conducted in nonresponders to current therapy showed wide genetic diversity, with many showing no common traits to predict nonresponse to IFN therapy.[25,38,43]

However, in 2009 several major studies were published associating a single-nucleotide polymorphism (SNP) just upstream from interleukin-28B gene (IL28B) with IFN response in patients with HCV genotype 1.[44–48] Additional evidence points to the fact that the IL28B polymorphism is also linked to spontaneous clearance of HCV.[48,49] The IL28B variant encodes for IFN-λ3, a type III IFN belonging to the interleukin (IL)-10 superfamily, which function in a manner similar to type I IFNs, resulting in IFN-stimulated gene induction.[49–51]

The genome-wide association study conducted by Ge and colleagues[45] evaluated more than 1600 treatment-naïve HCV genotype 1 patients, the majority of whom originated from the IDEAL study. Results from logistic regression showed that the IL28B polymorphism was a stronger predictor of SVR than baseline viral load, ethnicity, or degree of fibrosis. Further research in this area is needed to clearly identify a future role for genotype testing and further clarify whether it may influence response to therapy in other HCV genotypes.

A multicenter, randomized, controlled study by Mangia and colleagues[52] analyzed 268 Caucasian patients with HCV genotype 2 (n = 213) and 3 (n = 55). Out of 61% of patients who achieved rapid virologic response (RVR), IL28B genotype was not associated with SVR, whereas in those patients who did not achieve RVR a significant difference in SVR was noted based on IL28B genotype. At this time genotype testing for IL28B is not routinely recommended for all HCV patients planning to undergo treatment, but it may be in the future. If done, it should not be used as the only factor when choosing a treatment strategy.[49]

Investigational IFN Therapies

The complexity of viral defense mechanisms and subsequent effect on the host response has led not only to development of chronic infections but also to a lack of a viable vaccine. HCV viral polymerase lacks a proofreading capability, creating a more diverse target for vaccine development.[18] Additional challenges include the lack of a suitable animal model to mimic a human environment and medium for viral growth.[18]

One of the major limitations to IFN therapy is adverse effects. Malaise, gastrointestinal effects, neuropsychiatric effects, neutropenia, and anemia can all limit the effectiveness of treatment by necessitating dosage reductions or treatment discontinuation. For newer IFN therapies to be successful, they must induce an antiviral response while at the same time limiting adverse effects.

Albinterferon is a new IFN therapy currently in development for the treatment of chronic HCV. This product is a combination of IFN-α2b fused to recombinant human albumin. One of the advantages with this product is that it only requires once or twice monthly dosing.[53] Not much is known at this time about the immunomodulating effects of albinterferon in HCV. It has been shown to have similar SVR and adverse event rates to traditional pegIFN when used in combination with ribavirin.[54–56]

Research into IFN-λ as an agent to treat HCV has also been initiated. It is hypothesized that λ IFNs may be associated with less adverse effects than IFN-α because IFN-λ receptors are primarily found in hepatocytes.[49,57] Specifically, research into new investigational pharmacotherapy in the form of pegylated IL-29 (IFN-λ1) in patients with HCV genotype 1 who relapsed following traditional treatment with peg-IFN-α and ribavirin appears promising.[50,57] Both IFN-λ1 and IFN-λ3 share a common receptor and have a similar sequence identity.[57]

A 4-week, open-label study conducted in 56 patients with chronic HCV genotype 1 was designed to assess pegIFN-λ1 in combination with ribavirin.[57] It was a dose escalation study conducted in 3 parts. Parts 1 and 2 evaluated patients who relapsed following treatment with IFN-α, and part 3 included treatment-naïve patients. In part 1, pegIFN-λ monotherapy (1.5 μg/kg or 3 μg/kg) was administered subcutaneously every 2 weeks or weekly. In parts 2 and 3, a range of pegIFN-λ dosages (0.5 μg/kg, 0.75 μg/kg, 1.5 μg/kg, or 2.25 μg/kg) were administered weekly in combination with ribavirin twice daily (1000 mg if weight <75 kg and 1200 mg if weight ≥75 kg). The primary outcomes were safety and tolerability. Pharmacokinetics and viral load reduction were evaluated as secondary end points.

Commonly reported adverse effects with pegIFN-λ included fatigue (29%), nausea (12%), myalgia (11%), and headache (9%). Most adverse events were mild or moderate in severity. Four patients (7%) experienced treatment-related toxicity and required doses to be withheld. One patient experienced grade 3 thrombocytopenic purpura and another patient had elevated alanine aminotransferase, aspartate aminotransferase, and bilirubin levels. Both events were considered to be related to treatment with pegIFN-λ. Aminotransferase elevations occurred most often in patients who received high-dose (3 μg/kg) pegIFN-λ monotherapy. No clinically relevant decreases in absolute neutrophil count occurred. Also, hemoglobin values remained consistent with known effects in patients who received ribavirin therapy. Viral activity decreased in the majority of patients who relapsed with previous treatment, with 23 of 24 patients achieving at least a greater than 2-log reduction in HCV RNA. Six of 7 treatment-naïve patients achieved a similar reduction in viral load and 2 achieved undetectable HCV RNA levels. Kinetic data showed a linear relationship between dose and exposure independent of body weight, which may prompt future research to evaluate a fixed dose of pegIFN-λ.[57]

Larger, longer, controlled, and blinded studies of IFN-λ as a viable treatment option in HCV are needed to define its place in therapy and benefits over existing IFN therapy. Studies in other HCV genotypes are also needed. In addition, with the advent of protease inhibitors, more research will be necessary to evaluate how direct antivirals and IL28B genotyping interact in guiding treatment decisions.

Adjunctive therapy with agents that induce or restore IFN-stimulated gene expression has recently been evaluated in patients with HCV. S-Adenosylmethionine (SAMe) given orally was evaluated in an open-label study in 24 patients with chronic HCV, genotype 1 who were considered nonresponders to previous IFN and ribavirin treatment.[41] SAMe was administered at a dose of 800 mg twice daily in combination with pegIFN-α2a (180 μg/kg weekly) and weight-based ribavirin (1000 mg if weight <75 kg and 1200 mg if weight ≥75 kg). The primary outcome was change in first-phase and second-phase viral decline. Treatment response and IFN-stimulated gene expression were also evaluated after up to 72 weeks of treatment. Results showed significant improvement in second-phase viral decline assessed at 2 weeks. SVR was also evaluated; however, this study was not powered to detect differences in virologic response rates. Furthermore, at the time of publication not all patients had reached 24 weeks post treatment, so the full effects on SVR were not fully known.

The addition of SAMe showed greater induction of IFN-stimulated genes, including viperin, myxovirus resistance protein, and ISG15, compared with control. Adverse effects noted with SAMe were mild and mostly related to gastrointestinal upset, likely as a result of lactose in the tablet preparation.[41]

Additional research is aimed at investigating structure-activity relationships, and preliminary pharmacokinetic studies on oral IFN inducers that act on TLRs in the treatment of HCV.[58]

USE OF INTERFERONS FOR RESPIRATORY VIRUS INFECTION

Upper respiratory tract infection in the form of "the common cold" can be caused by a variety of viruses including rhinovirus, coronavirus, influenza, parainfluenza, respiratory syncytial virus, adenovirus, Coxsackie, and echovirus families among others.[59] Symptoms may include rhinorrhea, nasal obstruction, cough, fever, and sore throat. The disease is usually mild and self-limited, but several trials have addressed treatment or prevention of the common cold with therapeutic agents. IFNs were once one of the most popular prospects for this purpose, but the minor benefit that was derived from them was counteracted by the adverse effects inflicted.[60]

An early double-blind trial with IFN-α2b intranasal drops did demonstrate that with use for several days before experimentally induced rhinovirus infection, common cold symptoms were significantly fewer in study participants compared with placebo-drop users.[61] Administration of the drops 4 times daily was superior to a higher dose given once daily at preventing infection. Short-term use was well tolerated, but obviously it is not realistic for everyone to use intranasal drops 4 times daily throughout the entire cold season. In an attempt to prevent natural infection during the period of increased acute respiratory tract virus activity, a twice-daily nasal spray was studied in volunteers over 28 days.[62] There was a significant decrease in the number of rhinovirus infections noted, but not in any other types of viral respiratory tract infections including parainfluenza. Adverse events with the IFN formulation were common in this placebo-controlled trial. During the first week alone, 20% of participants receiving IFN spray reported nosebleeds. This number increased to 41% by the end of the study.

Providing IFN prophylaxis for family members of those infected with common cold viruses is a more targeted approach to therapy. Several studies have addressed the usefulness of IFN nasal sprays in this scenario. Seven days of use did significantly reduce rhinovirus infections in 2 different trials when compared with placebo for both individuals (7.9% vs 15.5%) and their families (3.3% vs 33.3%, both P<.05), but not in 2 other studies when lower doses were given for a shorter 5-day course.[63–66] Overall, the intranasal dose of IFN needed to protect against upper respiratory tract infection appears to cause significant unwanted effects.[67] Infection with coronavirus and respiratory syncytial virus has also been an object of investigation for IFN-α2b nasal sprays, but with little success.[68,69] A study of intranasal human lymphoblastoid IFN-αn1 (Wellferon) suggested lower prophylactic activity for influenza than it did for rhinovirus.[70]

Because results of prophylactic trials with IFNs for common cold viruses were not favorable, use in the treatment of infection seemed a logical application for this biological response modifier. Although some benefit was originally seen with twice-daily IFN-α2b intranasal drops for treatment of experimentally induced rhinovirus,[71] no advantage was clear when an intranasal spray was used once daily for 5 days to treat natural infection.[72] Increased rates of blood in the mucus were again noted for participants receiving the intervention, and the IFN group experienced more secondary complications requiring prescription of antibiotics. The investigators concluded that intranasal IFN was ineffective for treating the common cold and was associated with clinically significant side effects.

Similar trials with IFN-β–serine and IFN-γ formulations, although initially positive, have shown equally disappointing clinical results.[73–76] Even though the prospects of further study on IFNs for upper respiratory tract infection appear limited, one modern trial did demonstrate an added benefit of intranasal IFN-α2b in combination with an antihistamine (chlorpheniramine) and nonsteroidal anti-inflammatory drug (ibuprofen) at reducing common cold symptoms, showing that at least one group is still interested in studying the topic.[77] Investigators have also recently begun research on an alternative therapeutic approach for rhinovirus infections using the IFN and TNF-α inducer, imiquimod. Application of this intranasal cream in primates has shown promising results in terms of enhancing cytokine response, but human trials have not yet been published.[78]

USE OF INTERFERONS FOR GENITAL INFECTIONS AND WARTS

Human papillomaviruses (HPVs) are now known to be the cause of cervical cancer and are also responsible for genital warts. HPVs are nonenveloped, double-stranded DNA viruses that invade mucosal and epithelial tissues during sexual contact with an infected partner. It is estimated that more than 50% of the sexually active American population has been or will be infected with HPV at one point in their lives.[79] When hyperproliferation of infected cells occurs, this can lead to genital warts or cancer of the cervix, vagina, vulva, and penis, among others. There are more than 100 different types of HPV and approximately 40 of them infect genital mucosa. Fifteen carcinogenic types of HPV have been identified, but 2 of them are associated with 70% of cervical cancers.[80] Two vaccines have recently been introduced that prevent infection with these most common high-risk types of HPV, 16 and 18.[81] One of these vaccines can also induce protection against the most prevalent HPV types that have a low risk of malignancy, but instead cause genital warts: HPV-6 and HPV-11.

HPV has the ability to persist in stratified epithelia for decades because of mechanisms that avoid immune eradication. IFN plays a large role in this cycle.[82] IFNs are normally secreted by keratinocytes, but HPV reduces their expression. Introduction of low-level IFN can actually increase early gene transcription and HPV replication, which may explain why use of the agent therapeutically has had mixed results.[83] Overall outcomes have been positive more often for cases of genital warts than reduction of HPV lesions associated with cancers. A study comparing the in vitro activity of IFN-α2b and IFN-αn3 on oncogenic HPV-16, HPV-18, and HPV-31b demonstrated that increasing concentrations did not always correlate with a stepwise inhibition of HPV replication.[84] Meanwhile, a meta-analysis recently analyzed locally used and systemic IFN for genital warts.[85] Seven randomized studies of IFN intralesional injection or topical gel met criteria for inclusion, and overall there was a benefit in complete response rates over placebo (44.4% vs 16.15%, relative risk 2.68, 95% confidence interval 1.79–4.02). However, there was no difference in outcomes for trials comparing systemic IFNs with placebo. In comparison, clearance of genital and perianal warts occurs in 50% of patients with the topical IFN inducer imiquimod, usually after 8 to 10 weeks of use.[3] The 5% imiquimod cream (Aldara) should be applied to affected areas 3 times a week for up to 16 weeks, whereas the newer 3.75% cream (Zyclara) can be applied once daily for as little as 8 weeks to treat external genital warts caused by HPV.

Systemic IFN therapy may be useful when HPV affects areas of the body other than the anogenital region.[86] Successful treatment with systemic pegIFN-α and a topical retinoid has been reported for mucosal carcinomas from epidermodysplasia verruciformis, a genetic abnormality leading to persistent and widespread HPV infection of the skin.[87] Recurrent respiratory HPV infection has also been effectively treated with IFN-α (12 of 18 patients), although it had no effect on viral load or replication.[88] A 20-year follow-up of patients treated with IFN-α for recurrent respiratory papillomatosis confirmed better response rates for HPV-6 than HPV-11, which had a higher likelihood of malignant transformation.[89] For recurrent conjunctival papilloma, topical plus systemic or intralesional IFN has been effective with partial excision.[90,91] The rapid resolution of significant HPV-associated warts on the hand, foot, and face has also occurred in an HIV-infected patient on antiretrovirals while being treated for hepatitis C with pegIFN-α2b and ribavirin.[92]

Case reports of treatment with the topical IFN inducer, imiquimod, have shown promise for its use in focal epithelial hyperplasia (Heck disease), a rare disorder caused by specific types of HPV (13, 14, 32, and 55) affecting oral mucosa primarily in children.[93] In addition, imiquimod 5% cream has been used successfully in the treatment of plantar warts, a smoother, flatter manifestation of HPV-1, HPV-2, and HPV-4 on the foot.[94] Of interest, the oral H2-antagonist cimetidine, along with reducing stomach acid, also induces production of IFN-γ and IL-2, which eliminates viral warts in some patients.[95] In the future the improved application of more effective topical IFNs may become a reality,[96] which could provide a valuable treatment for HPV infections without the systemic side effects of current injectable formulations.

USE OF INTERFERONS AS VACCINE ADJUVANTS

Adjuvants (*adjuvare*, Latin for "to help") are substances that augment the immunogenicity of an antigen when mixed with the antigen for use in a vaccine. Adjuvants (1) stimulate granuloma (which is a macrophage-rich mass), (2) enhance costimulatory signals, (3) stimulate nonspecific lymphocyte production, (4) prolong the antigen concentration in a site for lymphocyte exposure,[97] and (5) induce cytokines.[2,98]

Research in vaccine development has shown that one of the most promising uses of IFNs is as an adjuvant with specific antigens in prophylactic vaccines.[99] Toporovski and colleagues[99] provide a current review of the use of IFN-α, IFN-β, IFN-γ, and IFN-λ in vaccine studies that focus primarily on murine, avian, porcine, and nonhuman species. Regardless of the species, the use of IFNs as adjuvants seems to improve the efficacy and safety of most vaccines while providing the immunomodulatory effect of stimulating the T-helper 1 response.

In humans, IFN-α, predominantly produced by plasmacytoid dendritic cells, plays a large role in the body's immune response against viruses.[100] It induces plasma cell differentiation from B cells causing an increase in the serum level of influenza-specific immunoglobulins, and channels antigen-presenting cells (APCs) to the site of infection.[101] Most research on IFN-α adjuvant activity and its subsequent use in approved vaccines seems to indicate that it is a potent adjuvant.[99] When mixed with the influenza vaccine and injected intramuscularly, it is a highly effective adjuvant.[100] Oromucosal administration of recombinant IFN-α, like that of natural oromucosal IFN production, has been shown to provide immunity against viral infection and tumor cell growth.[102] Nonresponders low responders to a previous vaccine showed an improved immunoglobulin response with a recombinant IFN-α and HBV vaccine.[103]

Although research is also focused on the other classes of IFNs as adjuvants, thus far they have not yielded results as promising as that of IFN-α. The use of IFN-β has yielded mixed results; IFN-γ has been used primarily in DNA vaccines; and even less is known about the use of IFN-λ in vaccines.[99] Nevertheless, the use of IFNs as adjuvants shows great promise in augmenting vaccine efficiency, and should continue to be a top priority in the development of vaccines.

SUMMARY

IFNs have been tested repeatedly against infectious diseases, but injections are used mostly for the treatment of viral hepatitis C and prevention of infections in patients with chronic granulomatous disease clinically. Intralesional IFN and topical inducers are effective in reducing the manifestations of genital warts, but they do not eliminate cancer-causing HPV from the body. IFN has not proved to be consistently effective for treatment of respiratory tract infections from the common cold or influenza viruses, and prophylactic use is not currently feasible. The severity and quantity of adverse effects from systemic IFN therapy make it unattractive for many uses. Several infections, including herpes simplex, herpes zoster, cytomegalovirus, and even viral hepatitis B have other effective pharmacologic treatments. IFN has been successfully used as a vaccine adjuvant, and further research may allow for its additional use for this application in the future.

REFERENCES

1. Goering RV, Dockrell HM, Zuckerman M, et al. Mim's medical microbiology. 4th edition. Philadelphia: Elsevier Limited; 2008.
2. Male D, Brostoff J, Roth D, et al. Immunology. 7th edition. Philadelphia: Elsevier Limited; 2006.
3. Hayden FG. Antiviral agents. In: Brunton LL, Lazo JS, Parker KL, editors. Goodman & Gilman's the pharmacological basis of therapeutics. 11th edition. New York: McGraw-Hill; 2006. p. 1225–42.
4. Mullangi P, Shahani L, Koirala J. Role of endogenous biological response modifiers in pathogenesis of infectious diseases. Infect Dis Clin North Am, in press.
5. Borden EC, Sen GC, Uze G, et al. Interferons at age 50: past, current and future impact on biomedicine. Nat Rev Drug Discov 2007;6(12):975–90.
6. Hodson EM, Jones CA, Strippoli GF, et al. Immunoglobulins, vaccines or interferon for preventing cytomegalovirus disease in solid organ transplant recipients. Cochrane Database Syst Rev 2007;2:CD005129.
7. Houglum JE. Interferon: mechanisms of action and clinical value. Clin Pharm 1983;2(1):20–8.
8. Sakai Y, Ohga S, Tonegawa Y, et al. Interferon-alpha therapy for chronic active Epstein-Barr virus infection: Potential effect on the development of T-lymphoproliferative disease. J Pediatr Hematol Oncol 1998;20(4):342–6.
9. FDA authorizes Alferon LDO clinical study for treatment and prevention of influenza. Hemispherx Biopharma, Inc. Press Release. Available at: http://www.drugs.com/news/fda-authorizes-alferon-ldo-clinical-study-prevention-influenza-28692.html. Accessed April 25, 2011.
10. Alston B, Ellenberg JH, Standiford HC, et al. A multicenter, randomized, controlled trial of three preparations of low-dose oral alpha-interferon in HIV-infected patients with CD4+ counts between 50 and 350 cells/mm(3). Division of aids treatment research initiative (DATRI) 022 study group. J Acquir Immune Defic Syndr 1999;22(4):348–57.
11. Fitzgibbon JE, John JF. In vitro activity of interferon-alpha n3 (Alferon n) against HIV-1. Interscience Conference on Antimicrobial Agents and Chemotherapy [abstract no: I-13] vol. 38. San Diego (CA): American Society of Microbiology; 1998. p. 367.

12. Hoffman-LaRoche inc [package insert]. Nutley, NJ: Pegasys® (peg-interferon alfa-2a); 2010.
13. Schering Corporation [package insert]. Kenilworth, NJ: Peg-Intron® (peginterferon alfa-2b); 2010.
14. A controlled trial of interferon gamma to prevent infection in chronic granulomatous disease. The International Chronic Granulomatous Disease Cooperative Study Group. N Engl J Med 1991;324(8):509–16.
15. Marciano BE, Wesley R, De Carlo ES, et al. Long-term interferon-gamma therapy for patients with chronic granulomatous disease. Clin Infect Dis 2004; 39(5):692–9.
16. Rao S, Blessman D, Koirala J, et al. Biological response modifiers as adjunct treatment for refractory localized Mycobacterium avium complex infections. J Invest Med 2005;53(S2):S398.
17. Hepatitis B. Fact sheet: World Health Organization. Available at: http://www.who. int/vaccine_research/diseases/viral_cancers/en/index2.html. Accessed March 24, 2011.
18. Initiative for vaccine research. Viral cancers: World Health Organization. Available at: http://www.who.int/vaccine_research/diseases/viral_cancers/en/index2.html. Accessed April 6, 2011.
19. Daniels D, Grytdal S, Wasley A. Surveillance for acute viral hepatitis—United States, 2007. MMWR Surveill Summ 2009;58(3):1–27.
20. Aoki FA, Hayden FG, Dolin R. Antiviral drugs (other than antiretrovirals). In: Mandell GL, Bennett JE, Dolin R, editors. Principles and practices of infectious diseases, vol. 1. Philadelphia: Churchill Livingstone Elsevier; 2010. p. 565–610.
21. Crotta S, Ronconi V, Ulivieri C, et al. Cytoskeleton rearrangement induced by tetraspanin engagement modulates the activation of T and NK cells. Eur J Immunol 2006;36(4):919–29.
22. Golden-Mason L, Rosen HR. Natural killer cells: primary target for hepatitis C virus immune evasion strategies? Liver Transpl 2006;12(3):363–72.
23. Stegmann KA, Bjorkstrom NK, Veber H, et al. Interferon-alpha-induced trail on natural killer cells is associated with control of hepatitis C virus infection. Gastroenterology 2010;138(5):1885–97.
24. Wedemeyer H, He XS, Nascimbeni M, et al. Impaired effector function of hepatitis C virus-specific CD8+ T cells in chronic hepatitis C virus infection. J Immunol 2002;169(6):3447–58.
25. Wada M, Marusawa H, Yamada R, et al. Association of genetic polymorphisms with interferon-induced haematologic adverse effects in chronic hepatitis C patients. J Viral Hepat 2009;16(6):388–96.
26. He XH, Shaw PC, Tam SC. Reducing the immunogenicity and improving the in vivo activity of trichosanthin by site-directed pegylation. Life Sci 1999;65(4): 355–68.
27. Shiffman ML. Pegylated interferons: what role will they play in the treatment of chronic hepatitis C? Curr Gastroenterol Rep 2001;3(1):30–7.
28. Feld JJ, Lutchman GA, Heller T, et al. Ribavirin improves early responses to peginterferon through improved interferon signaling. Gastroenterology 2010; 139(1):154–62 e4.
29. Bacon BR, Gordon SC, Lawitz E, et al. Boceprevir for previously treated chronic HCV genotype 1 infection. N Engl J Med 2011;364(13):1207–17.
30. Berman K, Kwo PY. Boceprevir, an NS3 protease inhibitor of HCV. Clin Liver Dis 2009;13(3):429–39.

31. Lawitz E, Rodriguez-Torres M, Muir AJ, et al. Antiviral effects and safety of telaprevir, peginterferon alfa-2a, and ribavirin for 28 days in hepatitis C patients. J Hepatol 2008;49(2):163–9.
32. Forestier N, Reesink HW, Weegink CJ, et al. Antiviral activity of telaprevir (VX-950) and peginterferon alfa-2a in patients with hepatitis C. Hepatology 2007; 46(3):640–8.
33. Sarrazin C, Rouzier R, Wagner F, et al. SCH 503034, a novel hepatitis C virus protease inhibitor, plus pegylated interferon alpha-2b for genotype 1 nonresponders. Gastroenterology 2007;132(4):1270–8.
34. McHutchison JG, Everson GT, Gordon SC, et al. Telaprevir with peginterferon and ribavirin for chronic HCV genotype 1 infection. N Engl J Med 2009; 360(18):1827–38.
35. Hezode C, Forestier N, Dusheiko G, et al. Telaprevir and peginterferon with or without ribavirin for chronic HCV infection. N Engl J Med 2009;360(18):1839–50.
36. Fitzgerald KA. The interferon inducible gene: Viperin. J Interferon Cytokine Res 2011;31(1):131–5.
37. Jiang D, Guo H, Xu C, et al. Identification of three interferon-inducible cellular enzymes that inhibit the replication of hepatitis C virus. J Virol 2008;82(4): 1665–78.
38. Pfeffer LM, Madey MA, Riely CA, et al. The induction of type I interferon production in hepatitis C-infected patients. J Interferon Cytokine Res 2009;29(5). 299–306.
39. Keeffe EB, Dieterich DT, Han SH, et al. A treatment algorithm for the management of chronic hepatitis B virus infection in the United States: 2008 update. Clin Gastroenterol Hepatol 2008;6(12):1315–41 [quiz: 286].
40. Herrmann E, Lee JH, Marinos G, et al. Effect of ribavirin on hepatitis C viral kinetics in patients treated with pegylated interferon. Hepatology 2003;37(6): 1351–8.
41. Feld JJ, Modi AA, El-Diwany R, et al. S-adenosyl methionine improves early viral responses and interferon-stimulated gene induction in hepatitis C nonresponders. Gastroenterology 2011;140(3):830–9.
42. Meurs EF, Breiman A. The interferon inducing pathways and the hepatitis C virus. World J Gastroenterol 2007;13(17):2446–54.
43. Cuevas JM, Torres-Puente M, Jimenez-Hernandez N, et al. Genetic variability of hepatitis C virus before and after combined therapy of interferon plus ribavirin. PLoS One 2008;3(8):e3058.
44. Jensen DM. A new era of hepatitis C therapy begins. N Engl J Med 2011; 364(13):1272–4.
45. Ge D, Fellay J, Thompson AJ, et al. Genetic variation in IL28b predicts hepatitis C treatment-induced viral clearance. Nature 2009;461(7262):399–401.
46. Suppiah V, Moldovan M, Ahlenstiel G, et al. IL28b is associated with response to chronic hepatitis C interferon-alpha and ribavirin therapy. Nat Genet 2009; 41(10):1100–4.
47. Tanaka Y, Nishida N, Sugiyama M, et al. Genome-wide association of IL28b with response to pegylated interferon-alpha and ribavirin therapy for chronic hepatitis C. Nat Genet 2009;41(10):1105–9.
48. Thomas DL, Thio CL, Martin MP, et al. Genetic variation in IL28b and spontaneous clearance of hepatitis C virus. Nature 2009;461(7265):798–801.
49. Afdhal NH, McHutchison JG, Zeuzem S, et al. Hepatitis C pharmacogenetics: state of the art in 2010. Hepatology 2011;53(1):336–45.

50. Liapakis A, Jacobson I. Pharmacogenetics of hepatitis C therapy. Pharmacogenomics 2010;11(2):135–9.
51. Shackel NA, Bowen DG, McCaughan GW. Snipping away at hepatitis C. Hepatology 2010;51(2):703–5.
52. Mangia A, Thompson AJ, Santoro R, et al. An IL28b polymorphism determines treatment response of hepatitis C virus genotype 2 or 3 patients who do not achieve a rapid virologic response. Gastroenterology 2010;139(3):821–7, 27. e1.
53. Zeuzem S, Yoshida EM, Benhamou Y, et al. Albinterferon alfa-2b dosed every two or four weeks in interferon-naive patients with genotype 1 chronic hepatitis C. Hepatology 2008;48(2):407–17.
54. Bain VG, Kaita KD, Marotta P, et al. Safety and antiviral activity of albinterferon alfa-2b dosed every four weeks in genotype 2/3 chronic hepatitis C patients. Clin Gastroenterol Hepatol 2008;6(6):701–6.
55. Nelson DR, Benhamou Y, Chuang WL, et al. Albinterferon alfa-2b was not inferior to pegylated interferon-alpha in a randomized trial of patients with chronic hepatitis C virus genotype 2 or 3. Gastroenterology 2010;139(4):1267–76.
56. Zeuzem S, Sulkowski MS, Lawitz EJ, et al. Albinterferon alfa-2b was not inferior to pegylated interferon-alpha in a randomized trial of patients with chronic hepatitis C virus genotype 1. Gastroenterology 2010;139(4):1257–66.
57. Muir AJ, Shiffman ML, Zaman A, et al. Phase 1b study of pegylated interferon lambda 1 with or without ribavirin in patients with chronic genotype 1 hepatitis C virus infection. Hepatology 2010;52(3):822–32.
58. Tran TD, Pryde DC, Jones P, et al. Design and optimisation of orally active TLR7 agonists for the treatment of hepatitis C virus infection. Bioorg Med Chem Lett 2011;21(8):2389–93.
59. Turner RB. The common cold. In: Mandell GL, Bennett JE, Dolin R, editors. Principles and practices of infectious diseases. Philadelphia: Churchill Livingston Elsevier; 2010. p. 803–13.
60. Enlow ML, Haley CJ. Alpha 2-interferon for the common cold. Ann Pharmacother 1992;26(3):345–7.
61. Hayden FG, Gwaltney JM Jr. Intranasal interferon alpha 2 for prevention of rhinovirus infection and illness. J Infect Dis 1983;148(3):543–50.
62. Monto AS, Shope TC, Schwartz SA, et al. Intranasal interferon-alpha 2b for seasonal prophylaxis of respiratory infection. J Infect Dis 1986;154(1):128–33.
63. Douglas RM, Moore BW, Miles HB, et al. Prophylactic efficacy of intranasal alpha 2-interferon against rhinovirus infections in the family setting. N Engl J Med 1986;314(2):65–70.
64. Hayden FG, Albrecht JK, Kaiser DL, et al. Prevention of natural colds by contact prophylaxis with intranasal alpha 2-interferon. N Engl J Med 1986;314(2):71–5.
65. Monto AS, Schwartz SA, Albrecht JK. Ineffectiveness of postexposure prophylaxis of rhinovirus infection with low-dose intranasal alpha 2b interferon in families. Antimicrob Agents Chemother 1989;33(3):387–90.
66. Herzog C, Berger R, Fernex M, et al. Intranasal interferon (rIFN-alpha a, Ro 22-8181) for contact prophylaxis against common cold: a randomized, double-blind and placebo-controlled field study. Antiviral Res 1986;6(3):171–6.
67. Scott GM, Onwubalili JK, Robinson JA, et al. Tolerance of one-month intranasal interferon. J Med Virol 1985;17(2):99–106.
68. Turner RB, Felton A, Kosak K, et al. Prevention of experimental coronavirus colds with intranasal alpha-2b interferon. J Infect Dis 1986;154(3):443–7.

69. Higgins PG, Barrow GI, Tyrrell DA, et al. The efficacy of intranasal interferon alpha-2a in respiratory syncytial virus infection in volunteers. Antiviral Res 1990;14(1):3–10.

70. Phillpotts RJ, Higgins PG, Willman JS, et al. Intranasal lymphoblastoid interferon ("Wellferon") prophylaxis against rhinovirus and influenza virus in volunteers. J Interferon Res 1984;4(4):535–41.

71. Hayden FG, Gwaltney JM Jr. Intranasal interferon-alpha 2 treatment of experimental rhinoviral colds. J Infect Dis 1984;150(2):174–80.

72. Hayden FG, Kaiser DL, Albrecht JK. Intranasal recombinant alfa-2b interferon treatment of naturally occurring common colds. Antimicrob Agents Chemother 1988;32(2):224–30.

73. Sperber SJ, Levine PA, Innes DJ, et al. Tolerance and efficacy of intranasal administration of recombinant beta serine interferon in healthy adults. J Infect Dis 1988;158(1):166–75.

74. Sperber SJ, Levine PA, Sorrentino JV, et al. Ineffectiveness of recombinant interferon-beta serine nasal drops for prophylaxis of natural colds. J Infect Dis 1989;160(4):700–5.

75. Higgins PG, Al-Nakib W, Willman J, et al. Interferon-beta ser as prophylaxis against experimental rhinovirus infection in volunteers. J Interferon Res 1986; 6(2):153–9.

76. Higgins PG, Al-Nakib W, Barrow GI, et al. Recombinant human interferon-gamma as prophylaxis against rhinovirus colds in volunteers. J Interferon Res 1988;8(5):591–6.

77. Gwaltney JM Jr, Winther B, Patrie JT, et al. Combined antiviral-antimediator treatment for the common cold. J Infect Dis 2002;186(2):147–54.

78. Clejan S, Mandrea E, Pandrea IV, et al. Immune responses induced by intranasal imiquimod and implications for therapeutics in rhinovirus infections. J Cell Mol Med 2005;9(2):457–61.

79. Genital HPV infection—fact sheet. Centers for Disease Control and Prevention. Available at: http://www.cdc.gov/std/HPV/STDFact-HPV.htm. Accessed April 25, 2011.

80. Munoz N, Bosch FX, de Sanjose S, et al. Epidemiologic classification of human papillomavirus types associated with cervical cancer. N Engl J Med 2003; 348(6):518–27.

81. Bergman SJ, Collins-Lucey E. Update on human papillomavirus vaccines: life saver or controversy magnet? Clin Microbiol Newslett, in press.

82. Beglin M, Melar-New M, Laimins L. Human papillomaviruses and the interferon response. J Interferon Cytokine Res 2009;29(9):629–35.

83. Lace MJ, Anson JR, Klingelhutz AJ, et al. Interferon-beta treatment increases human papillomavirus early gene transcription and viral plasmid genome replication by activating interferon regulatory factor (IRF)-1. Carcinogenesis 2009; 30(8):1336–44.

84. Sen E, McLaughlin-Drubin M, Meyers C. Efficacy of two commercial preparations of interferon-alpha on human papillomavirus replication. Anticancer Res 2005;25(2A):1091–100.

85. Yang J, Pu YG, Zeng ZM, et al. Interferon for the treatment of genital warts: a systematic review. BMC Infect Dis 2009;9(1):156.

86. Shrestha NK, Hamrock DJ. Successful treatment of disseminated human papillomavirus infection with pegylated interferon and ribavirin. Clin Infect Dis 2010; 51(1):e4–6.

87. Gubinelli E, Posteraro P, Cocuroccia B, et al. Epidermodysplasia verruciformis with multiple mucosal carcinomas treated with pegylated interferon alfa and acitretin. J Dermatolog Treat 2003;14(3):184–8.
88. Szeps M, Dahlgren L, Aaltonen LM, et al. Human papillomavirus, viral load and proliferation rate in recurrent respiratory papillomatosis in response to alpha interferon treatment. J Gen Virol 2005;86(Pt 6):1695–702.
89. Gerein V, Rastorguev E, Gerein J, et al. Use of interferon-alpha in recurrent respiratory papillomatosis: 20-year follow-up. Ann Otol Rhinol Laryngol 2005; 114(6):463–71.
90. de Keizer RJ, de Wolff-Rouendaal D. Topical alpha-interferon in recurrent conjunctival papilloma. Acta Ophthalmol Scand 2003;81(2):193–6.
91. Kothari M, Mody K, Chatterjee D. Resolution of recurrent conjunctival papilloma after topical and intralesional interferon alpha2b with partial excision in a child. J AAPOS 2009;13(5):523–5.
92. Pavan MH, Velho PE, Vigani AG, et al. Treatment of human papillomavirus with peg-interferon alfa-2b and ribavirin. Braz J Infect Dis 2007;11(3):383–4.
93. Yasar S, Mansur AT, Serdar ZA, et al. Treatment of focal epithelial hyperplasia with topical imiquimod: report of three cases. Pediatr Dermatol 2009;26(4): 465–8.
94. Zamiri M, Gupta G. Plantar warts treated with an immune response modifier: a report of two cases. Clin Exp Dermatol 2003;28(Suppl 1):45–7.
95. Mitsuishi T, Iida K, Kawana S. Cimetidine treatment for viral warts enhances IL-2 and IFN-gamma expression but not IL-18 expression in lesional skin. Eur J Dermatol 2003;13(5):445–8.
96. Foldvari M, Badea I, Kumar P, et al. Topical delivery of interferon alpha in human volunteers and treatment of patients with human papillomavirus infections. Curr Drug Deliv 2011;8(3):307–19.
97. Kuby J. Immunology. New York: W.H. Freeman and Co; 1997.
98. Singh M, O'Hagan D. Advances in vaccine adjuvants. Nat Biotechnol 1999; 17(11):1075–81.
99. Toporovski R, Morrow MP, Weiner DB. Interferons as potential adjuvants in prophylactic vaccines. Expert Opin Biol Ther 2010;10(10):1489–500.
100. Jego G, Palucka AK, Blanck JP, et al. Plasmacytoid dendritic cells induce plasma cell differentiation through type I interferon and interleukin 6. Immunity 2003;19(2):225–34.
101. Tovey MG, Lallemand C, Meritet JF, et al. Adjuvant activity of interferon alpha: mechanism(s) of action. Vaccine 2006;24(Suppl 2):46–7.
102. Tovey MG, Maury C. Oromucosal interferon therapy: marked antiviral and antitumor activity. J Interferon Cytokine Res 1999;19(2):145–55.
103. Goldwater PN. Randomized comparative trial of interferon-alpha versus placebo in hepatitis B vaccine non-responders and hyporesponders. Vaccine 1994; 12(5):410–4.

Mediators of Systemic Inflammatory Response Syndrome and the Role of Recombinant Activated Protein C in Sepsis Syndrome

Vivek Kak, MD

KEYWORDS

• Sepsis • Sepsis mediators • Activated protein C

The systemic inflammatory response syndrome (SIRS) is the clinical manifestation of the host-derived systemic inflammatory response to an invasive infection. SIRS often follows an infection but can also occur from multiple noninfectious causes, including trauma and ischemia. When this inflammatory response follows an infection it is defined as sepsis. The sepsis syndrome is a series of cascading events that follows this infectious insult. Severe sepsis is defined as organ dysfunction caused by an infection, and septic shock is defined as severe sepsis along with hypotension that does not respond to fluids.[1] This continuum of sepsis severity leads to major morbidity and mortality in the world, with mortality ranging from 10% to 36% in sepsis, 18% to 52% in severe sepsis, and 46% to 82% in septic shock.[2,3] The most frequent infection that leads to sepsis is pneumonia (44%), followed by primary bacteremias (17%); genitourinary infections (9%); abdominal infections (9%); and then other infections, such as skin infections and meningitis.[4] Although bacteria are the classic causes of sepsis, other organisms, such as fungi and viruses, can lead to sepsis, especially influenza A.[5] These syndromes develop when the host response to an infection becomes magnified and then dysregulated. The clinical presentation often includes fever, confusion, and hypotension. If unarrested, this often leads to renal failure, coagulopathy followed by severe hypotension, and ultimately death.[6] It is estimated that these syndromes are increasing in incidence across the world and may lead to death in a significant amount of patients, with mortality approaching 50% in patients with

The author is a member of the Speaker's Bureau for Cubist Pharmaceuticals.
Infectious Diseases, Allegiance Health, 1100 East Michigan Avenue, #305, Jackson, MI 49201, USA
E-mail address: vkak@yahoo.com

Infect Dis Clin N Am 25 (2011) 835–850
doi:10.1016/j.idc.2011.07.009
0891-5520/11/$ – see front matter © 2011 Elsevier Inc. All rights reserved.

septic shock.[3] The key to survival in patients with sepsis is often rapid resuscitation and the initiation of appropriate therapy in the initial hours.

This review presents an overview of the immunology of sepsis, the mediators that are responsible for the clinical picture associated with the SIRS. Later, the author examines the coagulopathy seen in sepsis syndrome, the role of activated protein C in this coagulopathy, and the therapeutic use of recombinant activated protein C in the clinical setting in patients with severe sepsis.

The phenomena that lead to the development of sepsis and septic shock are highly complex. A simplified overview of this process is shown in **Fig. 1**. The entry of bacteria or bacterial components leads to the activation of the immune system and a wide release of proinflammatory mediators that leads to the vasodilatation of blood vessels; upregulation of adhesion molecules that leads to extravasations of polymorphonuclear neutrophils and monocytes; and activation of cellular parts of the immune system, including leukocytes, monocytes, and endothelial cells. This whole process is accompanied by the activation of the coagulation system, which may lead to the development of a disseminated intravascular coagulopathy.[6,7]

RECOGNITION OF PATHOGEN

The immune system has baseline innate mechanisms to prevent entry of pathogens into the body. These mechanisms include the tight junctions on epithelium and the presence of cilia on mucous membranes that act as physical barriers to the entry of organisms.[8] Other measures include the presence of natural immunoglobulin (Ig)M that can recognize and bind conserved motifs on bacteria and the secretion of secretory IgA and surfactants on mucous membranes. Surfactants contain various antibacterial agents, such as defensins and cathelicidins, that can destroy both gram-positive

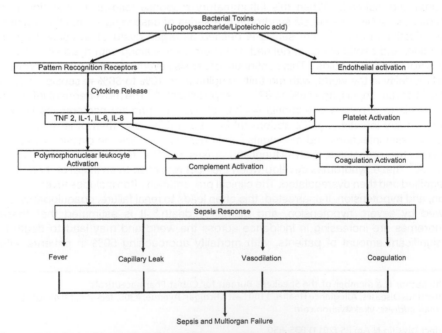

Fig. 1. Overview of systemic inflammatory response syndrome. IL, interleukin; TNF, tumor necrosis factor.

and gram-negative organisms by pore-forming activity.[9] The complement system is also important in the initial response to bacteria. The deposition of complement C3b (opsonin) on gram-positive or gram-negative bacteria facilitates neutrophil-mediated bacterial killing, whereas gram-negative bacteria can also be destroyed by the terminal complex formed by complements C5 to C9.[10] If a pathogen is able to evade these mechanisms, it is exposed to the immune cells that are able to recognize certain preserved bacterial motifs. These pathogen-associated molecular patterns (PAMPs) are recognized by pattern-recognition receptors on the immune cells, which then trigger the sepsis cascade.[11]

The most important PAMPs are bacterial cell surface components because they are often conserved motifs across various bacteria. One family of pattern-recognition receptors, the Toll-like receptors (TLRs), plays a central role in the initiation of the immune response. A variety of TLRs have been identified in humans, and these extracellular receptors recognize various microbial ligands.[12] Another important pattern-recognition receptor recognizes peptidoglycan, which is present in both gram-positive and gram-negative organisms. The recognition of a subunit of peptidoglycan (muramyl dipeptide) by receptors containing ligand-sensing leucine-rich repeat regions leads to the activation of the immune system through connected signaling components called nucleotide-binding oligomerization domains.[13]

The most well-studied microbial ligand that initiates sepsis in humans is lipopolysaccharide (LPS), also known as endotoxin, found in the outer cytoplasmic membrane of gram-negative bacteria.[14] The recognition of LPS by the pattern-recognition receptors of the immune system triggers sepsis in various gram-negative infections. The initiation of this process occurs when LPS is bound by the host-derived lipopolysaccharide-binding protein after the bacterial entry into the host. This protein transfers bound LPS to the opsonin receptor CD14 on the cell surface. The binding of LPS to CD14 leads to the association of CD14 with the Toll-like receptor TLR4 and then initiates TLR stimulation.[15] This stimulation leads to the initiation of the intracellular signaling cascade and recruitment of a signaling protein called myeloid differentiation primary response protein (MyD88). MyD88 subsequently leads to the release of transcription factors, such as nuclear factor-κB release, and the transcription of various inflammatory genes and the release of various cytokines and other molecules.[12] In addition, LPS can also bind to soluble CD14 in serum; and this complex can activate endothelial, epithelial, and smooth muscle cells.[16]

In contrast, the gram-positive infections involve recognition by TLRs of gram-positive cell wall components, lipoteichoic acid (LTA), and peptidoglycans. The lipoprotein components of LTA are recognized by Toll-like receptor 2 (TLR2), and the activation of TLR2 leads to signal transduction and the subsequent release of cytokines.[17,18] Another important feature of sepsis with gram-positive organisms is the production of potent exotoxins. These exotoxins have properties of superantigens and are able to bind to the major histocompatibility complex class II and T-lymphocyte receptors. This activity leads to a massive T-cell activation and release of various cytokines independent of the TLR pathways. Examples of these toxins include the toxic shock syndrome toxin 1 produced by certain strains of *Staphylococcus aureus*.[8]

A family of TLRs has been identified that can recognize various bacterial, fungal, and yeast proteins and, thus, initiate the inflammatory process from diverse microbial challenges.[19] The Toll-like receptor TLR2 can also recognize yeast, cell wall components of mycobacteria, lipoproteins from spirochetes, and mycoplasma, whereas TLR3 can recognize viral dsRNA.[19,20] It is also postulated that polymorphisms in the Toll-family proteins may explain the variability of the immune response among humans with a similar infective challenge.[21,22]

RELEASE OF INFLAMMATORY MEDIATORS
Overview

The activation of TLRs leads to the transcription of various proinflammatory cytokines and chemokines. The mononuclear cells play a central role in this by releasing the proinflammatory cytokines as well as other products, such as lipid mediators (tissue factor, prostaglandins, platelet activating factor) and nitric oxide.[23] The primary aim of this mediator release is the enhancement of leukocyte migration to the infective site to combat the infecting organism and to limit the area of infection. This release also involves endothelial activation, increased neutrophil migration, and neutrophil-mediated killing.[24] The release of tissue factor leads to the activation of the coagulation cascade and, in severe sepsis, can lead to the development of a consumptive coagulopathy.[25] The activation of the complement system leads to the production of complement C5a, which enhances cytokine and chemokine production in sepsis.[26] The release of nitric oxide causes local vasodilatation, which may lead to hypotension. These mediators are produced early in the onset of the inflammatory response to infection and reflect the overactive status of the immune response.[27] The effector phagocytic cells of the immune system (neutrophils and macrophages) respond to these mediators by releasing granular enzymes and producing reactive oxygen species, such as H_2O_2, to enhance the killing of the infecting bacteria. These products, such as H_2O_2, are also capable of causing tissue damage, which ultimately leads to increased vascular permeability and organ injury. Unchecked, this proinflammatory response can lead to refractory hypotension, endothelial leakage with severe edema, and, ultimately, organ failure and death.[11,28] In the later stages of sepsis, antiinflammatory mediators, such as interleukin (IL)-10, transforming growth factor-β, and IL-13, are produced; these lead to suppression in the production of many of the proinflammatory mediators.[24] This suppression, in turn, often leads to the suppression of the various functions of the immune function, especially the functions of neutrophils, leading to a depressed host defense system.[11]

INFLAMMATORY MEDIATORS
Cytokines and Chemokines

The cytokines play a central role in the development of the systemic inflammatory response to an infection. The activation of the TLRs by bacteria leads to the activation of nuclear factor (NF)-κB, which leads to the intracellular transcription of various proinflammatory cytokines, such as tumor necrosis factor-alpha (TNF-α); IL-1; IL-6; IL-8; and other cytokines, including IL-12, IL-15, and IL-18.

The cytokines TNF-α and IL-1 play a synergistic role in the development of the inflammatory response.[24,27,29] They activate neutrophils, lymphocytes, and vascular endothelial cells. They upregulate the expression of adhesion molecules and enhance the procoagulant activity of vascular endothelial cells. They also trigger the production of inducible nitric oxide (iNOS) in immune and vascular cells, which leads to the local production of nitric oxide (NO).[30] The NO-induced local vasodilatation slows the blood flow and, with the increased expression of adhesion molecules, leads to the enhanced adhesion of the neutrophils to the tissue wall.[6] They also induce synthesis of lipid mediators of sepsis (prostaglandins) and induce the production of acute phase proteins and induce fever.[14]

IL-8 is the prototypical chemokine that is produced locally at the site of infection. It is important as an activator and chemoattractant for neutrophils to marginate on the vessel wall and enter the area of infection.[31] The cytokine IL-6 is often elevated in patients with severe sepsis, and IL-6 levels, but not TNF-α levels, have been shown to predict a fatal outcome in patients with septic shock.[32,33] However, studies in humans and animals have not shown a causal role for this cytokine in septic shock. IL-6 is also considered by some to be an antiinflammatory cytokine because it can induce the release of IL-10, which is thought of as the classic antiinflammatory cytokine.[24] The cytokines IL-12 and IL-18 are important in the production of interferon (IFN)-γ.[29] IFN-γ enhances phagocytosis and free radical production and increases the bactericidal activity of macrophages and neutrophils. In animal models of sepsis, IFN-γ blockage is associated with decreased systemic inflammation and better prognosis.[34] IL-12 also plays a major role in the defense against polymicrobial sepsis, whereas IL-18 is important in infections caused by gram-negative organisms because its neutralization in an animal model of sepsis showed protection against endotoxemia.[35,36]

Other critical cytokine mediators in SIRS include macrophage migration inhibition factor (MIF) and high-mobility group box protein 1(HMGB1). MIF is preformed within leukocytes and is also secreted by the anterior pituitary, hypothalamus, and adrenal glands.[37] It was originally described during endotoxemia but also seems to mediate shock caused by gram-positive agents, such as toxic shock caused by S aureus.[38] In humans, high levels of MIF are associated with severe sepsis; and in animal models of sepsis, inhibition of MIF can protect from death. MIF functions by activating macrophages and T cells. It also upregulates the expression of TLR4 by phagocytes, which leads to amplification and development of a sustained inflammatory response in sepsis.[39] MIF also acts as a linkage between the immune system and the endocrine system because it can be induced by low doses of glucocorticoids; but once released, MIF acts as a proinflammatory agent and can override the immunosuppressive effects of glucocorticoids.[40,41] This finding is interesting in view of the studies that have suggested beneficial effects of low-dose steroids in patients with severe sepsis.[42,43]

HMGB1 is also recognized as a late mediator of sepsis.[44] It was originally described as a transcription factor, but later recognized as a late mediator of sepsis in endotoxemia. Its level rises much later than TNF-α in sepsis, and higher levels of HMGB1 in sepsis are associated with increased mortality.[45] HMGB1 is found in all cell types except those without a nucleus, but its main sources in SIRS are macrophages, monocytes, and neutrophils.[46] The release of HMGB1 promotes inflammation and disruption of epithelial barriers leading to tissue edema. It also increases the proinflammatory activity of other cytokines, such as IL-1. The peak release of HMGB1 occurs during later stages of sepsis; and its release is induced by cytokines, such as TNF-α, IL-1, and IFN-γ, as well as by the complement system.[47] HMGB1 secretion is also influenced by the autonomic nervous system, and the vagus nerve activation can downregulate the release of HMGB1.[48]

The IL-17A cytokine is another proinflammatory cytokine that is produced mainly by T helper (Th) 17 cells. It mediates SIRS by also triggering the production of other cytokines, such as IL-1, IL-6, and TNF-α.[49] Triggering receptor expressed on myeloid cells (TREM)-1, another proinflammatory mediator found in plasma during sepsis, is expressed by monocytes and neutrophils during sepsis and it amplifies other proinflammatory responses during sepsis.[50–52] It was thought that high levels of TREM-1 might be helpful as a marker of infection in patients with SIRS; however, recent studies have suggested that this cytokine may not be a specific marker for infection.[53]

This profound cytokine storm associated with SIRS and the effects on the vasculature and endothelium lead to the clinical manifestations of SIRS. There is the development of the acute phase response with fevers, leukocytosis, and vasodilatation along with the activation of the complement and the coagulation pathway.

COMPLEMENTS AND COMPLEMENT PATHWAY

The complement pathway and its products are important sepsis mediators.[54] The major purpose of the activation of this pathway through any of the 3 pathways (classic, alternate, and mannose-binding lectin [MBL]) is to damage and or remove infecting organisms. The classical pathway is activated by antigen-antibody complexes, whereas the alternate pathway is activated by LPS. The MBL pathway of complement activation is initiated by mannose sugars on the bacterial surface through the MBL protein and subsequent interaction with MBL-activated serine proteases. After that point, this pathway functions identically to the classical pathway. All pathways converge at the level of complement C3 and lead to the production of the complement cleavage products, C3a and C5a, as well as the terminal membrane attack complex, C5b-9, which forms pores in the membranes of bacteria causing their death.[54] Although the complement system is a vital part of the defense against invading pathogens, complement activation also contributes to the development of sepsis.[55] In clinical studies, increased levels of C3a, C4a, and C5a in serum are associated with a worse outcome in sepsis.[56]

Complement C5a, which is generated after the complement system is activated, exerts its effects after binding to its receptors C5a receptor and C5a-like receptor 2.[57] These receptors are upregulated during sepsis. C5a leads to the synthesis and release of the proinflammatory cytokines TNF-α, IL-1, IL-6, and IL-8 from leucocytes.[26] It also triggers the release of MIF and HMGB1, which can then amplify the inflammatory response in SIRS.[58] Early on in sepsis, C5a enhances phagocytosis and induces the oxidative burst and release of granular enzymes from neutrophils; but in later stages of sepsis, C5a causes neutrophil dysfunction, which, along with the C5a induced increased apoptosis of thymocytes and adrenal medullary cells, leads to the immunosuppression seen later in sepsis.[59–62] C5a also plays a vital role in connecting the complement system to the coagulation cascade. It causes the induction of tissue factor, which triggers the coagulation cascade and, thus, leads to the development of coagulopathy seen in sepsis.[63] Besides the previously mentioned roles, C5a also acts as a potent vasodilator along with increasing the expression of adhesion molecules on endothelium. It is also thought to play a major role in the development of sepsis-induced cardiomyopathy.[64] The appearance of C5a in blood in sepsis often indicates a loss of control over the complement pathway, and the blockade of C5a in animal models of sepsis prevents the development of multiple organ failure and is thought to be a promising target for intervention in treatment of sepsis.[26]

PROTEASES AND OTHER ENZYMES

After development of sepsis, cytokine-induced activated leukocytes release a variety of enzymes, including proteases. Among proteases, the matrix metalloproteinases are important in the inflammatory process.[65] The matrix metalloproteinase's MMP-9 levels increase in gram-negative sepsis and correlates with severity of sepsis.[66] Other proteases, such as elastase, are also associated with organ dysfunction.[29] These proteases cleave factors associated with the contact (Hageman factor) pathway of coagulation and activate the contact pathway leading to the release of bradykinin from high-molecular-weight kininogen (HMWK). The release of bradykinin leads to vasodilatation and endovascular fluid leakage into tissues and is ultimately another factor in the intravascular hypovolemia and hypotension seen in septic shock.[67] Many of the proinflammatory effects of bradykinin are mediated by the secondary release of other mediators, particularly NO and eicosanoids, such as platelet-activating factor (PAF).

Lipid Mediators/Lipoproteins and LPS Binding Proteins

The eicosanoids products are another group of important mediators in sepsis. Of these lipid products produced, proinflammatory cytokines (TNF-α, IL-1) lead to the synthesis of phospholipase A2 and the subsequent induction of cyclooxygenease-2, 5'lipooxygenase, and acetyltransferase enzymes.[27] These enzymes, in turn, lead to the production of various eicosanoids, such as leukotrienes, prostaglandins, thromboxane A$_2$, as well as the production of PAF. These factors promote inflammation, alter vasomotor tone, and change vascular permeability and blood flow and, thus, contribute to the inflammatory response in sepsis.

Thromboxane A2 is synthesized primarily by platelets, neutrophils, macrophages, and monocytes, and is a potent promoter of platelet aggregation, vasoconstriction, bronchoconstriction, and leukocyte adhesion. Prostacyclin tends to oppose the effects of thromboxane A2 and is a platelet antiaggregant and endothelium-independent vasodilator.[68]

PAF is produced by endothelial cells, leukocytes, and macrophages. It promotes the adhesion of neutrophils to the endothelium, increases vascular permeability, and also causes vasoconstriction. In animal models, PAF causes systemic arterial hypotension, pulmonary hypertension, diminished cardiac output, increased vascular permeability, and bronchoconstriction.[69] Although PAF can affect cells directly, most of its effects are caused by the release of secondary mediators, including thromboxane A2 and leukotrienes. The levels of PAF rise during sepsis, and the inhibition of PAF before endotoxin challenge in human studies does lead to decreased symptoms and lower levels of proinflammatory cytokines.[70]

Serum lipoproteins have been shown to have a role in binding endotoxins and neutralizing its proinflammatory effects. LPS is neutralized by lipoproteins and then transported to the liver where the Kupffer cells (liver macrophages) clear the portal circulation of various foreign and toxin materials, including the lipoprotein-bound LPS.[71] Apolipoprotein E, a lipoprotein, also acts as an immunomodulator in sepsis by inhibiting proliferation of mononuclear cells and lymphocyte activation. Animal studies have demonstrated that deficiencies of apolipoprotein A lead to an increase in susceptibility to LPS during septic shock.[72] Other proteins, such as lactoferrin, lysozyme, hemoglobin, and surfactant protein, can also bind to endotoxins and, thus, mitigate the development of SIRS.[10]

Nitric Oxide

The activation of Toll-like receptor TLR4 by endotoxins or the release of the proinflammatory cytokines, such as TNF-α and IL-1, leads to the production of iNOS in immune and vascular cells. This activity leads to the production of NO, which causes local vasodilatation and slows the blood flow. There follows an increased expression of adhesion molecules on endothelial cells and, thus, increased margination of neutrophils to vessels; however, paradoxically NO has also been shown to reduce neutrophil migration to infected tissues.[73,74] The ability of NO to alter epithelial tight junction can cause a loss of epithelial integrity, especially in lung and gut tissue, during sepsis.[75] In animal models of sepsis, inhibition of the production of NO by inhibiting iNOS has been associated with improvement in acidosis and hypotension; however, in human trial of sepsis, use of a nonselective NO synthase inhibitor increased mortality in patients with septic shock.[76,77]

Antiinflammatory Mediators

The proinflammatory response in sepsis initiated by pathogen recognition by TLRs has a counter regulatory response that attempts to downregulate the proinflammatory response. This antiinflammatory response involves the negative regulation of the TLR signaling pathway to decrease the production of the proinflammatory cytokines (TNF-α, IL1, IL-6) and also involves the production of antiinflammatory cytokines. Antiinflammatory or counter-inflammatory mediators include soluble TNF receptors and the IL-1 receptor antagonist; decoy receptors, such as IL-1 receptor type II; antiinflammatory cytokines, such as IL-10, IL-4, IL-13 and Interferon-α; and inactivators of the complement cascade.[6,18,24] These mediators lead to the suppression of immune response and are augmented by the development of lymphocyte apoptosis that can lead to T-cell hyporesponsiveness and anergy development. There is also extensive apoptosis of gastrointestinal epithelial cells and endothelial cells during sepsis. This activity may lead to the compromise of bowel wall integrity during sepsis, which leads to a possible increase in secondary bacteremias and candidemias from the translocation of bowel flora.[78]

Another physiologic antiinflammatory mediator in sepsis is the autonomic nervous system. The vagus nerve can downregulate inflammation by decreasing the release of TNF-α, IL1, IL-6, and HMGB1.[79] This antiinflammatory effect is mediated by the release of the neurotransmitter acetylcholine, interacting with the α7 nicotinic acetylcholine receptors on macrophages. In experimental animal models of sepsis, treatment with nicotine that binds to the α7 nicotinic acetylcholine receptor reduces circulating TNF-α and HMGB-1 levels and reduced mortality.[80]

Although this antiinflammatory response attempts to dampen the proinflammatory seen earlier in sepsis, it can also lead to a suppressed immune system and an inability to clear infection and a predisposition to nosocomial infection.

COAGULATION PATHWAY PRODUCTS

The coagulation pathway is intricately linked in the development of sepsis. The initial activation of the coagulation pathway with deposition of fibrin is the body's attempt to localize inflammation at the site of infection. However, dysregulation of the coagulation cascade can lead to the development of disseminated intravascular coagulation (DIC).[81] An overview of this process is shown in **Fig. 2**.

The entry of an infecting organism leads to release of the proinflammatory cytokines (TNF-α, IL1, IL-6) and the development of the acute phase response. The acute phase response leads to the increased concentrations of several coagulation components, including fibrinogen and HMWK, whereas the release of cytokines leads to an increased induction of tissue factor (TF) on mononuclear and endothelial cells. TF can also be induced directly by lipopolysaccharide in gram-negative infections. The presentation of TF activates a proteolytic cascade that leads to the formation of thrombin and a fibrin clot.[82] The development of activated thrombin can also cause increased generation of the proinflammatory cytokines TNF-α, IL1, and IL-6 as a form of a positive feedback loop that reinforces the coagulation cascade. It also leads to the generation of C5a, which, in turn, can also lead to the increased expression of TF. The ability of TF to activate coagulation by the extrinsic (factor VII) pathway is normally suppressed by inhibitors, such as tissue factor plasminogen inhibitor, antithrombin III, and protein C. However, these proteins are downregulated or consumed during sepsis. Concomitantly, the endogenous fibrinolytic pathways are impaired because of elevated serum levels of fibrinolysis inhibitors, such as plasminogen-activator inhibitor 1(PAI-1) and tissue-factor fibrinolysis inhibitor.[25,82] The complement system and the coagulation system also interact with each other during sepsis and often amplify both the inflammatory and the coagulation response. The coagulation factor XIIa can activate the classical complement pathway, whereas thrombin and

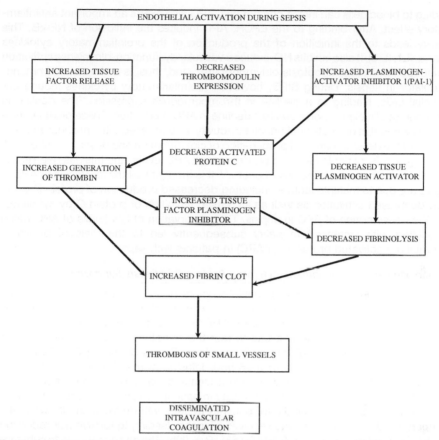

Fig. 2. Overview of coagulation in sepsis. PAI-1, plasminogen-activator inhibitor 1.

plasmin can cleave C3. Thrombin can also cleave C5 into C5a independently of the 3 complement activation pathways. The complement pathway also amplifies coagulation by the C5a-induced expression of TF and PAI-1 from leucocytes.[59] The procoagulant activity of complement is also augmented by the inhibition of protein S by the C4-binding protein of the complement system.[83]

The net result of this derangement of the coagulation cascade is the excess production and diminished removal of fibrin lead to the development of fibrin clots in blood vessels, causing microvascular hypoperfusion and multiorgan damage.

Anticoagulant Mechanisms and Protein C

Protein C, an endogenous vitamin K dependent serine protease, is an important modulator of the coagulation pathway. In the normal state, the activated form is formed by cleavage from soluble protein C after thrombin interacts with thrombomodulin.[84] Activated protein C (APC) has anticoagulant and profibrinolytic activity via the inhibition of activated factors V and VIII and plasminogen activator-inhibitor 1.[85] It also has antiinflammatory activity through its interaction with the endothelial protein C receptor (EPCR) that is found on endothelial cells, neutrophils, monocytes, and eosinophils.[86] The binding of APC to endothelial cells leads to a decrease in thrombin-induced endothelial permeability injury, possibly leading to a decrease in tissue edema, whereas its

binding to blood cells can inhibit chemotaxis. APC also exerts an important antiinflammatory effect. After binding to the EPCR, APC induces the inhibition of NF-κB. This
activity leads to the inhibition of the production of the proinflammatory cytokines
(TNF-α, IL1, IL-6). It also inhibits NO-induced vascular dysfunction, diminishes activation
of neutrophils, inhibits apoptosis of lymphocytes, and, thus, is an important immunomodulator in sepsis. During SIRS, however, proinflammatory cytokines induce endothelial cells, leading to a decline in thrombomodulin expression. The decline in
thrombomodulin expression leads to a decline in APC production. These proinflammatory cytokines also promote antifibrinolytic activity, as discussed in the previous section,
leading to the development and propagation of clot formation and development of DIC.

During sepsis, patients tend to have decreased APC levels, and this has been associated with an increase in the risk of death.[86] It is thought that the low levels of APC in
sepsis are due to multiple factors, including decreased production of protein C in the
liver, decreased activation as well as increased inhibition of protein C by cytokines,
and the consumption of APC in sepsis. This observation of low levels of APC being
associated with increased mortality subsequently led to the trials of providing
recombinant activated protein C (rhAPC) in patients with sepsis.

Human Studies of Recombinant Activated Protein C in Sepsis Syndrome

Activated protein C intervenes at multiple points during sepsis as previously discussed. Because patients with sepsis have low levels of APC, it was postulated that
supplementing endogenous APC with rhAPC in patients with sepsis may lead to
a decrease in mortality. The first trial to test this hypothesis was the Recombinant
Human Activated Protein C Worldwide Evaluation in Severe Sepsis (PROWESS) trial.[87]

This phase 3 multicenter trial of a 96-hour infusion of rhAPC (drotrecogin alfa) in
patients with severe sepsis involved 1690 patients. It was stopped early because of
a statistically significant reduction in mortality in patients who were treated with drotrecogin alfa. The all-cause mortality of patients treated with drotrecogin alfa was 24.7
compared with 30.8 in those who received placebo, leading to relative risk reduction
of 19.4% (confidence interval -6.6% to 30.5%; $P = .005$). The drug was noted to substantially reduce d-dimer levels and IL-6 levels, suggesting a diminished activation of the
coagulant pathway as well as reduced cytokine production. This study led to the
approval of drotrecogin alfa in the United States by the Food and Drug Administration
(FDA) for patients with severe sepsis and a high risk of death. A subsequent detailed
subgroup analysis suggested that patients with a higher acute risk of death as suggested
by a higher Acute Physiology and Chronic Health Evaluation (APACHE) II score (>25) and
a greater risk of death had a greater reduction in mortality with the use of the drug.[88]

The FDA required the manufacturer to study the efficacy of drotrecogin alfa for adults
with severe sepsis who had a low risk of death as defined by an APACHE II score of less
than 25 or single organ failure. The study addressing this question, the Administration of
Drotrecogin alfa (activated) in Early Severe Sepsis (ADDRESS) trial, involved 2613
patients and was terminated early because of a low likelihood of achieving the study
objective of demonstrating a reduction in mortality with drotrecogin alfa in patients
with severe sepsis but a low risk of death.[89] The mortality in the ADDRESS trial was
18.5% in the study group, whereas it was 17% in the placebo arm. Subgroup analysis
from the ADDRESS trial in 324 patients with APACHE score >25 or more than one organ
failure failed to show any observed benefit for use of drotrecogin alfa, however differences in the baseline characteristics in patients between the PROWESS and the
ADDRESS trials limit making any conclusions on this subgroup analysis. The REsearch-
ing severe Sepsis and Organ dysfunction in cHildren: a gLObal perspectiVE trial,
a placebo-controlled trial of the use of drotrecogin alfa in children with severe sepsis

and cardiovascular and respiratory organ dysfunction, also did not show any difference in mortality with the use of drotrecogin alfa as compared with placebo.[90]

In the major clinical trials, the use of drotrecogin alfa has increased the risk of bleeding compared with placebo. In the ADDRESS trial, mortality among surgical patients with single organ injury was higher with the use of drotrecogin alfa leading to a black box warning about its use in such a scenario. These uncertainties among the studies have led to controversy about its use in the clinical setting of severe sepsis. These uncertainties relate to the identification of the appropriate patients in sepsis who should be treated with this drug. Based on both the ADDRESS and the PROWESS trial, its use seems most appropriate in patients with severe sepsis who have both an APACHE II score of greater than 25 and dysfunction of more than one organ. It also should not be used in patients with contraindications that can increase the risk of bleeding.

Other Immunomodulatory Strategies in Treatment of Sepsis

Guidelines for the treatment of sepsis and septic shock have been developed under the aegis of the Surviving Sepsis Campaign.[91] These guidelines focus on a multifaceted approach and involve, among other modalities, early aggressive resuscitation, appropriate antimicrobials and drainage of pus, and supportive care of any life-threatening organ dysfunction. The recognition of patients developing sepsis is often the key to the initiation of aggressive resuscitation.[92] The Surviving Sepsis guidelines also suggest consideration of drotrecogin alfa in patients with severe sepsis. Besides drotrecogin alfa, the only other immunomodulating agent that has entered routine clinical practice in patients with sepsis is the use of stress dose steroids. In a large trail, and other small studies, administering hydrocortisone as 50mg to 100 mg 3 to 4 times a day for 1 week has been shown to be beneficial in patients with sepsis.[43,93] Other immunomodulating agents that seem beneficial in sepsis include preparation of polyclonal IVIG.[94,95] This beneficial effect is most noted when using preparations also containing IgM and IgA along with IgG and involves a possible increase in the opsonization of bacteria by the complement system and downregulation of the release of the proinflammatory cytokines and increase of antiinflammatory mediators, such as soluble decoy receptors for various cytokines.[96]

The presence of multiple mediators and pathways in the host response to sepsis has lead to studies of numerous therapeutic interventions in clinical trials of patients with sepsis. These trials have targeted the proinflammatory mediators in sepsis. Thus, LPS and TNF-α have been targeted using monoclonal antibodies; IL-1 was targeted using a recombinant Il-1 receptor antagonist. These interventions, despite showing promise in animal models, were not efficacious in human studies.[97–100] Other studies have aimed for inhibition of other proinflammatory mediators, including platelet-activating factor; lipid mediators, including thromboxane and prostaglandins; NO; bradykinin; and oxygen radicals, but most of these strategies have not shown any benefit other than the ones previously discussed.[101]

SUMMARY

The sepsis syndrome is a clinical syndrome that develops from the host response to an infecting organism. Although this syndrome initially tries to limit the damage caused by infection, it rapidly becomes amplified and dysregulated leading to damage to the host. It is a complex process that involves the interplay of various microbial proteins; endogenous mediators of sepsis, such as proinflammatory and antiinflammatory cytokines; complement system products; proteases; lipid mediators; and NO and coagulation system components. The dysregulation of these mediators often leads to increased mortality in sepsis. The central role of these mediators in the development of sepsis has lead to therapeutic trials targeting these sepsis mediators to improve survival in patients with sepsis. However, so far, other than the use of rhAPC in patients with severe sepsis and organ failure, none of these interventions on mediators of sepsis have been shown to improve mortality.

REFERENCES

1. Bone R, Balk RA, Cerra FB, et al. Definitions for sepsis and organ failure and guidelines for the use of innovative therapies in sepsis. Chest 1992;101:1644–55.
2. Pittet D, Thievent B, Wenzel RP, et al. Bedside prediction of mortality from bacteremic sepsis, a dynamic analysis of ICU patients. Am J Respir Crit Care Med 1996;153:684–93.
3. Salvo I, Decain W, Musicco M, et al. The Italian Sepsis Study, preliminary results on the incidence and evolution of SIRS, sepsis, severe sepsis and septic shock. Intensive Care Med 1995;21(Suppl 2):S244–9.
4. Angus DC, Linde-Zwirble WT, Lidicker J, et al. Epidemiology of severe sepsis in the United States: analysis of incidence, outcome, and associated costs of care. Crit Care Med 2001;29:1303–10.
5. Webb SA, Pettila V, Seppelt I, et al. ANZIC Influenza Investigators. Critical care services and 2009 H1N1 influenza in Australia and New Zealand. N Engl J Med 2009;361(20):1925–34.
6. Hotchkiss RS, Karl IE. The pathophysiology and treatment of sepsis. N Engl J Med 2003;348(2):138–50.
7. Remick DG. Pathophysiology of sepsis. Am J Pathol 2007;170:1435–44.
8. Sriskandan S, Altmann DM. The immunology of sepsis. J Pathol 2008;214:211–23.
9. Ganz T. Defensins: antimicrobial peptides of innate immunity. Nat Rev Immunol 2003;3:710–20.
10. Gasque P. Complement: a unique innate immune sensor for danger signals. Mol Immunol 2004;41:1089–98.
11. Rittirsch D, Flierl MA, Ward PA. Harmful molecular mechanisms in sepsis. Nat Rev Immunol 2008;8:776–87.
12. Van Amersfoort ES, Van Berkel TJ, Kuiper J. Receptors, mediators and mechanisms involved in bacterial sepsis and septic shock. Clin Microbiol Rev 2003; 16(3):379–414.
13. Inohara C, McDonald C, Nunez G. NOD-LRR proteins: role in host–microbial interactions and inflammatory disease. Annu Rev Biochem 2005;74:355–83.
14. Cohen J. The immunopathogenesis of sepsis. Nature 2002;420:885–91.
15. Poltorak A, He X, Smirnova I, et al. Defective LPS signaling in C3H/HeJ and C57BL/10ScCr mice: mutations in TLR4 gene. Science 1998;282:2085–8.
16. Ulevitch RJ, Tobias PS. Receptor-dependent mechanisms of cell stimulation by endotoxin. Annu Rev Immunol 1995;13:437–57.
17. Takeuchi O, Hoshino K, Kawai T, et al. Differential roles of TLR2 and TLR4 in recognition of gram-negative and gram- positive bacterial cell wall components. Immunity 1999;1:443–51.
18. Wiersinga WJ, van der Poll T. Is the septic response good or bad? Curr Infect Dis Rep 2007;9:366–73.
19. Aderem A, Ulevitch RJ. Toll-like receptors in the induction of the innate immune response. Nature 2000;406:782–7.
20. Vasselon T, Detmers PA. Toll receptors: a central element in innate immune responses. Infect Immun 2002;70:1033.

21. Lorenz E, Mira JP, Cornish KL, et al. A novel polymorphism in the Toll-like receptor 2 gene and its potential association with staphylococcal infection. Infect Immun 2000;68:6398–401.
22. Lorenz E, Mira JP, Frees KL, et al. Relevance of mutations in the TLR4 receptor in patients with gram-negative septic shock. Arch Intern Med 2002;162: 1028–32.
23. Haveman JW, Muller Kobold AC, Tervaert JW, et al. The central role of monocytes in pathogenesis of sepsis: consequences for immunomonitoring and treatment. Neth J Med 1999;55(3):132–41.
24. Dinarello CA. Proinflammatory and anti-inflammatory cytokines as mediators in the pathogenesis of septic shock. Chest 1997;112:321S–9S.
25. Wiersinga WJ, Levi M, van der Poll T. Coagulation in sepsis. In: Vincent JL, editor, Mechanisms of sepsis-induced organ dysfunction and recovery, vol. 44. Heidelberg (Germany): Springer-Verlag; 2007. p. 273–85.
26. Ward PA. The dark side of C5a in sepsis. Nat Rev Immunol 2004;4(2):133–42.
27. Dinarello CA. Proinflammatory cytokines. Chest 2000;118:503–8.
28. Cavaillon JM, Adib-conquy M, Fitting C, et al. Cytokine cascade in sepsis. Scand J Infect Dis 2003;35:535–44.
29. Philippart F, Cavaillon JM. Sepsis mediators. Curr Infect Dis Rep 2007;9(5):358–65.
30. Annane D, Bellissant E, Cavaillon JM. Septic shock. Lancet 2005;365:63–78.
31. Ley K, Laudanna C, Cybulsky MI, et al. Getting to the site of inflammation: the leucocyte adhesion cascade updated. Nat Rev Immunol 2007;7:678–89.
32. Casey LC, Balk RA, Bone RC. Plasma cytokines and endotoxin levels correlate with survival in patients with the sepsis syndrome. Ann Intern Med 1993;119:771–8.
33. Fisher CJJ, Opal SM, Dhainaut JF, et al. Influence of an anti-tumor necrosis factor monoclonal antibody on cytokine levels in patients with sepsis. Crit Care Med 1993;21:318–27.
34. Qiu G, Gribbin E, Harrison K, et al. Inhibition of gamma interferon decreases bacterial load in peritonitis by accelerated peritoneal fibrin deposition and tissue repair. Infect Immun 2003;71:2766–74.
35. Moreno SE, Alves-Filho JC, Alfaya TM, et al. IL-12, but not IL-18, is critical to neutrophil activation and resistance to polymicrobial sepsis induced by cecal ligation and puncture. J Immunol 2006;177:3218–24.
36. Hochholzer P, Lipford GB, Wagner H, et al. Role of interleukin-18 (IL-18) during lethal shock: decreased lipopolysaccharide sensitivity but normal superantigen reaction in IL-18-deficient mice. Infect Immun 2000;68:3502–8.
37. Calandra T, Roger T. Macrophage migration inhibitory factor: a regulator of innate immunity. Nat Rev Immunol 2003;3:791–800.
38. Calandra T, Spiegel LA, Metz CN, et al. Macrophage migration inhibitory factor is a critical mediator of the activation of immune cells by exotoxins of gram-positive bacteria. Proc Natl Acad Sci U S A 1998;95:11383–8.
39. Roger T, David J, Glauser MP, et al. MIF regulates innate immune response through modulation of Toll-like receptor 4. Nature 2001;414(6866):920–4.
40. Calandra T, Bernhagen J, Metz CN, et al. MIF as a glucocorticoid-induced modulator of cytokine production. Nature 1995;377:68–71.
41. Flaster H, Bernhagen J, Calandra T, et al. The macrophage migration inhibitory factor-glucocorticoid dyad: regulation of inflammation and immunity. Mol Endocrinol 2007;21:1267–80.
42. Annane D, Sebille V, Charpentier C, et al. Effect of treatment with low doses of hydrocortisone and fludrocortisone on mortality in patients with septic shock. JAMA 2002;288:862–71.

43. Oppert M, Schindler R, Husung C, et al. Low dose hydrocortisone improves shock reversal and reduces cytokine levels in early hyperdynamic septic shock. Crit Care Med 2005;33:2457–64.

44. Wang H, Bloom O, Zhang M, et al. HMG-1 as a late mediator of endotoxin lethality in mice. Science 1999;285:248–51.

45. Sunden-Cullberg J, Norrby-Teglund A, Rouhiainen A, et al. Persistent elevation of high mobility group box-1 protein (HMGB1) in patients with severe sepsis and septic shock. Crit Care Med 2005;33:564–73.

46. Lotze MT, Tracey KJ. High mobility group box 1 protein (hmgb1): nuclear weapon in the immune arsenal. Nat Rev Immunol 2005;5:331–42.

47. Yang H, Wang H, Tracey KJ. HMG-1 rediscovered as a cytokine. Shock 2001;15: 247–53.

48. Wang H, Liao H, Ochani M, et al. Cholinergic agonists inhibit HMGB1 release and improve survival in experimental sepsis. Nat Med 2004;10:1216–21.

49. Weaver CT, Hatton RD, Mangan PR, et al. Il-17 family cytokines and the expanding diversity of effector t-cell lineages. Annu Rev Immunol 2007;25: 821–52.

50. Bouchon A, Dietrich J, Colonna M. Inflammatory responses can be triggered by TREM-1, a novel receptor expressed on neutrophils and monocytes. J Immunol 2000;164:4991–5.

51. Gibot S, Kolopp-Sarda MN, Bene MC, et al. A soluble form of the triggering receptor expressed on myeloid cells-1 modulates the inflammatory response in murine sepsis. J Exp Med 2004;200:1419–26.

52. Bouchon A, Facchetti F, Weigand MA, et al. TREM-1 amplifies inflammation and is a crucial mediator of septic shock. Nature 2001;410:1103–7.

53. Adib-Conquy M, Goulenok M, Laurent C, et al. Enhanced plasma levels of soluble triggering expressed on myeloid cells-1 and procalcitonin after cardiac surgery and cardiac arrest in the absence of infection. Shock 2007;28(4):406–10.

54. Haeney MR. The role of the complement cascade in sepsis. J Antimicrob Chemother 1998;41:s41–6.

55. Huber-Lang MS. Complement-induced impairment of innate immunity during sepsis. J Immunol 2002;169:3223–31.

56. Nakae H. Serum complement levels and severity of sepsis. Res Commun Chem Pathol Pharmacol 1994;84:189–95.

57. Rittirsch D, Flierl MA, Nadeau BA, et al. Functional role for C5a receptors in sepsis. Nat Med 2008;14(5):551–7.

58. Riedemann NC. Regulatory role of c5a on macrophage migration inhibitory factor release from neutrophils. J Immunol 2004;173:1355–9.

59. Gerard C. Complement c5a in the sepsis syndrome– too much of a good thing? N Engl J Med 2003;348:167–9.

60. Huber-Lang M. Role of c5a in multiorgan failure during sepsis. J Immunol 2001; 166:1193–9.

61. Solomkin JS, Jenkins MK, Nelson RD, et al. Neutrophil dysfunction in sepsis. II. Evidence for the role of complement activation products in cellular deactivation. Surgery 1981;90:319–27.

62. Riedemann NC, Guo RF, Laudes IJ, et al. C5a receptor and thymocyte apoptosis in sepsis. FASEB J 2002;16:887–8.

63. Muhlfelder TW, Niemetz J, Kreutzer D, et al. C5 chemotactic fragment induces leukocyte production of tissue factor activity: a link between complement and coagulation. J Clin Invest 1979;63:147–50.

64. Niederbichler AD, Hoesel LM, Westfall MV, et al. An essential role for complement c5a in the pathogenesis of septic cardiac dysfunction. J Exp Med 2006; 203:53–61.
65. Renckens R, Roelofs JJ, Florquin S, et al. Matrix metalloproteinase-9 deficiency impairs host defense against abdominal sepsis. J Immunol 2006;176:3735–41.
66. Yassen KA, Galley HF, Webster NR. Matrix metalloproteinase-9 concentrations in critically ill patients. Anaesthesia 2001;56:729–32.
67. Frick IM, Bjorck L, Herwald H. The dual role of the contact system in bacterial infectious disease. Thromb Haemost 2007;98:497–502.
68. Fink MP. Therapeutic options directed against platelet activating factor, eicosanoids and bradykinin in sepsis. J Antimicrob Chemother 1998;41(Suppl A): 81–94.
69. Mozes T, Zijlstra FJ, Heiligers JPC. Interactions between platelet activating factor and eicosanoids during endotoxic shock in anaesthetized pigs. Mediators Inflamm 1992;1:183–90.
70. Gomes RN, Layne MD, Carvajal IM, et al. Exogenous platelet-activating factor acetylhydrolase reduces mortality in mice with systemic inflammatory response syndrome and sepsis. Shock 2006;26:41–9.
71. Pajkrt D, Doran JE, Koster F, et al. Antiinflammatory effects of reconstituted high-density lipoprotein during human endotoxemia. J Exp Med 1996;184:1601–8.
72. Imai T, Fujita T, Yamazaki Y. Beneficial effects of apolipoprotein A-I on endotoxemia. Surg Today 2003;33:684–7.
73. Kengatharan KM, De Kimpe SJ, Thiemermann C. Role of nitric oxide in the circulatory failure and organ injury in a rodent model of gram-positive shock. Br J Pharmacol 1996;119:1411–21.
74. Benjamin CF, Silva JS, Fortes ZB, et al. Inhibition of leukocyte rolling of nitric oxide during sepsis leads to reduced migration of active microbicidal neutrophils. Infect Immun 2002;70:3602–10.
75. Han X, Fink MP, Uchiyama T, et al. Increased iNOS activity is essential for pulmonary epithelial tight junction dysfunction in endotoxemic mice. Am J Physiol Lung Cell Mol Physiol 2004;286:L259–67.
76. Evans T, Carpenter A, Silva A, et al. Inhibition of nitric oxide synthase in experimental gram-negative sepsis. J Infect Dis 1994;169:343–9.
77. López A, Lorente JA, Steingrub J, et al. Multiple-center, randomized, placebo-controlled, double-blind study of the nitric oxide synthase inhibitor 546C88: effect on survival in patients with septic shock. Crit Care Med 2004;32:21–30.
78. Hotchkiss RS, Coppersmith CM, Karl IE. Prevention of lymphocyte apoptosis-a potential treatment of sepsis. Clin Infect Dis 2005;41(S7):S465–9.
79. Borovikova LV, Ivanova S, Zhang M, et al. Vagus nerve stimulation attenuates the systemic inflammatory response to endotoxin. Nature 2000;405:458–62.
80. Wang H, Yu M, Ochani M, et al. Nicotinic acetylcholine receptor [alpha]7 subunit is an essential regulator of inflammation. Nature 2003;421:384–8.
81. Levi M, Ten Cate H. Disseminated intravascular coagulation. N Engl J Med 1999;341:586–92.
82. Esmon CT. The impact of the inflammatory response on coagulation. Thromb Res 2004;114:321–7.
83. Levi M, de Jonge E, van der Poll T. New treatment strategies for disseminated intravascular coagulation based on current understanding of the pathophysiology. Ann Med 2004;36:41–9.
84. Esmon CT. The protein C pathway. Chest 2003;124:S26–32.

85. Levi M, van der Poll T. Recombinant human activated protein C: current insights into its mechanism of action. Crit Care 2007;11:S3.
86. Faust SN, Levin M, Harrison OB, et al. Dysfunction of endothelial protein C activation in meningococcal sepsis. N Engl J Med 2001;345(6):408–16.
87. Bernard GR, Vincent JL, Laterre PF, et al. Efficacy and safety of recombinant human activated protein C for severe sepsis. N Engl J Med 2001;344:699–709.
88. Ely EW, Laterre PF, Angus DC, et al. Drotrecogin alfa (activated) administration across clinically important subgroups of patients with severe sepsis. Crit Care Med 2003;31:12–9.
89. Abraham E, Laterre PF, Garg R, et al. Drotrecogin alfa (activated) for adults with severe sepsis and a low risk of death. N Engl J Med 2005;353:1332–41.
90. Nadel S, Goldstein B, Williams MD, et al. Drotrecogin alfa (activated) in children with severe sepsis: a multicentre phase III randomized controlled trial. Lancet 2007;369(9564):836–43.
91. Dellinger RP, Carlet JM, Masur H, et al. Surviving sepsis campaign management guidelines committee (2004) surviving sepsis campaign guidelines for management of severe sepsis and septic shock. Crit Care Med 2004;32:858–73.
92. Rivers E, Nguyen B, Havstad S, et al. Early goal-directed therapy in the treatment of severe sepsis and septic shock. N Engl J Med 2001;345:1368–77.
93. Keh D, Boehnke T, Weber-Cartens S, et al. Immunologic and hemodynamic effects of "low-dose" hydrocortisone in septic shock: a double-blind, randomized, placebo-controlled, crossover study. Am J Respir Crit Care Med 2003;167:512–20.
94. Laupland KB, Kirkpatrick AW, Delaney A. Polyclonal intravenous immunoglobulin for the treatment of severe sepsis and septic shock in critically ill adults: a systematic review and meta-analysis. Crit Care Med 2007;35(12):2686–92.
95. Alejandria MM, Lansang MA, Dans LF, et al. Intravenous immunoglobulin for treating sepsis and septic shock. Cochrane Database Syst Rev 2002;1:CD001090.
96. Berlot Giorgio, Bacer Barbara, Piva Marco, et al. Immunoglobulins in sepsis. Adv Sepsis 2007;6(2):41–6.
97. Bone RC, Balk RA, Fein AM, et al. A second large controlled study of E5, a monoclonal antibody to endotoxin: results of a prospective, multicenter, randomized, controlled trial. The E5 sepsis study group. Crit Care Med 1995;23:994–1006.
98. Ziegler EJ, Fischer CJ, Sprung CL, et al. Treatment of gram-negative bacteremia and shock with HA-1A human monoclonal antibody against endotoxin. A randomized, double-blind, placebo-controlled trial. The HA-1A sepsis study group. N Engl J Med 1991;324:429–36.
99. Reinhart K, Karzai W. Anti-tumor necrosis factor therapy in sepsis: update on clinical trials and lessons learned. Crit Care Med 2001;29:S121–5.
100. Fischer CJ, Dhainaut JF, Opal SM, et al. Recombinant human interleukin 1 receptor antagonist in the treatment of patients with sepsis syndrome. Results from a randomized, double-blind, placebo-controlled trial. Phase III rhIL-1ra sepsis syndrome study group. JAMA 1994;271:1836–43.
101. Vincent JL, Sun Q, Dubois MJ. Clinical trials of immunomodulatory therapies in severe sepsis and septic shock. Clin Infect Dis 2002;34:1084–93.

The Common Immunogenic Etiology of Chronic Fatigue Syndrome: From Infections to Vaccines via Adjuvants to the ASIA Syndrome

Hemda Rosenblum, MD[a,b], Yehuda Shoenfeld, MD, FRCP[b], Howard Amital, MD, MHA[a,b],*

KEYWORDS

- Chronic fatigue syndrome • Adjuvants • Vaccinations
- Autoimmunity • ASIA syndrome

DEFINITIONS AND DIAGNOSIS

Chronic fatigue syndrome (CFS), immune dysfunction syndrome, and myalgic encephalomyelitis are the terms generally accepted by scientists and clinicians to define a large range of complaints that patients commonly refer to as CFS. The illness is characterized by persistent and unexplained fatigue that severely impairs daily functioning.

Interest in CFS increased in the early 1980s with the recognition of myalgic encephalomyelitis, a term that had been introduced 30 years earlier for an epidemic of neurologic symptoms experienced by staff at the Royal Free Hospital in London. Apart from neurologic symptoms, chronic fatigue was the main symptom of myalgic encephalomyelitis. In the absence of a recognizable cause, myalgic encephalomyelitis was referred to as a psychiatric disorder, or a 20th century illness. Since then, practitioners have disagreed on whether the illness really exists.[1]

The prevalence of CFS is difficult to quantify because of the lack of validated diagnostic tests and the heterogeneity of the CSF population.[2] CFS is a heterogeneous

a Department of Medicine B, Sheba Medical Center, Sackler Faculty of Medicine, Tel Aviv University, Ramat Aviv, Tel-Hashomer 52621, Israel
b Zabludowicz Center for Autoimmune Diseases, Sheba Medical Center, Sackler Faculty of Medicine, Tel Aviv University, Ramat Aviv, Tel-Hashomer 52621, Israel
* Corresponding author. Sheba Medical Center, Tel Hashomer, 52621 Israel.
E-mail address: hamital@netvision.net.il

Infect Dis Clin N Am 25 (2011) 851–863
doi:10.1016/j.idc.2011.07.012
0891-5520/11/$ – see front matter © 2011 Elsevier Inc. All rights reserved.

disorder affecting more than 267 per 100,000 people. The reported prevalence of CFS is 0.2% to 2.6%, with women being affected almost twice as often as men. Demographic data show that in most studies, 75% or more patients with CFS are female. A similar prevalence was found in different geographic locations and in diverse ethnic groups, with higher rates in members of minority groups and among people with lower educational attainment and occupational status.[1,3]

The mean age at onset of CFS is between 29 and 35 years. The mean illness duration ranges from 3 to 9 years. Reyes and colleagues[4] found that among white women, the prevalence of CFS increased steadily with age, reaching a maximum among those aged 50 to 59 years, and decreasing in older populations. CFS is defined by the Centers for Disease Control and Prevention as a syndrome of severe, disabling physical and mental fatigue lasting for at least 6 months, exacerbated by minimal exertion, and unexplained by a conventional medical diagnosis. Therefore, CFS is a purely subjective condition and its diagnosis is based on exclusion because no diagnostic laboratory marker or pathognomonic biopsy specimen has been identified.[5]

The origin and pathophysiology of CFS are unknown, because it has no characteristic physical signs or diagnostic laboratory abnormalities. It is defined by self-reported symptoms and disability, but only approximately 1% of patients who are diagnosed in primary care settings meet the criteria for CSF.

Patients with CSF experience disabling fatigue, headaches, concentration difficulties, and memory deficits (90%). Additional symptoms are often observed, such as sore throat (85%), tender lymph nodes (80%), skeletal muscle pain, feverishness (75%), sleep disruption (70%), psychiatric problems (65%), and rapid pulse (10%).[3] Because of these complaints, patients often have familial, social, and vocational crises.

In 1994, Fukuda and colleagues[6] proposed a method for obtaining the correct diagnosis: a patient must present with four or more symptoms concurrently for at least 6 months. Characteristics excluding patients from CFS include active medications, past or current major depressive disorders, alcohol abuse, and morbid obesity. Patients with suspected CFS must be stratified based on four criteria: (1) coexisting medical or neuropsychiatric condition not explaining the chronic fatigue, (2) level of fatigue, (3) total duration of fatigue, and (4) level of overall functional performance.[6]

CAUSES
Personality and Lifestyle

Opinions differ about classifying chronic fatigue cases with a history of psychiatric illnesses.[7] In studies comparing patients with CFS and distinct control groups, psychiatric, especially depressive, disorders were found in a minority of patients with CFS. Fatigue is part of a wide spectrum of diagnoses, ranging from a symptom in depression, anxiety, seasonal affective disorder, and multiple other diagnoses, to being a full syndromal disorder in CFS. However, CFS is undiagnosed in 80% of cases and is often misdiagnosed as depression.[8]

In a review of personality characteristics, neuroticism and introversion have been reported as risk factors for the disorder. Inactivity in childhood and after infectious mononucleosis have been found to increase the risk of CFS in adults.[9–12] Serious life events, such as the loss of a loved one or a job, and other stressful situations have been found to precipitate the disorder.[1,13,14]

Viner and Hotopf[15] explored whether childhood risk factors were associated with a lifetime risk of developing CFS by the age of 30 years. Prematurity, birth order, obesity, atopy, chronic limiting conditions, high exercise levels, school factors, and psychological factors, including poor maternal mental health and childhood behavior problems, have all been proposed as possibly associated with the lifetime risk of CFS. The investigators found no association between childhood or adolescent behavioral or psychological morbidity and the risk of self-reported CFS by the age of 30 years. Children at greater risk for CFS had higher socioeconomic backgrounds, rarely played sports, and had longstanding, limiting physical or mental conditions other than CFS.

In contradistinction, Rangel and colleagues[16] found that CFS in childhood and adolescence was associated with higher levels of parental mental distress, emotional involvement, and family illness burden than those observed in association with juvenile rheumatoid arthritis, a chronic pediatric physical illness.

Endicott[17] described stressors, including earlier mortality and increased prevalence of cancer, autoimmune disorders, and CFS-like conditions, in parents of psychiatric patients with CFS compared with control groups. Childhood trauma was associated with a 3- to 8-fold increased risk for CFS across different trauma types in one study.[18] Sleep is also a causal factor, with many patients who have sleep disorders showing greater functional impairment independent of their psychiatric disorder.[19–21]

Infections

Many patients report an acute onset of symptoms after an infectious illness.[1] Three-quarters of patients with CFS reported an infection, such as a cold, flu-like illness, or infectious mononucleosis, as the trigger.[22] The sudden onset of the syndrome, and the symptoms of myalgia, arthralgia, sore throat, and tender lymphadenopathy, support theories of infection-related illness.[23,24] Infections have important causal roles, and have been considered predictors of better prognosis compared with CFS that has a noninfectious origin.[25]

CFS was first described in the 1980s and was thought to be the consequence of a viral or bacterial infection. One of the first suspected pathogens was Epstein-Barr virus (EBV). Various viruses have been shown to play a triggering or perpetuating role, or both, in this disease. Microbes that have been shown to trigger CFS include enteroviruses, EBV, *Chlamydia pneumoniae*, parvovirus B19, *Coxiella burnetii*, Borna disease virus, varicella-zoster virus, cytomegalovirus, and herpes virus type 6. Chronic microbial infections documented in patients with CFS include *C brunetii*, parvovirus B19, *C pneumonia*, hepatitis C, enterovirus, and human retroviruses. Virus reactivations include varicella zoster, herpes simplex, and EBV.[26–29]

Earlier studies showed raised antibody titers and viral RNA in blood and muscle biopsy specimens of patients with CFS compared with normal controls.[26,30–35] Chia and Chia[28] investigated the presence of enterovirus protein and RNA, and culturable viruses in stomach biopsies of patients with CFS. Of 165 patients with CFS who underwent upper gastrointestinal endoscopies and antrum biopsies, 135 biopsies (82%) stained positive for viral capsid protein 1 within parietal cells, whereas 7 of 34 (20%) of the controls stained positive ($P<.001$). EBV RNA was detected in 37% of samples, whereas fewer than 5% of controls had detectable enterovirus RNA ($P<.01$). A significant subset of patients with CFS may have a chronic, disseminated form of enteroviral infection, which could be diagnosed by stomach biopsy. These findings correlate with the high percentage of patients with CFS who have gastrointestinal complaints.

Recent implications indicated a possible linkage between a human gammaretrovirus—xenotropic murine leukemia virus–related virus (XMRV) infection—and CFS. A study of peripheral blood mononuclear cells from patients with CFS showed viral DNA in 68 of 101 patients (67%) compared with 8 of 218 (3.7%) healthy controls. Additionally, patient-derived XMRV was shown to be infectious, and both cell-associated and cell-free transmission of the virus were shown to be possible.[36]

Gene Expression

No clear association between gene expression and individual symptom domains has been found, suggesting that CFS symptomatology probably cannot be elucidated by individual laboratory tests or gene expression.[37]

Twin studies have shown a familial predisposition. The concordance rate was higher in monozygotic than in dizygotic female twins for chronic fatigue[38]; but no genetic abnormalities have been found.[1] Hickie and colleagues[39] evaluated genetic and environmental determinants of prolonged fatigue in a twin study and found that 44% (95% CI, 25–60) of the genetic variance for fatigue was not shared by other forms of psychological distress, and also that environmental factors made negligible contributions to fatigue. On the other hand, Cho and colleagues[40] found evidence of a partly genetic influence, but environmental effects continued to predominate.

A study by Smith and colleagues[41] that did not include twins found that CFS might be associated with human leukocyte antigen (HLA)-DQA1*01, but this needs to be confirmed in a larger and independent cohort. Ortega-Hernandez and colleagues[42] showed that in CFS, like other autoimmune diseases, different genetic features are likely related to age at onset and symptoms. For example, age at CFS onset during the third decade of life was associated with the serotonin receptor AA genotype and the HLA-DRB1*03 allele, whereas episodes of unexplained fever were associated with myalgia.

Immune System

Patients with CFS have an immune imbalance represented by decreased functioning of K cells and macrophages, reduced mitogenic response of lymphocytes, IgG subclass deficiencies, and decreased complement levels, including studies in monozygotic twins.[43,44] However no evidence of a clear link between abnormal immunity and CFS has been established.[45,46] Other abnormal findings identified in patients with CFS include abnormal natural killer cell cytotoxicity, increased immune activation markers, greater numbers of CD16/CD3 natural killer cells, and the presence of interferon in serum and CSF. Clues also suggest that a loss of immunologic tolerance to vasoactive neuropeptides or their receptors occurs after infection, either as part as other immune mediated disorders or as a de novo mechanism.[24,47–50]

Nishikai[51] showed that patients with CFS have specific antinuclear antibodies against the anti-68/48kD protein. Some groups of young patients with CFS (age, 18–29 years) were shown to present with antibodies to single-stranded DNA. However, no association was found between CFS and Sm, U1-RNP, SS-A/Ro, SS-B/Ro, Scl-70, and centromere antibodies.[52]

Neuroendocrine Factors

Evaluation of (HPA) axis abnormalities have been studied as potential biologic tests to diagnose CFS. Neuroendocrine challenge tests among patients with CFS have found a lower than normal cortisol response to increased corticotrophin concentrations and up-regulation of the serotonergic system. Studies also showed higher chronic adrenocorticotropic hormone (ACTH) autoantibody levels as significant pathologic factors in CFS.[25,53–55] The low cortisol levels may be secondary to the physical inactivity and sleep disturbances found with long-standing CFS.[56]

Reduced area under the ACTH response curve in patients with CFS undergoing insulin tolerance testing was significantly associated with the duration of CFS symptoms ($P = .05$) and the severity of fatigue symptomatology.[57] Other studies have suggested up-regulation of hypothalamic 5-hydroxytryptamine receptors in patients with postviral fatigue syndrome but not in those with primary depression.[58]

Abnormalities in the stress response have been identified as potential triggers or mediators of CFS symptoms. Hence, Fletcher and colleagues[27] studied the stress mediator neuropeptide (NPY), assuming that it would be a useful biomarker for CFS. NPY is found in both the central and peripheral nervous systems. In the peripheral system, it is concentrated in and released from sympathetic nerve endings, either alone or with catecholamines. In the peripheral nervous system, NPY activates and stimulates the stress response, but in the brain, it is anxiolytic, inhibits sympathetic activity, and decreases blood pressure and heart rate.[59,60] The investigators showed that NPY in the plasma of patients with CFS is significantly elevated over that of healthy controls, and this elevation is associated with severity of stress, negative mood, and clinical symptoms.

Exercise

Patients with CFS have increased fatigue after physical exertion and cannot exercise as much as healthy controls.[61] Cytokines have been hypothesized to mediate some of the symptoms and immunologic disturbances,[49,62] but this has not been proven, except for one cytokine, transforming growth factor ß (TGF-ß). Higher levels of TGF-ß were found in patients with CFS immediately and within 40 minutes after mild exercise.[63] In addition, studies showed alterations in muscle excitability, which can cause postexercise oxidative stress, explaining muscle pain and postexertional malaise reported by the patients. The oxidative stress can be generated by a lower maximal aerobic capacity and a reduced baseline oxygen uptake by tissues in patients with CFS.[64–66] MacDonald and colleagues[67] also suggested that higher levels of routine exercise may precipitate or exacerbate CFS.

On the other hand, Viner and Hotopf[15] found that children who routinely played more sports in their spare time had a significantly lower risk of CFS, a finding that was independent of potential confounding by limiting chronic illness or obesity and was also robust to adjustments for sex and socioeconomic status. Children who were sedentary at 10 years of age had approximately twice the risk for lifetime CFS. Hours of sports played at school were not associated with risk of CFS, suggesting that the protective effect of exercise lies within the individual and family rather than timed school activities.

THERAPY AND PROGNOSIS

The duration of follow-up of prognostic studies ranged from 1 to 5 years. The median recovery rate was 5% (range, 0%–31%) and the median improvement rate 39.5% (range, 8%–63%). Less-severe fatigue at baseline and the patient's not attributing the illness to physical causes were predictive of better outcome, whereas psychiatric disorders predicted poorer outcomes.[1]

Cognitive behavioral therapy (CBT) and graded exercise therapy (GET) are the only interventions found to be beneficial, especially in conjunction with other treatment modalities and compared with other relaxation procedures as controls.[68–71]

CBT is a general form of psychotherapy directed at changing condition-related cognitions and behaviors. It has been effective in treating symptoms of fatigue, mood, and physical fitness; some studies showed limited effect on pain.[72] CBT for depression has not been effective for patients with CFS, nor did it show improvement in cognitive function or quality of life.

Central CBT components for CFS include explanation of the causal model, motivation for CBT, challenging and changing fatigue-related cognitions, achievement and maintenance of a basic amount of physical activity, gradual increase in physical activity, and planning work rehabilitation among other personal activities. CBT teaches patients with CFS how to acquire control over symptoms.

GET is a form of physical therapy. CBT for CFS is based on a behavioral model of avoidance and always includes a graded activity program. GET is based on a physiologic model of deconditioning and has no intention to explicitly treat cognitions. In a few GET studies, cognitions to encourage graded exercise have been modified. CBT is generally a more complex treatment than GET, which might explain why CBT studies show better improvement rates (approximately 70%) than those with GET (approximately 55%).

Pacing is an energy management strategy that encourages behavioral change while acknowledging patient fluctuations in symptom severity and delayed exercise recovery. Patients are advised to set manageable daily activity/exercise goals and balance activity and rest to avoid overexertion, which may worsen symptoms. Those able to function within their individual limits are encouraged to gradually increase activity and exercise levels while maintaining established energy management techniques. The goal is to gradually increase the individual's level of routine functioning.

The subtle changes found in the HPA axis have led to two randomized controlled trials involving adding low-dose steroids, which provided no clinical benefit. Based on these, researchers have not concluded that steroids are the preferred treatment.[73,74]

Antidepressants are the most common medications used in this regard. Selegiline had a small but significant therapeutic effect independent of its antidepressant effect. Fluoxetine was shown to improve overall symptoms and measures of immune function in one study but not in others.[75–77] Moclobemide showed significant but small reductions in fatigue, depression, anxiety, and somatic amplification, and a modest overall improvement.[78]

For immunologic interventions, such as intravenous immunoglobulin administration, the evidence has been inconclusive.[79] No therapeutic effects were found for natural killer cell stimulant and antiviral substances.[80,81]

Hence, the big challenge is to develop an effective and holistic model therapy for CFS based on the biopsychosocial model that integrates strategies such as CBT and GET and molecular and biologic treatments.

ASIA: AUTOIMMUNE/INFLAMMATORY SYNDROME INDUCED BY ADJUVANTS

The characterization of the ASIA syndrome (auto-inflammatory syndrome induced by adjuvants) is an attempt to classify the ill-defined collection of signs and symptoms that often occur together in certain individuals after exposure to adjuvants. An immunologic adjuvant is a substance that enhances antigen-specific immune response, preferably without triggering one on its own.[82] This new syndrome subsumes four well-known medical conditions, namely postvaccination adverse events, exposure to silicone implants, the Gulf War syndrome, and macrophagic myofasciitis, all of which share similar clinical manifestations and involve previous exposure to immune adjuvants.[82]

The activation of an autoimmune mechanism by infectious agents is common, and on rare occasions, similar to infectious agents, vaccines can induce the appearance of autoantibodies, enigmatic inflammatory conditions, and overt autoimmune disease.[82,83] The same mechanisms may trigger an autoimmune response in some susceptible individuals, regardless of whether exposure was to an infectious agent or a vaccine.[84,85]

In the past decade, the plausible association between vaccines, silicone, and other environmental factors with immune-mediated conditions has raised concerns addressed by the medical and legal communities.[83] Despite the numerous publications covering this issue, a clear cause-and-effect relationship between vaccinations and autoinflammatory disorders has been difficult to prove.[86–89]

Vaccine administration has been reported to precede the development of CFS and fibromyalgia. Fatigue has been observed in a third of people vaccinated against hepatitis B virus, and at least 30 cases of CFS were associated with hepatitis B vaccine within 3 months of vaccination.[90,91]

Silicone may be considered an adjuvant to the immune system. Adverse events related to silicone were termed in the 1990s *the adjuvant disease* and included weakness, fatigue, myalgia, arthralgia, and loss of myelinated nerve fibers.[92] The relationship among silicone breast implants, autoimmunity, and CFS has been the focus of considerable debate. Although the association between silicone exposure and a definite connective tissue disorder was difficult to establish, the induction of silicon-associated disease that combines autoimmune manifestations and central sensitivity syndromes has been strongly supported by numerous studies. These adverse events are further aggravated by silicone leaks beyond the capsular boundaries.[85] CFS is documented in up to 71% of women with silicone breast implants, and most women with silicone-associated disorder have CFS or fibromyalgia-like syndrome.[93]

Another epidemiologic obstacle to recognizing this potential association is the time between exposure to a plausible trigger and the appearance or diagnosis of a medical condition. Latency periods of several weeks are commonly accepted based on the classical time from the diagnosis of a streptococcal infection to the emergence of rheumatic fever.[94] However, reports indicating periods lasting months and even years after exposure have been published.[94,95]

The most evaluated postvaccination condition is the macrophagic myofasciitis syndrome, a rare immune-mediated condition.[96] It is caused by deposition of aluminum used to adjuvant different vaccines, which cause an immune-mediated muscle disease. Macrophagic myofasciitis syndrome is characterized by systemic signs and symptoms and an active lesion at the site of inoculation.[97,98] Systemic manifestations include myalgias, arthralgia, marked asthenia, muscle weakness, chronic fatigue, fever, and sometimes the appearance of a demyelinating disorder. Additionally, elevated creatine kinase and the appearance of autoantibodies and myopathic electromyogram changes have been documented.[97,98]

Also implicated in the adjuvant effect is the Gulf War syndrome. Hotopf and colleagues[99] postulated that Gulf War syndrome, which combines CFS and other manifestations, is the result of multiple vaccinations that induced a chronic Th-2 immune response.

The mechanisms through which ASIA-related symptoms are triggered (ie, cognitive impairment, joint pain) are not fully understood. Epidemiologic studies have shown poor performance in cognitive tests and a higher abundance of neurologic symptoms among workers who were occupationally exposed to aluminum.[100,101]

Adjuvants may play a major role in inducing the ASIA manifestations. However, whether concomitant exposure to adjuvants or infections fulfill a "second hit" that triggers this mechanism is unknown. The author (Y.S.) suggests a set of criteria that helps determine a possible role of adjuvant/vaccination-induced symptomatology, the ASIA syndrome (**Fig. 1**).

Criteria suggested by Shoenfeld for ASIA diagnosis

Major criteria:
- Exposure to an external stimuli (infection, vaccine, silicone, or adjuvant) prior to clinical manifestations
- Appearance of one of the clinical manifestations listed below:
  - Myalgia, myositis, or muscular weakness
  - Arthralgia and/or arthritis
  - Chronic fatigue, non-restful sleep, or sleep disturbances
  - Neurological manifestations (especially those associated with demyelization)
  - Cognitive alterations and loss of memory
  - Fever and dry mouth
- Removal of the initiating agent induces improvement
- Typical biopsy of the involved organs

Minor criteria:
- Appearance of autoantibodies directed against the suspected adjuvant
- Other clinical manifestations (e.g., irritable bowel syndrome)
- Specific HLA (e.g., HLA DRB1, HLA DQB1)
- Initiation of an autoimmune illness (e.g., multiple sclerosis or systemic sclerosis)

Fig. 1. For the diagnosis of ASIA, the presence of at least two major or one major and two minor criteria must be apparent.

REFERENCES

1. Prins JB, van der Meer JW, Bleijenberg G. Chronic fatigue syndrome. Lancet 2006;367:346–55.
2. Michiels V, Cluydts R. Neuropsychological functioning in chronic fatigue syndrome: a review. Acta Psychiatr Scand 2001;103:84–93.
3. Bassi N, Amital D, Amital H, et al. Chronic fatigue syndrome: characteristics and possible causes for its pathogenesis. Isr Med Assoc J 2008;10:79–82.
4. Reyes M, Nisenbaum R, Hoaglin DC, et al. Prevalence and incidence of chronic fatigue syndrome in Wichita, Kansas. Arch Intern Med 2003;163:1530–6.
5. Working Group of the Royal Australasian College of Physicians. Chronic fatigue syndrome. Clinical practice guidelines—2002. Med J Aust 2002;176(Suppl): S23–56.
6. Fukuda K, Straus SE, Hickie I, et al. The chronic fatigue syndrome: a comprehensive approach to its definition and study. International Chronic Fatigue Syndrome Study Group. Ann Intern Med 1994;121:953–9.
7. Matthews DA, Lane TJ, Manu P. Definition of the chronic fatigue syndrome. Ann Intern Med 1988;109:511–2.
8. Griffith JP, Zarrouf FA. A systematic review of chronic fatigue syndrome: don't assume it's depression. Prim Care Companion J Clin Psychiatry 2008;10:120–8.
9. Candy B, Chalder T, Cleare AJ, et al. A randomised controlled trial of a psycho-educational intervention to aid recovery in infectious mononucleosis. J Psychosom Res 2004;57:89–94.
10. Katz BZ, Shiraishi Y, Mears CJ, et al. Chronic fatigue syndrome after infectious mononucleosis in adolescents. Pediatrics 2009;124:189–93.
11. Moss-Morris R, Spence MJ, Hou R. The pathway from glandular fever to chronic fatigue syndrome: can the cognitive behavioural model provide the map? Psychol Med 2011;41:1099–107.
12. Vollmer-Conna U. Chronic fatigue syndrome in adolescence: where to from here? Arch Pediatr Adolesc Med 2010;164:880–1.

13. Harvey SB, Wessely S, Kuh D, et al. The relationship between fatigue and psychiatric disorders: evidence for the concept of neurasthenia. J Psychosom Res 2009;66:445–54.
14. Hatcher S, House A. Life events, difficulties and dilemmas in the onset of chronic fatigue syndrome: a case-control study. Psychol Med 2003;33:1185–92.
15. Viner R, Hotopf M. Childhood predictors of self reported chronic fatigue syndrome/myalgic encephalomyelitis in adults: national birth cohort study. BMJ 2004;329:941.
16. Rangel L, Garralda ME, Jeffs J, et al. Family health and characteristics in chronic fatigue syndrome, juvenile rheumatoid arthritis, and emotional disorders of childhood. J Am Acad Child Adolesc Psychiatry 2005;44:150–8.
17. Endicott NA. Chronic fatigue syndrome in private practice psychiatry: family history of physical and mental health. J Psychosom Res 1999;47:343–54.
18. Heim C, Wagner D, Maloney E, et al. Early adverse experience and risk for chronic fatigue syndrome: results from a population-based study. Arch Gen Psychiatry 2006;63:1258–66.
19. Morriss R, Sharpe M, Sharpley AL, et al. Abnormalities of sleep in patients with the chronic fatigue syndrome. BMJ 1993;306:1161–4.
20. Morriss RK, Wearden AJ, Battersby L. The relation of sleep difficulties to fatigue, mood and disability in chronic fatigue syndrome. J Psychosom Res 1997;42:597–605.
21. Friedlander AH, Mahler ME, Yagiela JA. Restless legs syndrome: manifestations, treatment and dental implications. J Am Dent Assoc 2006;137:755–61.
22. Salit IE. Precipitating factors for the chronic fatigue syndrome. J Psychiatr Res 1997;31:59–65.
23. Evengard B, Jonzon E, Sandberg A, et al. Differences between patients with chronic fatigue syndrome and with chronic fatigue at an infectious disease clinic in Stockholm, Sweden. Psychiatry Clin Neurosci 2003;57:361–8.
24. Klimas NG, Salvato FR, Morgan R, et al. Immunologic abnormalities in chronic fatigue syndrome. J Clin Microbiol 1990;28:1403–10.
25. Masuda A, Nakayama T, Yamanaka T, et al. The prognosis after multidisciplinary treatment for patients with postinfectious chronic fatigue syndrome and noninfectious chronic fatigue syndrome. J Behav Med 2002;25:487–97.
26. Lane RJ, Soteriou BA, Zhang H, et al. Enterovirus related metabolic myopathy: a postviral fatigue syndrome. J Neurol Neurosurg Psychiatry 2003;74:1382–6.
27. Fletcher MA, Rosenthal M, Antoni M, et al. Plasma neuropeptide Y: a biomarker for symptom severity in chronic fatigue syndrome. Behav Brain Funct 2010;6:76.
28. Chia JK, Chia AY. Chronic fatigue syndrome is associated with chronic enterovirus infection of the stomach. J Clin Pathol 2008;61:43–8.
29. Appel S, Chapman J, Shoenfeld Y. Infection and vaccination in chronic fatigue syndrome: myth or reality? Autoimmunity 2007;40:48–53.
30. Chia JK. The role of enterovirus in chronic fatigue syndrome. J Clin Pathol 2005;58:1126–32.
31. Yousef GE, Bell EJ, Mann GF, et al. Chronic enterovirus infection in patients with postviral fatigue syndrome. Lancet 1988;1:146–50.
32. Cunningham L, Bowles NE, Lane RJ, et al. Persistence of enteroviral RNA in chronic fatigue syndrome is associated with the abnormal production of equal amounts of positive and negative strands of enteroviral RNA. J Gen Virol 1990;71(Pt 6):1399–402.

33. Galbraith DN, Nairn C, Clements GB. Phylogenetic analysis of short enteroviral sequences from patients with chronic fatigue syndrome. J Gen Virol 1995; 76(Pt 7):1701–7.

34. Douche-Aourik F, Berlier W, Feasson L, et al. Detection of enterovirus in human skeletal muscle from patients with chronic inflammatory muscle disease or fibromyalgia and healthy subjects. J Med Virol 2003;71:540–7.

35. Kerr JR. Enterovirus infection of the stomach in chronic fatigue syndrome/myalgic encephalomyelitis. J Clin Pathol 2008;61:1–2.

36. Lombardi VC, Ruscetti FW, Das GJ, et al. Detection of an infectious retrovirus, XMRV, in blood cells of patients with chronic fatigue syndrome. Science 2009; 326:585–9.

37. Fostel J, Boneva R, Lloyd A. Exploration of the gene expression correlates of chronic unexplained fatigue using factor analysis. Pharmacogenomics 2006;7: 441–54.

38. Buchwald D, Herrell R, Ashton S, et al. A twin study of chronic fatigue. Psychosom Med 2001;63:936–43.

39. Hickie I, Kirk K, Martin N. Unique genetic and environmental determinants of prolonged fatigue: a twin study. Psychol Med 1999;29:259–68.

40. Cho HJ, Skowera A, Cleare A, et al. Chronic fatigue syndrome: an update focusing on phenomenology and pathophysiology. Curr Opin Psychiatry 2006; 19:67–73.

41. Smith J, Fritz EL, Kerr JR, et al. Association of chronic fatigue syndrome with human leucocyte antigen class II alleles. J Clin Pathol 2005;58:860–3.

42. Ortega-Hernandez OD, Cuccia M, Bozzini S, et al. Autoantibodies, polymorphisms in the serotonin pathway, and human leukocyte antigen class II alleles in chronic fatigue syndrome: are they associated with age at onset and specific symptoms? Ann N Y Acad Sci 2009;1173:589–99.

43. Bates DW, Buchwald D, Lee J, et al. Clinical laboratory test findings in patients with chronic fatigue syndrome. Arch Intern Med 1995;155:97–103.

44. Sabath DE, Barcy S, Koelle DM, et al. Cellular immunity in monozygotic twins discordant for chronic fatigue syndrome. J Infect Dis 2002;185:828–32.

45. Lorusso L, Mikhaylova SV, Capelli E, et al. Immunological aspects of chronic fatigue syndrome. Autoimmun Rev 2009;8:287–91.

46. Rasmussen AK, Nielsen H, Andersen V, et al. Chronic fatigue syndrome– a controlled cross sectional study. J Rheumatol 1994;21:1527–31.

47. Landay AL, Jessop C, Lennette ET, et al. Chronic fatigue syndrome: clinical condition associated with immune activation. Lancet 1991;338:707–12.

48. Robertson MJ, Schacterle RS, Mackin GA, et al. Lymphocyte subset differences in patients with chronic fatigue syndrome, multiple sclerosis and major depression. Clin Exp Immunol 2005;141:326–32.

49. Lloyd A, Hickie I, Brockman A, et al. Cytokine levels in serum and cerebrospinal fluid in patients with chronic fatigue syndrome and control subjects. J Infect Dis 1991;164:1023–4.

50. Staines DR. Postulated vasoactive neuropeptide autoimmunity in fatigue-related conditions: a brief review and hypothesis. Clin Dev Immunol 2006; 13:25–39.

51. Nishikai M. Antinuclear antibodies in patients with chronic fatigue syndrome. Nippon Rinsho 2007;65:1067–70 [in Japanese].

52. Vernon SD, Reeves WC. Evaluation of autoantibodies to common and neuronal cell antigens in Chronic Fatigue Syndrome. J Autoimmune Dis 2005;2:5.

53. Wheatland R. Chronic ACTH autoantibodies are a significant pathological factor in the disruption of the hypothalamic-pituitary-adrenal axis in chronic fatigue syndrome, anorexia nervosa and major depression. Med Hypotheses 2005; 65:287–95.

54. Gottschalk M, Kumpfel T, Flachenecker P, et al. Fatigue and regulation of the hypothalamo-pituitary-adrenal axis in multiple sclerosis. Arch Neurol 2005;62: 277–80.

55. Wessely S. The neuropsychiatry of chronic fatigue syndrome. Ciba Found Symp 1993;173:212–29.

56. Cleare AJ. The HPA axis and the genesis of chronic fatigue syndrome. Trends Endocrinol Metab 2004;15:55–9.

57. Gaab J, Engert V, Heitz V, et al. Associations between neuroendocrine responses to the Insulin Tolerance Test and patient characteristics in chronic fatigue syndrome. J Psychosom Res 2004;56:419–24.

58. Bakheit AM, Behan PO, Dinan TG, et al. Possible upregulation of hypothalamic 5-hydroxytryptamine receptors in patients with postviral fatigue syndrome. BMJ 1992;304:1010–2.

59. Kuo LE, Abe K, Zukowska Z. Stress, NPY and vascular remodeling: implications for stress-related diseases. Peptides 2007;28:435–40.

60. Kuo LE, Kitlinska JB, Tilan JU, et al. Neuropeptide Y acts directly in the periphery on fat tissue and mediates stress-induced obesity and metabolic syndrome. Nat Med 2007;13:803–11.

61. Peterson PK, Schenck CH, Sherman R. Chronic fatigue syndrome in Minnesota. Minn Med 1991;74:21–6.

62. Holmes GP, Kaplan JE, Gantz NM, et al. Chronic fatigue syndrome: a working case definition. Ann Intern Med 1988;108:387–9.

63. Peterson PK, Sirr SA, Grammith FC, et al. Effects of mild exercise on cytokines and cerebral blood flow in chronic fatigue syndrome patients. Clin Diagn Lab Immunol 1994;1:222–6.

64. Fulle S, Belia S, Vecchiet J, et al. Modification of the functional capacity of sarco-plasmic reticulum membranes in patients suffering from chronic fatigue syndrome. Neuromuscul Disord 2003;13:479–84.

65. Murphy ME, Kehrer JP. Oxidative stress and muscular dystrophy. Chem Biol Interact 1989;69:101–73.

66. Jammes Y, Steinberg JG, Mambrini O, et al. Chronic fatigue syndrome: assessment of increased oxidative stress and altered muscle excitability in response to incremental exercise. J Intern Med 2005;257:299–310.

67. MacDonald KL, Osterholm MT, LeDell KH, et al. A case-control study to assess possible triggers and cofactors in chronic fatigue syndrome. Am J Med 1996; 100:548–54.

68. Price JR, Couper J. Cognitive behaviour therapy for adults with chronic fatigue syndrome. Cochrane Database Syst Rev 2000;2:CD001027.

69. Akagi H, Klimes I, Bass C. Cognitive behavioral therapy for chronic fatigue syndrome in a general hospital–feasible and effective. Gen Hosp Psychiatry 2001;23:254–60.

70. Deale A, Husain K, Chalder T, et al. Long-term outcome of cognitive behavior therapy versus relaxation therapy for chronic fatigue syndrome: a 5-year follow-up study. Am J Psychiatry 2001;158:2038–42.

71. Deale A, Chalder T, Marks I, et al. Cognitive behavior therapy for chronic fatigue syndrome: a randomized controlled trial. Am J Psychiatry 1997;154:408–14.

72. O'Dowd H, Gladwell P, Rogers CA, et al. Cognitive behavioural therapy in chronic fatigue syndrome: a randomised controlled trial of an outpatient group programme. Health Technol Assess 2006;10:iii–iix, 1.
73. Cleare AJ, Heap E, Malhi GS, et al. Low-dose hydrocortisone in chronic fatigue syndrome: a randomised crossover trial. Lancet 1999;353:455–8.
74. McKenzie R, O'Fallon A, Dale J, et al. Low-dose hydrocortisone for treatment of chronic fatigue syndrome: a randomized controlled trial. JAMA 1998;280: 1061–6.
75. Vercoulen JH, Swanink CM, Zitman FG, et al. Randomised, double-blind, placebo-controlled study of fluoxetine in chronic fatigue syndrome. Lancet 1996;347:858–61.
76. Natelson BH, Cheu J, Hill N, et al. Single-blind, placebo phase-in trial of two escalating doses of selegiline in the chronic fatigue syndrome. Neuropsychobiology 1998;37:150–4.
77. Wearden AJ, Morriss RK, Mullis R, et al. Randomised, double-blind, placebo-controlled treatment trial of fluoxetine and graded exercise for chronic fatigue syndrome. Br J Psychiatry 1998;172:485–90.
78. White PD, Cleary KJ. An open study of the efficacy and adverse effects of moclobemide in patients with the chronic fatigue syndrome. Int Clin Psychopharmacol 1997;12:47–52.
79. Vollmer-Conna U, Hickie I, Hadzi-Pavlovic D, et al. Intravenous immunoglobulin is ineffective in the treatment of patients with chronic fatigue syndrome. Am J Med 1997;103:38–43.
80. Williams G, Waterhouse J, Mugarza J, et al. Therapy of circadian rhythm disorders in chronic fatigue syndrome: no symptomatic improvement with melatonin or phototherapy. Eur J Clin Invest 2002;32:831–7.
81. McDermott C, Richards SC, Thomas PW, et al. A placebo-controlled, double-blind, randomized controlled trial of a natural killer cell stimulant (BioBran MGN-3) in chronic fatigue syndrome. QJM 2006;99:461–8.
82. Shoenfeld Y, gmon-Levin N. 'ASIA' – autoimmune/inflammatory syndrome induced by adjuvants. J Autoimmun 2011;36:4–8.
83. gmon-Levin N, Zafrir Y, Paz Z, et al. Ten cases of systemic lupus erythematosus related to hepatitis B vaccine. Lupus 2009;18:1192–7.
84. Altman A, Szyper-Kravitz M, Shoenfeld Y. HBV vaccine and dermatomyositis: is there an association? Rheumatol Int 2008;28:609–12.
85. Nancy AL, Shoenfeld Y. Chronic fatigue syndrome with autoantibodies–the result of an augmented adjuvant effect of hepatitis-B vaccine and silicone implant. Autoimmun Rev 2008;8:52–5.
86. Sanchez-Guerrero J, Colditz GA, Karlson EW, et al. Silicone breast implants and the risk of connective-tissue diseases and symptoms. N Engl J Med 1995;332: 1666–70.
87. Bryant H, Brasher P. Breast implants and breast cancer–reanalysis of a linkage study. N Engl J Med 1995;332:1535–9.
88. Angell M. Do breast implants cause systemic disease? Science in the courtroom. N Engl J Med 1994;330:1748–9.
89. Kessler DA. The basis of the FDA's decision on breast implants. N Engl J Med 1992;326:1713–5.
90. House A. Alleged link between hepatitis B vaccine and chronic fatigue syndrome. CMAJ 1992;146:1145.
91. Halperin SA, Dobson S, McNeil S, et al. Comparison of the safety and immunogenicity of hepatitis B virus surface antigen co-administered with an

immunostimulatory phosphorothioate oligonucleotide and a licensed hepatitis B vaccine in healthy young adults. Vaccine 2006;24:20–6.

92. Shoaib BO, Patten BM. Human adjuvant disease: presentation as a multiple sclerosis-like syndrome. South Med J 1996;89:179–88.

93. Vasey FB, Zarabadi SA, Seleznick M, et al. Where there's smoke there's fire: the silicone breast implant controversy continues to flicker: a new disease that needs to be defined. J Rheumatol 2003;30:2092–4.

94. Kivity S, Fireman E, Greif J, et al. Effect of budesonide on bronchial hyperresponsiveness and pulmonary function in patients with mild to moderate asthma. Ann Allergy 1994;72:333–6.

95. Arbuckle MR, McClain MT, Rubertone MV, et al. Development of autoantibodies before the clinical onset of systemic lupus erythematosus. N Engl J Med 2003; 349:1526–33.

96. Gherardi RK, Coquet M, Cherin P, et al. Macrophagic myofasciitis: an emerging entity. Groupe d'Etudes et Recherche sur les Maladies Musculaires Acquises et Dysimmunitaires (GERMMAD) de l'Association Francaise contre les Myopathies (AFM). Lancet 1998;352:347–52.

97. Exley C, Swarbrick L, Gherardi RK, et al. A role for the body burden of aluminium in vaccine-associated macrophagic myofasciitis and chronic fatigue syndrome. Med Hypotheses 2009;72:135–9.

98. Gherardi RK, Coquet M, Cherin P, et al. Macrophagic myofasciitic lesions assess long-term persistence of vaccine-derived aluminium hydroxide in muscle. Brain 2001;124:1821–31.

99. Hotopf M, David A, Hull L, et al. Role of vaccinations as risk factors for ill health in veterans of the Gulf war: cross sectional study. BMJ 2000;320:1363–7.

100. Kumar V, Bal A, Gill KD. Impairment of mitochondrial energy metabolism in different regions of rat brain following chronic exposure to aluminium. Brain Res 2008;1232:94–103.

101. Kumar V, Gill KD. Aluminium neurotoxicity: neurobehavioural and oxidative aspects. Arch Toxicol 2009;83:965–78.

Mycobacteria and Biological Response Modifiers: Two Sides of the Relationship

Vidya Sundareshan, MD, MPH[a],*, Jignesh Modi, MD[a],
Nancy Misri Khardori, MD, PhD[b]

KEYWORDS

- Mycobacteria • Biological response modifiers • Reactivation
- Adjunct therapy

Tuberculosis (TB) is one of the oldest diseases known to mankind; humans have adapted to the disease as advances in medicine have been made. Because of its complex immunology, involving the organism and the host, newer treatment modalities in various fields of medicine have affected the outcome of this infection and have caused resurgence of the disease. What makes tuberculosis unique from an epidemiologic standpoint is the large reservoir of infection, consisting of approximately one-third of the world's population.[1] A recent study from Boston showed that overall rates of reactivation TB in that area have declined from 0.10 to 0.16 cases per 100 person-years in the 1950s to 0.040 cases per 100 person-years recently, but reactivation has increased among those individuals older than 50 years (rate ratio [RR], 3.8) and among those born in the United States (RR, 3.2).[2] About 9.2 million new cases of active disease arise every year (roughly 10% of the infected reservoir), many of which are believed to be reactivation disease.[3,4] Some of the causes for reactivation due to immunocompromise include HIV infection, advancing age, use of corticosteroids, organ transplantation (renal, cardiac, liver, and allogenic stem cell), and, more recently, increasing worldwide use of biological response modifiers (BRMs) for the treatment of systemic inflammatory diseases with tissue destruction, particularly rheumatoid arthritis.[5–8] Although BRMs are effective drugs that have revolutionized the treatment of these diseases, there exist considerable adverse effects of BRMs including reactivation of several latent infections. Therefore, their efficacy in disease control needs to be balanced against the risk of development of serious infections,

The authors have nothing to disclose.

[a] Division of Infectious Diseases, Southern Illinois University School of Medicine, 801 North Rutledge, PO 9636, Springfield, IL-62794, USA

[b] Division of Infectious Disease, Eastern Virginia Medical School, 825 Fairfox Avenue, Norfolk, VA 23507, USA

* Corresponding author.

E-mail address: vsundareshan@siumed.edu

Infect Dis Clin N Am 25 (2011) 865–893

doi:10.1016/j.idc.2011.07.010

0891-5520/11/$ – see front matter Published by Elsevier Inc.

id.theclinics.com

particularly TB.[9] The future in treatment of inflammatory diseases includes increased use of recombinant human antiinflammatory cytokines, agents targeting proinflammatory cytokines, and granulocyte-macrophage colony-stimulating factors. The risk of developing reactivation disease with the increased and improved or newer treatment modalities for inflammatory conditions needs to be considered. However, many in vitro and a few in vivo studies have reported benefits of certain BRMs in treatment of TB as adjuncts.[10,11] This article summarizes the different aspects of the relationship between mycobacterial infections and the use of various BRMs (**Table 1**).

IMMUNOLOGY OF TUBERCULOSIS

Only 10% of people infected with *Mycobacterium tuberculosis* develop active disease.[3] For this effective control, innate and adaptive immune responses of the host are operative in mycobacterial infections. Multiple bacterial and host factors determine the outcome of either latent tuberculosis infection (LTBI) or active disease.[12] The immunology of early disease is still not well understood. Mouse studies indicate that the cell type infected initially with *M tuberculosis* is the myeloid dendritic cell (**Fig. 1**).[13]

Macrophages and Mycobacteria

M tuberculosis (an obligatory aerobic and intracellular organism) is acquired by the host through inhalation and infects macrophages early. On infecting the macrophages, multiple macrophage-Mycobacterium interactions occur to evade early intracellular killing. These include binding of *M tuberculosis* to macrophages via surface receptors, inhibition of phagosome-lysosome fusion, inhibition of acidification of the lysosomes, recruitment of accessory immune cells for local inflammatory response, and presentation and modulation of antigens to T cells for development of acquired immunity.[14–16] Mycobacterial growth inhibition and killing can be mediated via free radicals such as reactive oxygen and nitrogen intermediates and cytokines.[17] Within 2 to 6 weeks of infection, cell-mediated immunity develops and a granuloma forms with an influx of lymphocytes and activated macrophages at that site.[18] *M tuberculosis*–infected macrophages have decreased ability to present antigens by major histocompatibility complex (MHC) class II molecules to CD4+ T cells and this can lead to persistent infection.[19] Virulent mycobacteria can escape from fused phagosomes and multiply. Antigen-presenting cells (APCs) contribute further to defective T-cell proliferation and function by the production of cytokines such as transforming growth factor β (TGF-β), interleukin (IL)-10, or IL-6.[20]

Table 1	
Mycobacteria: classification of species and primary host	
Species oF M TB Complex	**Primary Target/Reservoir**
M tuberculosis	Human (world wide)
M africanum	Human (mostly in African countries)
M canetti	Human (mostly in African countries)
M caprae	Cattle
M bovis	Cattle
M microti	Rodents
M pinnipedii	Seals

Data from Geyer M, Müller-Ladner U. Rationale of using different biological therapies in rheumatoid arthritis. Arthritis Res Ther 2010;12(4):214.

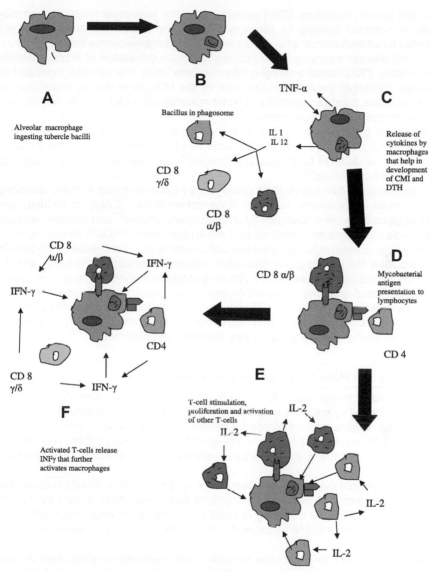

Fig. 1. Early immune response in tuberculosis. (*Adapted from* Iseman MD. Immunity and pathogenesis Iseman MD. A clinician's guide to tuberculosis. Philadelphia: Lippincott Williams & Wilkins; 2000. p. 63–91.)

Complement receptors (CR1, CR2, CR3, and CR4), mannose receptors (MR), and other cell surface receptor molecules are important in binding of tubercle bacilli to monocytes and phagocytes.[21] The interaction between mycobacteria and the MR on phagocytes are believed to be mediated through the mycobacterial surface glyco-protein lipoarabinomannan (LAM),[22] prostaglandin E2 (PGE2), and IL-4, a Th2-type cytokine, which upregulate complement and mannose receptor expression as well as function. Mannosylated LAM has also been shown to protect macrophages from apoptosis.[23] Interferon (IFN)-γ decreases the receptor expression, therefore decreasing the adherence of bacteria to the macrophages. Other receptors such as surfactant protein receptors, CD14 receptor, and the scavenger receptors can play a role in bacterial binding to phagocytes.[24,25] The phagocytosed bacteria are degraded by intralysosomal acidic hydrolases after phagolysosome fusion.[15] Antimycobacterial effector functions of macrophages include generation of reactive oxygen intermediates (ROI), reactive nitrogen intermediates (RNI), mechanisms mediated by cytokines. Hydrogen peroxide (H_2O_2), one of the ROI generated by macrophages via the oxidative burst produced by alveolar macrophages (not specific for TB), can mediate mononuclear phagocytosis.[26,27]

Phagocytes generate nitric oxide (NO) and RNI on activation by IFN-γ and tumor necrosis factor (TNF)-α. Animal studies show that inducible nitrogen oxide sulfatase (iNOS) can slow down M tuberculosis replication[28] but does not alter the intracellular viability of M tuberculosis.[29]

M tuberculosis in turn has multiple strategies for evasion of host immune response. Mycobacterial components such as lipoarabinomannan (LAM), sulfatides, and phenolic glycolipids are scavengers for oxygen intermediates[30] and secreted proteins (superoxide dismutase and catalase) and are antagonistic to ROI.[31] The cyclopropanated mycolic acids in mycobacterial cell walls resist H_2O_2[32] and hence killing by ROI. M tuberculosis cell wall lipids are important in early interaction of the bacilli with the host immune response as well as by effecting cytokine responses, determining virulence and clinical outcomes.[33] Both Mycobacterium avium and M tuberculosis can inhibit vacuolar acidification.[34,35] Other hypervirulence factors include the presence of a glycolipid trehalose dimycolate (TDM; or cord factor) in the organism, which elicits distinct host immune responses and may alter clinical outcomes.[36]

Role of IFN-γ and TNF-α in Mycobacterial Infection

The role of INF-γ in mycobacterial killing is uncertain. Some studies show that cells incubated with INF-γ enhance intracellular proliferation of mycobacteria,[37] whereas other in vitro studies show that coadministration with calcitriol caused monocytic maturation with enhanced intracellular killing of M tuberculosis.[38] Case reports have shown benefit of IFN-γ as an adjunct treatment of refractory mycobacterial infections.[39]

Another important cytokine in M tuberculosis control is TNF-α. Its role in controlling latent infection with M tuberculosis in humans has been amply shown by multiple reports of reactivation TB occurring in individuals treated for rheumatoid arthritis or Crohn disease with anti–TNF-α antibody (infliximab) or TNF-α receptor antibodies (etanercept).[40–42]

TNF-α is important for granuloma formation and maintenance (described in detail later). Mice treated with neutralizing anti–TNF-α antibody develop disorganized granuloma, which can eventually kill the mice.[43] Mice deficient in this cytokine or TNF-α receptor are highly susceptible to M tuberculosis infection.[44,45]

Innate Immune Mechanisms Against Mycobacteria

Apart from phagocytosis, other components of innate immunity are natural resistance–associated macrophage protein (Nramp), neutrophils, and natural killer (NK) cells.

Nramp
Nramp is crucial in transporting nitrite intracellularly for conversion to NO. Defects in this protein may increase susceptibility to pulmonary tuberculosis.

Neutrophils

Neutrophils are part of granulomas. Neutrophils are first to arrive at the site of bacillary multiplication, followed by NK cells, γ/δ cells, and α/β cells. Neutrophils can also cause mycobacterial killing via agents such as defensins.[46]

NK cells

NK cells are effector cells of innate immunity. These cells may directly lyse the pathogens or can lyse infected monocytes. During early infection, NK cells activate phagocytic cells at the site of infection. IL-2–activated NK cells can bring about mycobactericidal activity in macrophages infected with M avium complex (MAC).[47] Apoptosis is a likely mechanism of NK cytotoxicity. NK cells also produce IFN-γ. Depressed NK activity is seen in multidrug-resistant TB (MDR-TB) infections. Augmenting NK activity with cytokines may find a role as potential adjunct to TB chemotherapy.[48]

Toll-like Receptors in Mycobacterial Infections

Toll-like receptors (TLRs) are a family of transmembrane proteins in mammalian cells that mediate immune response in infections eliciting a proinflammatory response via the NF-kB pathway.[49] TLRs exhibit pattern recognition of organism group characteristic molecules.[50] TLR2 and TLR4 are important for the recognition of M tuberculosis products.[51,52] In humans, TLR2 activation by the 19-kD lipoprotein (independent of intracellular nitric oxide pathway) kills M tuberculosis. TLR1/2 activation upregulates expression of the vitamin D receptor, as well as vitamin D-1-hydroxylase.[53] The expression of vitamin D receptor–related genes increases expression of peptides such as cathelicidin that inhibit mycobacterial growth.

TLR2 and TLR4 can induce early innate immune response to pathogens via intracellular adapter protein pathways (MyD88).[54]

Cell-mediated Immunity

Cell-mediated immunity (CMI) plays a crucial role in the host's protective response against M tuberculosis. It has been noted from the mouse model that, within 1 week of infection, there is an increase in the number of activated CD4 and CD8 cells in the lymph nodes draining the lungs. These activated T cells migrate to the site of infection in the lungs and interact with the APCs. The tuberculous granulomas consist of both CD4+ and CD8+ T cells and both are involved in arresting the infection within the granuloma.[55] The bacilli are contained in a macrophage and antigens are presented to CD4+ cells through MHC class II.

The primary effector function of CD4+ T cells is the production of IFN-γ and possibly other cytokines that activate macrophages. In vitro, CD4 and MHC class II deficiency causes diminished levels of IFN-γ early in infection,[56] delayed NOS2 expression by macrophages, and rapid reactivation of disease.

CD8+ cells can also secrete cytokines such as IFN-γ and IL-4, regulating the interplay between proinflammatory and antiinflammatory responses in TB.[57,58] They can help decrease bacterial burden[59] and effect intracellular bacterial killing by perforin/granulysin.[60] TB bacilli can also cause T-cell hyporesponsiveness by inducing apoptosis (from mycobacterial antigens or spontaneously), thereby attenuating cell-mediated immunity.[61,62] Apoptosis is associated with diminished IFN-γ and IL-2 production. Apoptotic cells are also found in granulomas, especially those with necrotic centers.[63,64]

These T-cell responses are shown clinically by the development of a delayed-type hypersensitivity (DTH) response to intradermal injection of tuberculin or protein purified derivative purified protein derivative (PPD). Development of DTH does not confer protection against TB.[65] As a result, the protective T-cell response is distinct from the T-cell response associated with DTH.

In vitro, whole blood–based tests have been designed to assess T-cell activation by measuring IFN-γ released into blood from T cells by M tuberculosis antigens.[58,59] The mycobacterial antigens used in such assays include early secretory antigenic target 6 (ESAT-6) and culture filtrate protein (CFP-10).[66,67] These proteins are encoded by genes located within the region of difference 1 (RD1) of the M tuberculosis genome. They are not present in the bacillus Calmette-Guérin (BCG) vaccine used in many countries. This information defines a new role for a BRMs in the diagnosis of latent TB infection in patients, thus differentiating them from those vaccinated with BCG.

A study conducted in Ethiopia showed that high blood levels of IFN-γ in healthy contacts of active cases of TB were associated with progression to active disease, suggesting a role for cytokine response assay as a marker of disease progression.[68]

Th1 and Th2 responses in TB

T cells are described as Th1 type and Th2 type, based on the type of cytokines they secrete on antigen stimulation. Th1 cells secrete IL-2 and IFN-γ and have a protective role in intracellular infections. Th2-type cells secrete IL-4, IL-5, and IL-10, and may potentiate disease. The differentiation into Th1 and Th2 types from precursor cells is probably mediated by certain cytokines such as IL-12.

Cytokines

IL-12 is induced with phagocytosis of M tuberculosis bacilli by macrophages and dendritic cells and produced by monocytes and macrophages, which causes development of a Th1 response with production of IFN-γ and TNF-α. It can suppress IL-4, IL-5, and IL-10 by inhibiting the Th2 responses. IL-12 is important for development of immunity to TB bacteria by promoting differentiation and proliferation of CD4 Th1 cells and production of INF-γ from these cells as well as NK cells. Mice deficient in the gene for IL12 were noted to be more susceptible to infection and had increased bacterial burden, and decreased survival time.[69] Humans with mutations in IL-12 p40 gene or the IL-12R genes present with reduced IFN-γ production from T cells and seem to be more susceptible to disseminated BCG and M avium infections.[70] Patients with MDR-TB had less secretion of IL-2 and IFN-γ from peripheral blood monocytes. If these cells were supplemented with IL12, IFN-γ production could be restored.[71]

IFN-γ

IFN-γ is one of the most important cytokines in TB immunology and functions in a protective role. It is produced by CD4+, CD8+ T cells, and NK cells. The role of IFN-γ is believed to be multifold: increasing antigen presentation, recruitment of CD4+ T lymphocytes, and cytotoxic T lymphocytes (CTL) for bacterial killing.[72]

IFN-γ activates macrophages and, in mice, has even been known to inhibit growth of M tuberculosis.[73] INF-γ can act in synergy with IL-4, IL-6, and granulocyte-macrophage colony-stimulating factor to cause killing of mycobacteria by macrophages.[74] Patients with defective genes for IFN-γ or the IFN-γ receptor can get serious mycobacterial infections, including M tuberculosis.[75] In active TB, the levels of INF-γ can be low. Moreover, the response of macrophages to INF-γ may be decreased as well.[76,77] Studies have shown that IFN-γ production was severely depressed in patients with advanced pulmonary TB and in malnourished patients.[78]

TNF-α

TNF-α is another important cytokine involved in TB immunology. TNF-α is produced by macrophages, dendritic cells, and T cells in response to mycobacterial infection.

TNF-α is important for granuloma formation and helps to wall off the infection and prevent dissemination.[44,79] TNF-α has multiple functions in cell migration and localization of infection, expression of adhesion molecules, chemokines, and chemokine receptors. It can also cause host-mediated pulmonary tissue destruction with infection.

IL-1

IL-1, along with TNF-α, is an acute-phase reactant causing the clinical syndrome typical of tuberculosis comprising pyrexia and cachexia. These cytokines are triggered by the mycobacterial antigen. IL-1 has immunosuppressive functions.[80] It can stimulate release of IL-2 by T cells.

IL-2

IL-2 helps in proliferation of lymphocytes specific to the antigenic stimulus.

IL-4

Th2 responses and IL-4 in TB are not believed to be associated strongly with TB disease in humans.

IL-6

IL-6 has also been implicated in inflammation, hematopoiesis, and differentiation of T cells in the initial innate response to mycobacteria.[81]

IL-10

IL-10 is an antiinflammatory cytokine countering the macrophage-activating function of INF-γ. This cytokine, produced by macrophages and T cells, can deactivate macrophages by downregulating IL-12 and, in turn, INF-γ production. IL-10 inhibits CD4+ T cells directly as well as by inhibition of the antigen-presenting function of cells.[82]

TGF-β

TGF-β is found in the granulomas of patients with TB. It is produced by human monocytes after stimulation with tubercle bacilli or lipoarabinomannan[83] TGF-β has antiinflammatory properties. It can deactivate macrophage production of reactive oxygen and nitrogen species,[84] inhibition of T-cell proliferation,[85] interference with NK and CTL function, and downregulate release of IFN-γ, TNF-α, and IL-1.[86]

Granuloma Formation

Multiple steps are involved in the walling off of tubercle bacilli successfully by the host. The first step is recruitment of intravascular cells to extravasate near the site of infection. This process is controlled by adhesion molecules and chemokines. Chemokines help with cell migration and localization. They play a role in priming and differentiation of T-cell responses.[87] CD4+ T cells and CD8+ T cells are important lymphocytic cells around the granuloma. Intracellular adhesion molecules-1 (ICAM-1), extracellular matrix proteins, and integrin molecules are involved in maintaining the structure of granulomas. Dendritic cells with long filopodia are present in conjunction with epithelioid cells, many of which are apoptotic.[88,89] Proliferation of mycobacteria in situ occurs in both the lymphocyte and macrophage-derived cells in the granuloma.[90]

Chemokines

Chemokines lead to attraction and activation of inflammatory effector cells such as lymphocytes.

IL-8

IL-8 attracts neutrophils, T lymphocytes, and basophils in response to stimuli. It is mainly released by monocytes/macrophages, but it can also be expressed by fibroblasts, keratinocytes, and lymphocytes.[91] IL-8 is the neutrophil-activating factor.

Other chemokines

Other chemokines important in host responses to TB include monocyte chemoattractant protein-1 (MCP-1), regulated on activation, normal T cell expressed and secreted (RANTES), and macrophage inflammatory proteins (MIP-1, MIP2, MCP-1, MCP-3, MCP-5, and interferon-gamma inducible protein).[92] Upregulation of many chemokines and chemokine receptor expression help in formation and maintenance of granuloma in TB.

Pathogenesis of Tuberculosis

M tuberculosis complex comprises 7 species: *M tuberculosis*, *Mycobacterium africanum*, *Mycobacterium canetti*, *Mycobacterium caprae*, *Mycobacterium bovis*, *Mycobacterium microti*, and *Mycobacterium pinnipedii*. *M tuberculosis*, *M africanum*, and *M canetti* can cause disease in humans. *M tuberculosis* is the most common of the mycobacteria. Humans are the only reservoir for *M tuberculosis* species, although there are case reports of various zoonotic species causing human disease as well[93] (see **Table 2**).

With exposure to the tubercle bacilli, the immune responses that prevent development of active disease are also responsible for local tissue damage. Humoral

Table 2
Biological therapies used in rheumatoid arthritis

Biological Agent	Structure	Approved Indications
Etanercept	soluble TNF-alpha receptor fusion protein	Monotherapy, combination therapy
Adalimumab	A fully human monoclonal anti-TNF-alpha antibody	Monotherapy, combination therapy
Infliximab	chimeric (mouse/human) anti-TNF-alpha monoclonal antibody	Only in combination with MTX
Certolizumab	pegylated Fab fragment of a humanized monoclonal antibody	Monotherapy, combination therapy
Golimumab	A human monoclonal anti-TNF-alpha antibody	Only in combination with Methotrexate
Rituximab	CD20-directed cytolytic antibody	With or without Methotrexate
Abatacept	fusion protein composed of an immunoglobulin fused to a molecule capable of binding B7protein.	With or without Methotrexate
Tocilizumab	Human monoclonal antibody against the interleukin 6-receptor (IL-6R)	Monotherapy, combination therapy
Anakinra	Recombinant human Interleukin-1 receptor antagonist protein	With or without Methotrexate

Adapted from Geyer M, Müller-Ladner U. Rationale of using different biological therapies in rheumatoid arthritis. Arthritis Res Ther 2010;12(4):214.

immunity, which is of paramount importance in bacterial infections, plays a negligible role in pathogenesis of mycobacterial infections. Cell-mediated immunity and the complement system are vital in almost every step of pathogenesis of tuberculosis.[93,94]

It is known that tubercle bacilli are transmitted mostly via inhalation of infected particles. High-velocity exhalation maneuvers like coughing, sneezing, and singing generate droplets that can survive for several hours.[95] These droplets vary in size. Droplets of 1 to 5 μm diameter serve as vehicles that may contain up to several hundreds of the bacilli and are able to reach distal part of airways. Particles larger than 10 μm only reach the larger airways. Animal models have shown that particles reaching distal airways can cause infection whereas particles that lodge in the proximal airways rarely cause infection.

On deposition in the alveoli, these bacilli are engulfed by alveolar macrophages that then undergo various morphologic, biochemical, and functional changes to inhibit bacillary proliferation and to kill the phagocytosed bacilli. These changes are described in detail earlier. Various ILs along with IFN-γ play a central role in acquired resistance as well as attracting other cell lines, including their activation and maturation. TNF-α and granulocyte-macrophage colony-stimulating factor attract and activate monocytes, endothelial cells, fibroblasts, and T lymphocytes. They play an active role in granuloma formation, which is an attempt to quarantine the bacteria that have not been killed. These granulomas are characterized by central caseation, which is caused by intense local inflammatory mediators released by various cells and may contains viable bacilli killed by macrophages and surrounded by fibrous tissue. Based on the organization and composition of the granuloma on lymph node biopsy specimens from patients with history of TB, the disease has been classified into 4 groups: (1) hyperplastic (22.4%), a well-formed epithelioid cell granuloma with little necrosis; (2) reactive (54.3%), a well-formed granuloma consisting of epithelioid cells, macrophages, lymphocytes, and plasma cells with fine, eosinophilic caseation necrosis; (3) hyporeactive (17.7%), a poorly organized granuloma with macrophages, immature epithelioid cells, lymphocytes, and plasma cells, and coarse, predominantly basophilic, caseation necrosis; and (4) nonreactive (3.6%), unorganized granuloma with macrophages, lymphocytes, plasma cells, and polymorphs with noncaseating necrosis. This spectrum is reflective of different pathogenic mechanisms underlying the disease.[96]

Animal studies have shown that lack of TNF-α leads to poor granuloma formation and inability to contain infected macrophages that later serve as vehicles for the infection itself, causing disseminated or miliary tuberculosis. TNF-α can also cause liquefaction of the granuloma because of its procoagulant activity by inhibiting protein C.[44,95]

The innate immunity is usually effective if the infectious load of the bacilli is low. However, mycobacteria have also evolved to protect themselves from host immune response by various mechanisms, as described earlier. However, if the bacillary load is higher, these nonspecific intracellular mechanisms are usually ineffective and the bacilli cause further tissue invasion via blood stream or lymphatics.[93] Organs with high oxygen tension like apical lung zones, vertebra, and kidney are the most favored location for persistence and proliferation for the tubercle bacilli compared with cardiac or splenic tissue. When exposed to the tubercle bacilli during childhood, the disease mostly involves midlung zones but may occur anywhere. Patients might develop fever, lassitude, or erythema nodusum, which are present transiently and are often missed and represent tuberculin conversion.[95] Children also have a tendency to develop extensive regional lymphadenopathy that may cause cough/segmental atelectasis because of local effect. Most of the infections in childhood are nonprogressive and may be seen as calcified lymph nodes on radiographs at a later age. In some individuals, it can disseminate by either lymphatic or hematogenous route and, in some, it can spread locally by rupture of lymph nodes that have undergone caseating necrosis and liquefy, spilling a large bacillary load into the bronchial tree.[95]

Most individuals are infected at later age and may not show any sign of infection and may produce typical primary complex in which granulomas are formed in apical lobes. When these granulomas liquefy, they leave behind an inelastic fibrous capsule that is seen as a cavity on radiographs. These cavities contain large numbers of viable bacilli and also provide a site for superinfection with nontuberculous mycobacteria and fungi. The liquefied material in the bronchial tree also contains large numbers of bacilli and can cause pneumonia of the distal lung zones or may cause endobronchial lesions that may extend up to the larynx and cause ulcerations.[97]

In current clinical practice, HIV infection and anti–TNF-α therapy are considered the most important risk factors for TB disease. In patients with advanced AIDS, TB is characterized by middle/lower lung field location, absence of cavitation, higher incidence of extrapulmonary disease, and negative tuberculin test. In patients who are on anti–TNF-α therapy, reactivation of latent tuberculosis has been observed, which suggests a role of TNF in maintaining integrity of the granuloma even years after it has been formed.

BRM Therapy and Mycobacteria

BRMs target key proinflammatory cytokines and cellular functions causing inflammation in several inflammatory conditions, such as rheumatoid arthritis, seronegative spondyloarthropathies, psoriasis, ankylosing spondylosis, and inflammatory bowel disease. Current options in biologics include not only agents against TNF-α but also directed against IL-1 or IL-6 and modulators of B-cell or T-cell activity, thereby abolishing disease progression and persistent residual activity.

Inhibitors of TNF-α represent important treatment advances, but are also associated with multiple complications and adverse effects of targeted TNF-α inhibition. These effects include reactivation of mycobacterial infection (particularly tuberculosis) and other infections such as listeriosis, histoplasmosis, nocardiosis, aspergillosis, coccidiomycosis, hepatitis B/C, herpes zoster,[98] injection site reactions, infusion reactions, induction of autoimmunity, demyelinating disease, heart failure, and malignancy are among the noninfectious complications.[99] The association between TNF-α inhibitor use and TB and nontuberculous mycobacterial infections has now been well established (**Table 3**). As discussed earlier, formation and maintenance of granulomas are essential for control of *M tuberculosis* infection and are regulated partly by the proinflammatory cytokine, TNF-α. Studies using murine models have shown that the organization of immune cells within a TB granuloma, as well as TNF-α receptor binding and intracellular modulation, are important factors that control availability of the cytokine and coordinate immunologic functions induced by TNF-α within a granuloma. TNF-α, an essential component of the host's innate immunity, has both advantages and disadvantages, because of its role in controlling the tuberculosis infection, and also because of the severe tissue damage it causes.[11]

TNF-α Inhibitors

As discussed earlier, TNF-α is a proinflammatory cytokine that is expressed mainly by activated macrophages and B and T lymphocytes. Its biological effects are mainly in sepsis and systemic inflammation, macrophage recruitment and activation, and granuloma formation/maintenance.[100] In addition, certain soluble TNF receptors (P-55 and

P-75) play a role in granuloma formation and are targets for action of certain TNF-α inhibitors.[101]

The United States Food and Drug Administration (FDA) has at present approved 5 TNF-α antagonists that are available for the treatment of inflammatory illnesses like rheumatoid arthritis: etanercept, adalimumab, infliximab, certolizumab, and golimumab. Their introduction has revolutionized the treatment of rheumatoid arthritis. Off-label uses of these agents also include uveitis, sarcoidosis, Wegener granulomatosis, polymyositis, and dermatomyositis.

Infliximab is a chimeric (mouse/human) anti–TNF-α monoclonal antibody, adalimumab is a fully human monoclonal anti–TNF-α antibody, etanercept is a soluble TNF-α receptor fusion protein, certolizumab is a pegylated Fab fragment of a humanized monoclonal antibody, and golimumab is a human monoclonal anti–TNF-α antibody.

Etanercept, adalimumab, and certolizumab are approved as monotherapy for rheumatoid arthritis, but infliximab and golimumab are only approved in combination with methotrexate. Data derived from various studies show that using TNF inhibitor alone or together with methotrexate might be superior to combinations of traditional disease-modifying agents used for rheumatoid arthritis.[102] Although TNF inhibitors exhibit differences in their composition, pharmacokinetic properties, and pharmacodynamic properties, there is no evidence suggesting that any one of these TNF-blocking agents is more effective than the other in rheumatoid arthritis. These agents, when administered, show response in rheumatoid arthritis as early as 2 to 4 weeks of starting treatment in some patients, but significant improvement of disease may take 12 to 24 weeks, as shown by improvement in clinical and laboratory parameters.[103]

In vitro studies show that TNF-α is protective for the host against in several mycobacterial infections, including M tuberculosis, M avium, M bovis, and BCG.[104–107] Granulomas have sequestered mycobacteria in a central core of macrophages, surrounded by multinucleated giant cells and lymphocytes.[104] TNF-α not only functions to recruit these cells but also helps with sustained maintenance of the structure of granulomas.[40,104] TNF-α inhibitors can increase the risk of reactivation of LTBI.[42,102,108–110] The risk of reactivation is greater for infliximab and adalimumab than for etanercept.[111,112] Certolizumab is a newer drug and evidence of reactivation disease with it is limited.[113] The first report of this increased risk was published by Keane and colleagues.[42] Most of the data for increased risk of TB with use of TNF-α inhibitors come from databases for drug safety monitoring. The FDA Adverse Event Reporting System (AERS) database established for postmarketing surveillance of adverse drug events with TNF-α inhibitors is an important database that showed that, between 1998 and 2002, patients in the United States treated with infliximab or etanercept respectively had an estimated TB rate of 54 and 28 per 100,000 patients respectively.[102,114] The baseline rate of TB in the United States during the same period was 5.2 to 6.8 cases per 100,000 without the use of TNF-α inhibitors.[115] This database showed that a large number of patients had extrapulmonary disease or disseminated disease as one may expect considering the biological function of TNF-α.[116] The mean time to reactivation with infliximab was 12 weeks.[42] Similarly, the Spanish Society of Rheumatology Database on Biologic Products (BIOBADASER), an active surveillance registry for assessing the safety of TNF-α inhibitors in patients with rheumatic disease, showed about a 50-fold higher rate of TB in patients receiving TNF-A inhibitors.[108] Data to April 2008 from the British Society for Rheumatology Biologics Register (a national prospective and observational study), have recorded TB rates in 100,000 patients on TNF-Aα inhibitors (infliximab, etanercept, and adalimumab).[112] They found a higher rate of TB in patients receiving adalimumab (144 events per 100,000 person-years) compared with infliximab (136 events per 100,000 person-years) and

Table 3
Summary of relationship between biological response modifiers (brms) and mycobacterial infections cytokines

Cytokine	Source	Role in Pathogenesis	Role as an Immunotherapeutic Agent
IFN-γ	CD4 (Th 1) lymphocytes CD8 lymphocytes γδ lymphocytes NK cells	• Principle mediator for Th 1 immune response. Acts primarily on macrophage • Is a macrophage activating factor and along with Cytotoxic T lymphocytes is involved in granule mediated lysis of infected macrophage and death of contained organism • Stimulates macrophage to convert Vit D2 to calcitriol	When used as an immunotherapeutic agent: • Adverse Outcomes -flu like symptoms, myelosuppression • Required daily dose • Expensive • Currently used for MDR-TB cases in phase I/II trials
TNF-α	Macrophages Monocytes T and B Lymphocytes NK cells	• Important mediator of Th 2 immune response. • Plays central role in granuloma formation, where tubercle bacilli live in a latent phase. • Chemotactic factor for monocytes and involved in activation and differentiation of macrophages • Procoagulant by blocking protein C	(A) soluble TNF-α receptors (Etanercept) • In phase I trials has shown earlier sputum conversion • Trials are done on weekly dosing • Can cause lymphoproliferative disorders and demyelineting diseases. • Can worsen congestive heart failure and also can reactivate latent tuberculosis (though less than infliximab) • Expensive (B) TNF-α inhibitors (thalidomide) • Showed decrease in granuloma size and faster clearance of bacteria in latent TB cases when combined with isoniazid compared to isoniazid alone.
TGF-β	Activated macrophages release TGF-b when stimulated by LAM(lipoarabinomannan) in tubercle bacillus cell wall.	• Down regulates/suppress CD4 lymphocyte function • Interferes with IL-2, IL-12 and IFNγ	• TGF-β inhibitors in murine models caused decrease in IL-4 level and increase IFN-γ and IL-2 level thereby up regulating Th 1 response • Significant reduction of bacillary load • Cox-2 inhibitors were added to decrease pulmonary inflammation
IL-4	Macrophages Mast Cells and Basophils T and B lymphocytes Bone Marrow and stromal cells	• Principle mediator in Th 2 response • Down regulation of cytotoxic T cells • Promotes B cell proliferation and differentiation • Increases IgE production from B cells	• Anti-IL-4 antibody administered as a pulse during the early or late stages of murine infection has shown decreased bacillary burden • Currently unavailable for clinical use

Interleukin 1	Monocytes and Macrophages Neutrophils T and B lymphocytes	• Endogenous pyrogen • Activates NK cells, promotes T and B lymphocyte proliferation	Not established yet
Interleukin 2	T lymphocytes	• Autocrine stimulation of T lymphocytes • Stimulates proliferation and Immunoglobulin production by B lymphocytes	Not established yet
Interleukin 8	Monocytes and macrophages T lymphocytes Other Somatic cells	• Plays a role in chemotaxis and activation for monotyes, neutrophils and T lymphocytes	Not established yet
Interleukin 10	Activated Macrophages B and T lymphocytes	• Decreases cytokine production by monocytes and macrophages.	Not established yet
Interleukin 12	Macrophages B lymphocytes	• Promotes Th 1 response by CTL, NK and macrophages • Increases IFN-γ production • Stimulates differentiation of uncommitted CD4 T lymphocytes into Th 1 cells	Not established yet
GM CSF	Monocytes T lymphocytes Endothelial cells Fibroblasts	• Promotes growth and differentiation of hematopoietic progenitor cells • Enhances Th1 response by stimulating monocytes-macrophages and neutrophils Also attracts macrophages to granulomas to inhibit mycobacterial growth	Not established yet
MCAF	B lymphocytes Other Somatic Cells Monocytes Macrophages	• Regulates cytokine production in monocytes • Stimulates histamine release from basophils	Not established yet
MIP 1a and 1b	T and B lymphocytes Monocytes Mast Cells Fibroblasts	• Acts as a chemotactic factor for monocytes and T lymphocytes • MIP-1a is an endogenous pyrogen	Not established yet

(continued on next page)

Table 3
(continued)

Vaccines	Content/Preparation	Dose/Storage/Schedule/Cold Chain (Looking for a Better Word to Describe them)	Role as an Adjunct Immunotherapeutic Agent
DNA vaccine	Various DNA vaccines which contain various antigens likeHsp 65, Ag85A, Ag85 N, Hsp70/80, ESAT-6	• May require multiple dose • Long shelf life • Toxicity unknown currently • No human trials are done	• Used in experimental models • Shown to enhance IFN-γ production and CD8 + CTL activity. Also down regulates production of IL-4 • Synergy between chemotherapy and DNA vaccine in BCG immunized TB challenged mice and role as a booster vaccine in previously BCG immunized mice
Mycobacterium vaccae	Mycobacterium vaccae is a saprophytic environmental mycobacterium which has many antigens like Hsp65 that cross react with Mycobacterium tuberculosis	• Available as oral and injectable form • Trials have shown equal efficacy when given as a single injectable dose early in treatment, three injectable dose monthly or when given as ten oral dose during the treatment	• Has shown earlier bacillary clearance, faster clinical and radiological improvement • Effective as an addition to chemotherapy in drug susceptible or drug resistant TB, with or without contomitant HIV • Upregulates Th1 and CD8 CTL response and down regulates IL-4 and there by Th 2 response
RUTI	RUTI is made of detoxified, fragmented mycobacterium tuberculosis which contains Hsp65	Detoxified fragmented M tuberculosis cells.	• In mice when given after one month of chemotherapy it caused mixed Th1 and Th2 response and local accumulation of specific CD8 T lymphocytes • So far tried in mice only where when given after one month of chemotherapy it showed protective effect towards regrowth of latent bacilli
Mycobacterium w	Saprophytic cultivable organism which shares T cell and B cell antigenic determinants with M tuberculosis and M leprae	Only one study in human tuberculosis where it was given intradermally every 15 days while on conventional anti TB therapy	• Shown to enhance Th 1 response by production of IFN-γ and IL 2 • Earlier sputum bacillary clearance. • Licensed in India as an immunomodulator for leprosy

etanercept (39 events per 100,000 person-years).They also found that patients of nonwhite ethnicity had a sixfold increased risk of TB compared with white people.[112] Other studies from other European countries with similar or higher baseline burden of TB disease have also shown an increased risk of reactivation of TB in patients receiving TNF-α inhibitors.[111,112,117,118] However, most of these studies are large registries or voluntary reporting systems and not randomized clinical trials. These studies are also complicated by the lack of a gold standard test for latent TB infection.[119] Current tests for latent TB infection include tuberculin skin test (TST) and whole-blood IFN-γ release assays (IGRAs), which may be falsely positive where they do not distinguish between persistence and immunologic memory when the infection has been sufficiently eradicated by the host response.[120] These tests may also be falsely negative (estimated at 20%–25%[124]) in patients with immunosuppression and with inflammatory conditions either caused by the underlying disease or treatment.[121] The new-generation tests involving IGRAs consist of incubating whole blood overnight in the presence of 2 antigens that are present in M tuberculosis but not in BCG or in most nontuberculous mycobacteria (early secretary antigen-6 and culture filtrate protein-10). After overnight incubation, the assay calculates the amount of IFN-γ (QuantiFERON) or the number of IFN-γ–producing cells.[119] It is clear from the studies that there are differences among the TNF-α inhibitors in increasing the risk of TB reactivation, the risk being higher with the use of infliximab and adalimumab than with etanercept. There are multiple explanations offered for this. Infliximab has high blood levels shortly after infusion.[122] Blood levels of etanercept are low, with little variation in relation to dosing. The second hypothesis to explain the difference is presence of antibody-dependent mechanisms of the TNF-α antibodies causing death of cells expressing TNF-α that results in reactivation of TB. Infliximab, binding to soluble trimeric TNF-α, forms large immune complexes that activate complement and cause cell lysis. Infliximab and adalimumab can cause cell death because of apoptosis in lamina propria T cells in patients with Crohn disease downregulating proinflammatory cytokines, both in vitro and in vivo.[123] Third, T-cell dysfunction may occur without cell death, as has been observed in whole-blood cultures treated with TNF-α inhibitors.[124] In this study, infliximab and adalimumab reduced the proportion of TB-responsive CD4 cells by 70% and 49%, respectively, and suppressed antigen-induced IFN-γ production by 70% and 64%. Etanercept had no significant effect on these parameters.[124]

Most of the TB disease associated with the use of TNF-α inhibitors seems to be reactivation disease caused by immune suppression. However, patients living in areas endemic for TB or with high-risk exposure as close contacts of patients with active TB could be at increased risk of newly acquired infection. If disease occurs soon after the initiation of TNF-α inhibitor, it suggests reactivation of latent TB infection. Disease occurring later may be either delayed reactivation or new TB infection. Once again, median time to onset of disease with use of TNF-α inhibitor seems to be shortest for infliximab (5.5 months) compared with etanercept (13.4 months) and adalimumab (18.5 months).[112] Because much of reactivation disease is preventable, it is important to appropriately identify and treat patients with LTBI who require TNF-α inhibitor therapy. Studies show that manifestations of TB disease with use of TNF-α inhibitors often involve extrapulmonary sites and may be disseminated.[116,119,125] Symptoms could include fever, malaise, cough, weight loss, night sweats, and lymphadenopathy. If symptomatic, these patients require immediate attention.

The United States Centers for Disease Control and Prevention recommends that, before receiving TNF-α inhibitors, all patients must be screened for LTBI.[125] Patients with evidence of LTBI should be treated before starting a TNF-α inhibitor. Screening includes a full medical history, physical examination, tuberculin skin test, or IGRA, although rates of indeterminate IGRA results are higher in patients with rheumatoid arthritis.[126,127] This screening should be followed by chest radiograph in those with a positive TST or IGRA or a history or physical examination suggestive of TB.[126,128] A positive skin TST for these patients requiring TNF-α is ≥5 mm of induration.[128] Treatment of LTBI should be considered even with negative TST or IGRA in patients with regional fibrosis with or without hilar lymphadenopathy on chest radiograph or evidence of prior TB exposure as a close contact of a patient with TB case or having resided in a TB-endemic country.[119] A Spanish observational study showed the advantage of screening for tuberculosis. It noted a 74% reduction in case rates of TB because of effective screening and treatment in patients with rheumatoid arthritis treated with infliximab.[108] Treatment of LTBI in these patients prevents reactivation but may not be prophylaxis against acquiring a new infection with M tuberculosis. Preventive measures in patients on TNF-α inhibitors include avoiding occupational exposures such as health care facilities with high TB prevalence, homeless shelters, and prisons; and travel to high-prevalence regions for TB.[129] If active TB is diagnosed in these patient, the TNF-α inhibitor therapy should be discontinued and treatment of TB disease should be started.[119,126] Before TNF-α inhibitor treatment, patients with latent TB infection should receive standard treatment with isoniazid for 9 months.[129] The duration of LTBI therapy before starting a TNF-α inhibitor is not clear, but most experts suggest that patients receive at least 1 month of LTBI treatment before starting anti–TNF-α therapy whenever possible.[130] For active TB infection when diagnosed in a patient receiving a TNF-α inhibitor, anti–TNF-α therapy should be discontinued, at least temporarily, along with a 4-drug regimen for tuberculosis. Some experts suggest that TNF-α inhibitor treatment may be resumed after drug susceptibility results for M tuberculosis are known and clinical improvement is evident.[130] Discontinuation of a TNF-α inhibitor in the setting of active TB may be associated with a paradoxic worsening of TB, which is hypothesized to be an immune reconstitution inflammatory syndrome (IRIS).[131,132] Short term glucocorticoid therapy can be used in this situation.

Risk of Nontuberculous Mycobacterial Infections with the Use of TNF-α Inhibitors

Although many studies suggest that TNF-α inhibitors confer a 5 to 10 times greater risk of TB than of nontuberculous mycobacterial (NTM) infections,[133] a study of the US FDA MedWatch database and a survey of Infectious Diseases Society of America physicians of the Emerging Infections Network in 2007 suggested otherwise.[133] In the survey, infections caused by NTM were reported nearly twice as often as TB. MAC was the most frequently reported NTM species, followed by Mycobacterium chelonae, Mycobacterium abscessus, Mycobacterium marinum, and others. In the MedWatch study, of the 239 cases reported, 105 (44%) met NTM disease criteria. Again, MAC was the most commonly occurring species. The mean age of the patients was 62 years and there was a preponderance of NTM infections in women (65%), occurring most commonly with infliximab, then etanercept, and least commonly with adalimumab. Many of the patients were concurrently on prednisone (65%) and methotrexate (55%). Mainly extrapulmonary disease was reported in NTM infections as well (44%), which included the skin and soft tissues (26%), bones or joints (9%), disseminated disease (8%), and the eye (1%).

In the United States, among the patients at risk for mycobacterial disease, NTM infections are more common in individuals born in the United States, and TB is more common in those from TB-endemic countries. Prospective studies need to be done to establish the risk of NTM infection following TNF-α inhibitor use. If this risk is found to be substantially greater than is presently appreciated, preventive strategies may be required for NTM infections.[134]

Steroids

Anecdotal reports suggest immune suppression with corticosteroids predisposes to tuberculosis, but retrospective studies on patients taking low doses of prednisone have not confirmed any increased risk.[109]

BRMs in the Treatment of Tuberculosis

In a healthy host, with latent infection, bacteriostatic immune responses are operative in a granuloma, forming a physical barrier to contain the infection. Mycobacteria undergo certain biochemical changes as well. Various immunotherapeutic agents have been tried with a goal of improving success rates for treatment of MDR-TB, shortening the treatment, and improving the efficacy of chemotherapeutic agents but so far the only success has been in the form of earlier sputum clearance by few days. This article reviews the potential role of BRMs in the treatment of TB based on experimental and limited clinical studies (see **Table 4**).

DNA vaccine

Various DNA vaccines have been studied, primarily in mice that have shown an increase in bacterial clearance when combined with antitubercular chemotherapy compared with antitubercular chemotherapy alone. These DNA vaccines are presumed to increase IFN-γ levels and decrease levels of IL-4, thereby increasing bactericidal activity.[135–137]

RUTI: therapeutic vaccine

It has been hypothesized that the foamy macrophages in granulomas serve as an escape for the latent bacilli that survive in the granuloma and may disseminate later. RUTI, a therapeutic vaccine was made of detoxified, fragmented *M tuberculosis* cells and delivered in liposomes. In mice, when given after 1 month of chemotherapy, it caused induction of a mixed Th1/Th2/Th3 and polyantigenic response with no local or systemic toxicity. Local accumulation of specific CD8 T cells and a strong humoral

Table 4
Immune response in tuberculosis

Type 1 Immune Response	Type 2 Immune Response
Characterized by phagocytosis and killing	Characterized by granuloma formation as it cannot kill the bacteria
Source – CD4 lymphocyte (Th 1), CD8 lymphocyte, NK cells	T lymphocyte – Th 2, macrophage, mast cells, basophils, B lymphocytes, Bone marrow and stromal cells
Principal cytokine - IFN-γ	IL-4
IFN-γ is a macrophage activating factor which along with Cytotoxic T Lymphocytes plays a central role in protective immunity. Cytotoxic T Lymphocytes – are responsible for granule mediated lysis of infected macrophages and death of contained organisms	IL-4 stimulates macrophages to produce TGF-β, and down regulates Cytotoxic T Lymphocytes response, decreases microbicidal activity of macrophages, increases cellular infiltration, increases TNF-α production, decreases IFN-γ and decreases killing of bacilli which are then contained by granuloma in the latent form

response were characteristic features of RUTI that explain its protective properties toward regrowth of remaining latent bacilli.

TGF-β inhibitors

Studies in mice have shown that TGF-β inhibitors in combination with cyclooxygenase-2 (COX-2) inhibitors increase expression of IFN-γ and IL-2, and decrease levels of IL-4, thereby upregulating Th1 response and downregulating Th2 response, resulting in significant reduction of bacillary load. When combined with chemotherapy, they were even more efficacious. COX-2 inhibitors are added to decrease pulmonary inflammation.[138]

High-dose intravenous immunoglobulin

High-dose intravenous immunoglobulin (IVIG) given alone in infected mice showed dose-related sustained reduction in bacterial counts, and this protective effect persisted beyond its half-life. The effect was presumed to be mediated through conventional T-cell responses, cytokine production, and effects on regulatory T cells. A similar effect was seen whether IVIG was added early or late in the treatment.[139]

Mycobacterium vaccae

M vaccae is a saprophytic mycobacterium that has antigenic cross-reactivity with M tuberculosis. Vaccination with M vaccae has been tried by oral and injectable routes and both of them have shown not only improved bacillary clearance but faster clinical and radiological improvement as well when combined with standard chemotherapy. The mechanism is mostly by increase in IFN-γ and CTL, thereby upregulating Th1 response and downregulation of Th2 by decreasing TLR-4 regulatory T cells. M vaccae vaccination has shown promising results in patients with MDR-TB when combined with chemotherapy.[140–144]

IFN

IFN is a principle cytokine involved in Th1 immune response, so several trials have used IFN-α and IFN-γ by inhalational and IFN-γ subcutaneously to improve response to treatment in tuberculosis. Most of the studies showed decreased bacillary burden but failed to clear infection. IFN-γ by subcutaneous route did not show any benefit. Grahmann and Braun[145] showed that patients given aerosolized recombinant IFN-γ twice weekly for an initial 2 months while on chemotherapy showed sputum clearance within 6 to 8 weeks and persistent radiological signs of recovery for several years of follow-up. Several other studies showed decreases in bacillary load and radiological improvement with aerosolized IFN therapy. Most of these studies were done in patients with patients with MDR-TB.[146–150]

IL-2

Contrary to initial smaller studies showing decrease in sputum bacillary load, a double-blind placebo-controlled trial of IL-2 in HIV-infected, drug-sensitive Ugandan patients with TB did not show any symptomatic improvement compared with the placebo arm. There were significant delays in clearance of viable M tuberculosis and conversion of sputum culture to negative in the IL-2 arm. These results could be interpreted as antagonism between immunotherapy and chemotherapy.[151]

Mycobacterium w

Mycobacterium w, which has been approved for its immunomodulatory properties in leprosy, for which it has shown clinical improvement, accelerated bacterial clearance and increased immune response to Mycobacterium leprae. It has also been studied as an alternative to M bovis for vaccination against M tuberculosis. When given by both parenteral and inhalational routes, it was more efficacious than BCG in murine model of tuberculosis. Largest human studies have been done in Kanpur, India, where 28,948 people were vaccinated with *Mycobacterium w* to investigate its effectiveness against leprosy. Data analysis later showed that *Mycobacterium w* had a protective effect against tuberculosis.[151,152]

Role of thalidomide in treatment
In a murine model of mice infected with *M tuberculosis*, addition of thalidomide resulted in smaller granulomas with apoptotic cells and no central caseation. It did not affect other cytokines.[153,154] Immunomodulatory effect of thalidomide by inhibition of TNF-α has shown faster clearance of bacteria in latent TB cases when combined with isoniazid compared with isoniazid alone.[155]

Studies of central nervous system tuberculosis in a rabbit model showed higher levels of TNF-α in cerebrospinal fluid.[153] This evidence is supported by several isolated case reports and smaller case studies that showed that thalidomide was helpful as salvage therapy in patients with TB meningitis with tuberculomas or optic neuritis that did not responded to standard TB drugs and high-dose corticosteroids.[155–158]

3-Hydroxy-3-methylglutaryl coenzyme A inhibitors
In vitro studies by Lu and Li[159] showed that lovastatin and fluvastatin were able to inhibit tyrosine phosphorylation and expression of glycoprotein metabolite-1 (lipid raft marker), and CD69 (activation marker) in γ/δ T cells sensitized by mycobacterial tuberculosis antigens.[139,159]

Steroids
Various prospective studies have shown the role of corticosteroids as adjuncts to chemotherapy with antituberculous drugs in tuberculous meningitis, pericardial and pleural disease, endobronchial disease, especially in pediatric patients, and extensive lung disease. Corticosteroids are especially useful with documented adrenal suppression and in cases of drug-related fever. In TB, the recommended dose is 40 to 60 mg of prednisone orally daily for 4 to 6 weeks depending on the site of disease, followed by tapering doses. Topical corticosteroid therapy for fierce reactions with BCG (keloid formation) or PPD (skin reaction) is useful.[160]

Vitamins A and D
In the preantibiotic era, treatment of tuberculosis in the setting of sanatoria consisted of plenty of sunlight, fresh air, and adequate nutrition. Vitamin D in its active form, calcitriol, is reported to play an important part in intracellular bacillary killing by induction of cathelicidin and also by induction of reactive oxygen and nitrogen metabolites. The effect of vitamin D is affected by polymorphism in the vitamin D receptor gene. The human vitamin D receptor carrying the t allele of the Taq I vitamin D receptor polymorphism was associated with increase in calcitriol-induced phagocytosis, enhanced intracellular killing by cathelicidin, induction of reactive oxygen and nitrogen metabolites, and rapid sputum conversion, whereas the f allele of the Fok I vitamin D receptor polymorphism was associated with decreased calcitriol-induced phagocytosis and slower sputum conversion.[161]

Few studies of the role of vitamin A as an adjunct in the treatment of tuberculosis report improved outcomes.[162–164]

Minerals
Two iron compounds showed in vitro growth inhibitory activity on *M tuberculosis* H(37) Rv (ATCC 27,294), together with very low unspecific cytotoxicity on eukaryotic cells (cultured murine cell line J774). Both complexes showed higher inhibitory effects on

M tuberculosis than the second-line therapeutic drugs. Zinc had been tried as a coadjuvant to chemotherapy but did not show any benefit.[161]

In conclusion, the immunology and pathogenesis of mycobacteria is complex and involves many networks and components. Because of its complexity, it is extremely difficult to identify the specific mechanisms in disease development. A clear understanding of the network of immune responses involved with this pathogen and their effector functions becomes crucial as newer treatment modalities become available for noninfectious diseases operating via this immunologic network. Continued research in animal models and human subjects, as well as technical advances in immunogenetics, is necessary to be able to use BRMs effectively and appropriately in the treatment of various diseases including mycobacterial infections.

REFERENCES

1. Lönnroth K, Raviglione M. Global epidemiology of tuberculosis: prospects for control. Semin Respir Crit Care Med 2008;29(5):481–91.
2. Horsburgh CR Jr, O'Donnell M, Chamblee S, et al. Revisiting rates of reactivation tuberculosis: a population-based approach. Am J Respir Crit Care Med 2010;182(3):420–5.
3. Comstock GW. Epidemiology of tuberculosis. Am Rev Respir Dis 1982;125:8.
4. Dye C, Floyd K, Uplekar M. Global tuberculosis control. WHO/HTM/TB/2008.393. Geneva (Switzerland): World Health Organization; 2008.
5. Guelar A, Gatell JM, Verdejo J, et al. A prospective study of the risk of tuberculosis among HIV-infected patients. AIDS 1993;7:1345.
6. Antonucci G, Girardi E, Raviglione MC, et al. Risk factors for tuberculosis in HIV-infected persons. A prospective cohort study. The Gruppo Italiano di Studio Tubercolosi e AIDS (GISTA). JAMA 1995;274:143.
7. Jick SS, Lieberman ES, Rahman MU, et al. Glucocorticoid use, other associated factors, and the risk of tuberculosis. Arthritis Rheum 2006;55(1):19.
8. Lichtenstein IH, MacGregor RR. Mycobacterial infections in renal transplant recipients: report of five cases and review of the literature. Rev Infect Dis 1983;5(2):216.
9. Malaviya AN, Nigil H. Infections associated with the use of biologic response modifiers in rheumatic diseases: a critical appraisal. Indian Journal of Rheumatology 2011;6(1 Suppl):99–112.
10. Tomioka H, Namba K. Development of antituberculous drugs: current status and future prospects [review]. Kekkaku 2006;81(12):753–74 [in Japanese].
11. Mootoo A, Stylianou E, Arias MA, et al. TNF-alpha in tuberculosis: a cytokine with a split personality. Inflamm Allergy Drug Targets 2009;8(1):53–62.
12. Flynn JL, Chan J. Immunology of tuberculosis. Annu Rev Immunol 2001;19:93–129.
13. Wolf AJ, Linas B, Trevejo-Nuñez GJ, et al. *Mycobacterium tuberculosis* infects dendritic cells with high frequency and impairs their function in vivo. J Immunol 2007;179:2509–19.
14. Hart PD, Armstrong JA, Brown CA, et al. Ultrastructural study of the behaviour of macrophages toward parasitic mycobacteria. Infect Immun 1972;5:803–7.
15. Cohn ZA. The fate of bacteria within phagocytic cells. I. The degradation of isotopically labeled bacteria by polymorphonuclear leucocytes and macrophages. J Exp Med 1963;117:27–42.
16. Chan J, Xing Y, Magliozzo RS, et al. Killing of virulent *Mycobacterium tuberculosis* by reactive nitrogen intermediates produced by activated murine macrophages. J Exp Med 1992;175(4):1111.

17. Armstrong JA, Hart PD. Response of cultured macrophages to *Mycobacterium tuberculosis*, with observations on fusion of lysosomes with phagosomes. J Exp Med 1971;134:713.
18. Raja A. Immunology of tuberculosis. Indian J Med Res 2004;120:213–32.
19. Pancholi P, Mirza A, Schauf V, et al. Presentation of mycobacterial antigens by human dendritic cells: lack of transfer from infected macrophages. Infect Immun 1993;61(12):5326.
20. Armstrong JA, Hart PD. Phagosome-lysosome interactions in cultured macrophages infected with virulent tubercle bacilli. Reversal of the usual nonfusion pattern and observations on bacterial survival. J Exp Med 1975;142(1):1.
21. Schlesinger LS. Role of mononuclear phagocytes in *M. tuberculosis* pathogenesis. J Investig Med 1996;44:312–23.
22. Schlesinger LS, Hull SR, Kaufman TM. Binding of the terminal mannosyl units of lipoarabinomannan from a virulent strain of *Mycobacterium tuberculosis* to human macrophages. J Immunol 1994;152:4070–9.
23. Wojtas B, Fijalkowska B, Wlodarczyk A, et al. Mannosylated lipoarabinomannan balances apoptosis and inflammatory state in mycobacteria-infected and uninfected bystander macrophages. Microb Pathog 2011;51(1–2):9–21.
24. Barnes PF, Modlin RL, Ellner JJ. T-cell responses and cytokines. In: Bloom BR, editor. Tuberculosis: pathogenesis, protection and control. Washington, DC: ASM Press; 1994. p. 417–35, 225.
25. Hoheisel G, Zheng L, Teschler H, et al. Increased soluble CD14 levels in BAL fluid in pulmonary tuberculosis. Chest 1995;108:1614–6.
26. Walker L, Lowrie DB. Killing of *Mycobacterium microti* by immunologically activated macrophages. Nature 1981;293:69–70.
27. Selvaraj P, Swamy R, Vijayan VK, et al. Hydrogen peroxide producing potential of alveolar macrophages and blood monocytes in pulmonary tuberculosis. Indian J Med Res 1988;88:124–9.
28. MacMicking JD, North RJ, LaCourse R, et al. Identification of nitric oxide synthase as a protective locus against tuberculosis. Proc Natl Acad Sci U S A 1997;94:5243–8.
29. Vishwanath V, Meera R, Puvanakrishnan R, et al. Fate of *Mycobacterium tuberculosis* inside rat peritoneal macrophages in vitro. Mol Cell Biochem 1997;175:169–75.
30. Chan J, Fan XD, Hunter SW, et al. Lipoarabinomannan, a possible virulence factor involved in persistence of *Mycobacterium tuberculosis* within macrophages. Infect Immun 1991;59(5):1755.
31. Schlesinger LS. Macrophage phagocytosis of virulent but not attenuated strains of *Mycobacterium tuberculosis* is mediated by mannose receptors in addition to complement receptors. J Immunol 1993;150(7):2920.
32. Yuan Y, Lee RE, Besra GS, et al. Identification of a gene involved in the biosynthesis of cyclopropanated mycolic acids in *Mycobacterium tuberculosis*. Proc Natl Acad Sci U S A 1995;92(14):6630.
33. Manca C, Tsenova L, Barry CE 3rd, et al. *Mycobacterium tuberculosis* CDC1551 induces a more vigorous host response in vivo and in vitro, but is not more virulent than other clinical isolates. J Immunol 1999;162(11):6740.
34. Sturgill-Koszycki S, Schlesinger PH, Chakraborty P, et al. Lack of acidification in *Mycobacterium* phagosomes produced by exclusion of the vesicular proton-ATPase. Science 1994;263(5147):678.
35. Xu S, Cooper A, Sturgill-Koszycki S, et al. Intracellular trafficking in *Mycobacterium tuberculosis* and *Mycobacterium avium*-infected macrophages. J Immunol 1994;153(6):2568.

36. Noll H, Bloch H, Asselinea UJ, et al. The chemical structure of the cord factor of *Mycobacterium tuberculosis*. Biochim Biophys Acta 1956;20(2):299.
37. Douvas GS, Looker DL, Vatter AE, et al. Gamma interferon activates human macrophages to become tumoricidal and leishmanicidal but enhances replication of macrophage-associated mycobacteria. Infect Immun 1985;50(1):1.
38. Rook GA, Steele J, Fraher L, et al. Vitamin D3, gamma interferon, and control of proliferation of *Mycobacterium tuberculosis* by human monocytes. Immunology 1986;57(1):159.
39. Rao S, Koirala J, Khardori N, et al. Biological response modifiers as adjunct treatment for refractory localized mycobacterium avium complex infection. J Investig Med 2005;53(Suppl 2):S398.
40. Gardam MA, Keystone EC, Menzies R, et al. Anti-tumour necrosis factor agents and tuberculosis risk: mechanisms of action and clinical management. Lancet Infect Dis 2003;3(3):148.
41. Long R, Gardam M. Tumour necrosis factor-alpha inhibitors and the reactivation of latent tuberculosis infection. CMAJ 2003;168(9):1153.
42. Keane J, Gershon S, Wise RP, et al. Tuberculosis associated with infliximab, a tumor necrosis factor alpha-neutralizing agent. N Engl J Med 2001;345(15):1098.
43. Mohan VP, Scanga CA, Yu K, et al. Effects of tumor necrosis factor alpha on host immune response in chronic persistent tuberculosis: possible role for limiting pathology. Infect Immun 2001;69:1847–55.
44. Flynn JL, Goldstein MM, Chan J, et al. Tumor necrosis factor-alpha is required in the protective immune response against *Mycobacterium tuberculosis* in mice. Immunity 1995;2(6):561–72.
45. Bean AG, Roach DR, Briscoe H, et al. Structural deficiencies in granuloma formation in TNF gene-targeted mice underlie the heightened susceptibility to aerosol *Mycobacterium tuberculosis* infection, which is not compensated for by lymphotoxin. J Immunol 1999;162:3504.
46. Ogata K, Linzer BA, Zuberi RI, et al. Activity of defensins from human neutrophilic granulocytes against *Mycobacterium avium-Mycobacterium intracellulare*. Infect Immun 1992;60:4720–5.
47. Bermudez LE, Young LS. Natural killer cell-dependent mycobacteriostatic and mycobactericidal activity in human macrophages. J Immunol 1991;146: 265–70.
48. Nirmala R, Narayanan PR, Mathew R, et al. Reduced NK activity in pulmonary tuberculosis patients with/without HIV infection: Identifying the defective stage and studying the effect of interleukins on NK activity. Tuberculosis 2001;81: 343–52.
49. Medzhitov R, Preston-Hurlburt P, Janeway CA Jr. A human homologue of the *Drosophila* toll protein signals activation of adaptive immunity. Nature 1997; 388(6640):394.
50. Edwards D, Kirkpatrick CH. The immunology of mycobacterial diseases. Am Rev Respir Dis 1986;134:1062–71.
51. Means TK, Wang S, Lien E, et al. Human toll-like receptors mediate cellular activation by *Mycobacterium tuberculosis*. J Immunol 1999;163(7):3920.
52. Underhill DM, Ozinsky A, Smith KD, et al. Toll-like receptor-2 mediates mycobacteria-induced proinflammatory signaling in macrophages. Proc Natl Acad Sci U S A 1999;96(25):14459.
53. Liu PT, Stenger S, Li H, et al. Toll-like receptor triggering of a vitamin D-mediated human antimicrobial response. Science 2006;311:1770.
54. Takeda K, Kaisho T, Akira S. Toll-like receptors. Annu Rev Immunol 2003;21:335.

55. Uma Devi KR, Ramalingam B, Raja A. Qualitative and quantitative analysis of antibody response in childhood tuberculosis against antigens of *Mycobacterium tuberculosis*. Indian J Med Microbiol 2002;20:145–9.
56. Randhawa PS. Lymphocyte subsets in granulomas of human tuberculosis: an in situ immunofluorescence study using monoclonal antibodies. Pathology 1990; 22:153–5.
57. Yu CT, Wang CH, Huang TJ, et al. Relation of bronchoalveolar lavage T lymphocyte subpopulations to rate of regression of active pulmonary tuberculosis. Thorax 1995;50:869–74.
58. Taha RA, Kotsimbos TC, Song YL, et al. IFN-gamma and IL-12 are increased in active compared with inactive tuberculosis. Am J Respir Crit Care Med 1997; 155:1135–9.
59. Stenger S, Mazzaccaro RJ, Uyemura K, et al. Differential effects of cytolytic T cell subsets on intracellular infection. Science 1997;276:1684–7.
60. Uma Devi KR, Ramalingam B, Raja A. Antibody response to *Mycobacterium tuberculosis* 30 and 16kDa antigens in pulmonary tuberculosis with human immunodeficiency virus coinfection. Diagn Microbiol Infect Dis 2003;46:205–9.
61. Hirsch CS, Toossi Z, Johnson JL, et al. Augmentation of apoptosis and interferon G production at sites of active *Mycobacterium tuberculosis* infection in human tuberculosis. J Infect Dis 2001;183:779–88.
62. Hirsch CS, Ioossl Z, Vanham G, et al. Apoptosis and T cell hyporesponsiveness in pulmonary tuberculosis. J Infect Dis 1999;179:945–53, 64.
63. Sulochana D, Deepa S, Prabha C. Cell proliferation and apoptosis: dual-signal hypothesis tested in tuberculous pleuritis using mycobacterial antigens. FEMS Immunol Med Microbiol 2004;41:85–92.
64. Varadhachary AS, Perdow SN, Hu C, et al. Differential ability of T cell subsets to undergo activation-induced cell death. Proc Natl Acad Sci U S A 1997;94: 5778–83.
65. McKinney JD, Jacobs WR, Bloom BR. Persisting problems in tuberculosis. In: Krause RM, editor. Emerging infections. San Diego (CA): Academic Press; 1998. p. 51–146.
66. Andersen P, Munk ME, Pollock JM, et al. Specific immune-based diagnosis of tuberculosis. Lancet 2000;356(9235):1099.
67. Barnes PF. Diagnosing latent tuberculosis infection: turning glitter to gold. Am J Respir Crit Care Med 2004;170(1):5.
68. Doherty TM, Demissie A, Olobo J, et al. Immune responses to the *Mycobacterium tuberculosis*-specific antigen ESAT-6 signal subclinical infection among contacts of tuberculosis patients. J Clin Microbiol 2002;40(2):704.
69. Ladel CH, Szalay G, Riedel D, et al. Interleukin-12 secretion by *Mycobacterium tuberculosis* infected macrophages. Infect Immun 1997;65:1936–8.
70. Cooper AM, Magram J, Ferrante J, et al. Interleukin 12 (IL-12) is crucial to the development of protective immunity in mice intravenously infected with *Mycobacterium tuberculosis*. J Exp Med 1997;186:39–45.
71. Ottenhof TH, Kumararatne D, Casanova JL. Novel human immunodeficiencies reveal the essential role of type-1 cytokines in immunity to intracellular bacteria. Immunol Today 1998;19:491–4.
72. Flesch I, Kaufmann SH. Mycobacterial growth inhibition by interferon-gamma-activated bone marrow macrophages and differential susceptibility among strains of *Mycobacterium tuberculosis*. J Immunol 1987;138:4408–13.
73. Cooper AM, Dalton DK, Stewart TA, et al. Disseminated tuberculosis in interferon gamma gene-disrupted mice. J Exp Med 1993;178:2243–7.

74. Blanchard DK, Michelini-Norris MB, Pearson CA, et al. Production of granulocyte-macrophage colony-stimulating factor (GM-CSF) by monocytes and large granular lymphocytes stimulated with *Mycobacterium avium-M. intracellulare*: activation of bactericidal activity by GM-CSF. Infect Immun 1991;59: 2396–402.

75. Jouanguy E, Altare F, Lamhamedi S, et al. Interferon-γ-receptor deficiency in an infant with fatal bacille Calmette-Guérin infection. N Engl J Med 1996;335: 1956–61.

76. Lin Y, Zhang M, Hofman FM, et al. Absence of a prominent Th2 cytokine response in human tuberculosis. Infect Immun 1996;64:1351–6.

77. Zhang M, Lin Y, Iyer DV, et al. T cell cytokine responses in human infection with *Mycobacterium tuberculosis*. Infect Immun 1995;63:3231–4.

78. Sodhi A, Gong J, Silva C, et al. Clinical correlates of interferon gamma production in patients with tuberculosis. Clin Infect Dis 1997;25:617–20.

79. Garcia I, Miyazaki Y, Marchal G, et al. High sensitivity of transgenic mice expressing soluble TNFR1 fusion protein to mycobacterial infections: synergistic action of TNF and IFN-gamma in the differentiation of protective granulomas. Eur J Immunol 1997;27:3182–90.

80. Fujiwara H, Kleinhenz ME, Wallis RS, et al. Increased interleukin-1 production and monocyte suppressor cell activity associated with human tuberculosis. Am Rev Respir Dis 1986;133:73–7.

81. Saunders BM, Frank AA, Orme IM, et al. Interleukin-6 induces early gamma interferon production in the infected lung but is not required for generation of specific immunity to *Mycobacterium tuberculosis* infection. Infect Immun 2000; 68:3322–6.

82. Rojas M, Olivier M, Gros P, et al. TNFa and IL-10 modulate the induction of apoptosis by virulent *Mycobacterium tuberculosis* in murine macrophages. J Immunol 1999;162:6122–31.

83. Dahl KE, Shiratsuchi H, Hamilton BD, et al. Selective induction of transforming growth factor β in human monocytes by lipoarabinomannan of *Mycobacterium tuberculosis*. Infect Immun 1996;64:399–405.

84. Ding A, Nathan CF, Graycar J, et al. Macrophage deactivating factor and transforming growth factor beta 1-beta 2 and beta 3 inhibit induction of macrophage nitrogen oxide synthesis by IFN-gamma. J Immunol 1990;145:940–4.

85. Rojas RE, Balaji KN, Subramanian A, et al. Regulation of human CD4+ αβ T cell receptor positive (TCR+) and γδ TCR+ T-cell responses to *Mycobacterium tuberculosis* by transforming growth factor β. Infect Immun 1999;67:6461–72.

86. Ruscetti F, Varesio L, Ochoa A, et al. Pleiotropic effects of transforming growth factor-beta on cells of the immune system. Ann N Y Acad Sci 1993;685: 488–500.

87. Bonecchi R, Bianchi G, Bordignon PP, et al. Differential expression of chemokine receptors and chemotactic responsiveness of type 1 T helper cells (Th1s) and Th2s. J Exp Med 1998;187:129–34.

88. Lopez Ramirez GM, Rom WN, Ciotoli C, et al. *Mycobacterium tuberculosis* alters expression of adhesion molecules on monocytic cells. Infect Immun 1994;62: 2515–20.

89. Nau GJ, Guilfoile P, Chupp GL, et al. A chemoattractant cytokine associated with granulomas in tuberculosis and silicosis. Proc Natl Acad Sci U S A 1997; 94:6414–9.

90. Spector WG, Lykke AW. The cellular evolution of inflammatory granulomata. J Pathol Bacteriol 1966;92:163–77.

91. Orme IM, Roberts AD, Griffin JP, et al. Cytokine secretion by CD4 T lymphocytes acquired in response to *Mycobacterium tuberculosis* infection. J Immunol 1993; 151:518–25.
92. Rhoades ER, Cooper AM, Orme IM. Chemokine response in mice infected with *Mycobacterium tuberculosis*. Infect Immun 1995;63:3871–7.
93. Fitzgerald D, Sterlin T, Haas D. *Mycobacterium tuberculosis*. In: Mandell GL, Bennett JE, Dolin R, editors. 7th edition. Principles and practice of infectious diseases, vol. 2. Philadelphia: Elsevier; 2010. p. 3129.
94. Sai Baba KS, Moudgil KD, Jain RC, et al. Complement activation in pulmonary tuberculosis. Tubercle 1990;71:103–7.
95. Iseman MD. Immunity and pathogenesis Iseman MD. A clinician's guide to tuberculosis. Philadelphia: Lippincott Williams & Wilkins; 2000. p. 63–91.
96. Ramanathan VD, Jawahar MS, Paramasivan CN, et al. A histological spectrum of host responses in tuberculous lymphadenitis. Indian J Med Res 1999;109: 212–20.
97. Hopewell PC, Kato-Maeda M, Mason RJ, et al. Tuberculosis. In: Mason RJ, Broaddus VC, Martin T, et al, editors. 5th edition. Murray and Nadel's textbook of respiratory medicine, vol. 1. Philadelphia: Saunders; 2010. p. 754–92. (Chapter: 34).
98. Mohan AK, Cote TR, Siegel JN, et al. Infectious complications of biologic treatments of rheumatoid arthritis. Curr Opin Rheumatol 2003;15:179–84.
99. Kwon HJ, Coté TR, Cuffe MS, et al. Case reports of heart failure after therapy with a tumor necrosis factor antagonist. Ann Intern Med 2003;138(10):807–11.
100. Tappy L, Chioléro R. Substrate utilization in sepsis and multiple organ failure. Crit Care Med 2007;35(Suppl 9):S531–4.
101. Fallahi-Sichani M, Schaller MA, Kirschner DE, et al. Identification of key processes that control tumor necrosis factor availability in a tuberculosis granuloma. PLoS Comput Biol 2010;6(5):e1000778.
102. Wallis RS, Broder MS, Wong JY, et al. Granulomatous infectious diseases associated with tumor necrosis factor antagonists. Clin Infect Dis 2004;38(9): 1261.
103. Geyer M, Müller-Ladner U. Rationale of using different biological therapies in rheumatoid arthritis. Arthritis Res Ther 2010;12(4):214.
104. Kindler V, Sappino AP, Grau GE, et al. The inducing role of tumor necrosis factor in the development of bactericidal granulomas during BCG infection. Cell 1989; 56(5):731.
105. Algood HM, Lin PL, Flynn JL. Tumor necrosis factor and chemokine interactions in the formation and maintenance of granulomas in tuberculosis. Clin Infect Dis 2005;41(Suppl 3):S189.
106. Benini J, Ehlers EM, Ehlers S. Different types of pulmonary granuloma necrosis in immunocompetent vs. TNFRp55-gene-deficient mice aerogenically infected with highly virulent Mycobacterium avium. J Pathol 1999;189(1):127.
107. Bopst M, Garcia I, Guler R, et al. Differential effects of TNF and LTalpha in the host defense against *M. bovis* BCG. Eur J Immunol 2001;31(6):1935.
108. Gómez-Reino JJ, Carmona L, Valverde VR, et al, BIOBADASER Group. Treatment of rheumatoid arthritis with tumor necrosis factor inhibitors may predispose to significant increase in tuberculosis risk: a multicenter active-surveillance report. Arthritis Rheum 2003;48(8):2122.
109. Brassard P, Kezouh A, Suissa S. Antirheumatic drugs and the risk of tuberculosis. Clin Infect Dis 2006;43(6):717.
110. Wallis RS. Reconsidering adjuvant immunotherapy for tuberculosis. Clin Infect Dis 2005;41(2):201–8.

111. Tubach F, Salmon D, Ravaud P, et al, Research Axed on Tolerance of Biotherapies Group. Risk of tuberculosis is higher with anti-tumor necrosis factor monoclonal antibody therapy than with soluble tumor necrosis factor receptor therapy: the three-year prospective French Research Axed on Tolerance of Biotherapies registry. Arthritis Rheum 2009;60(7):1884.

112. Dixon WG, Hyrich KL, Watson KD, et al. Drug-specific risk of tuberculosis in patients with rheumatoid arthritis treated with anti-TNF therapy: results from the British Society for Rheumatology Biologics Register (BSRBR). Ann Rheum Dis 2010;69(3):522.

113. Smolen J, Brezezicki J, Mason D, et al. Efficacy and safety of certolizumab pegol in combination with methotrexate (MTX) in patients with active rheumatoid arthritis despite MTX therapy: results from the RAPID 2 study. Ann Rheum Dis 2007;66(Suppl 2):187.

114. Wallis RS, Broder M, Wong J, et al. Granulomatous infections due to tumor necrosis factor blockade: correction. Clin Infect Dis 2004;39(8):1254.

115. Centers for Disease Control Prevention (CDC). Trends in tuberculosis–United States, 1998-2003. MMWR Morb Mortal Wkly Rep 2004;53(10):209.

116. Mohan AK, Coté TR, Block JA, et al. Tuberculosis following the use of etanercept, a tumor necrosis factor inhibitor. Clin Infect Dis 2004;39(3):295–9.

117. Fonseca JE, Canhão H, Silva C, et al. Tuberculosis in rheumatic patients treated with tumour necrosis factor alpha antagonists: the Portuguese experience. Acta Reumatol Port 2006;31(3):247 [in Portuguese].

118. Askling J, Fored CM, Brandt L, et al. Risk and case characteristics of tuberculosis in rheumatoid arthritis associated with tumor necrosis factor antagonists in Sweden. Arthritis Rheum 2005;52(7):1986.

119. Iseman MD. Mycobacterial infections in the era of modern biologic agents. Am J Med Sci 2011;341(4):278–80.

120. Nardell EA, Wallis RS. Here today–gone tomorrow: the case for transient acute tuberculosis infection. Am J Respir Crit Care Med 2006;174(7):734.

121. Coaccioli S, Di Cato L, Marioli D, et al. Impaired cutaneous cell-mediated immunity in newly diagnosed rheumatoid arthritis. Panminerva Med 2000;42(4):263.

122. Nestorov I. Clinical pharmacokinetics of TNF antagonists: how do they differ? Semin Arthritis Rheum 2005;34(5 Suppl 1):12.

123. Ringheanu M, Daum F, Markowitz J, et al. Effects of infliximab on apoptosis and reverse signaling of monocytes from healthy individuals and patients with Crohn's disease. Inflamm Bowel Dis 2004;10(6):801.

124. Saliu OY, Sofer C, Stein DS, et al. Tumor-necrosis-factor blockers: differential effects on mycobacterial immunity. J Infect Dis 2006;194(4):486.

125. Centers for Disease Control Prevention (CDC). Tuberculosis associated with blocking agents against tumor necrosis factor-alpha–California, 2002-2003. MMWR Morb Mortal Wkly Rep 2004;53(30):683.

126. Hill PC, Brookes RH, Fox A, et al. Large-scale evaluation of enzyme-linked immunospot assay and skin test for diagnosis of Mycobacterium tuberculosis infection against a gradient of exposure in The Gambia. Clin Infect Dis 2004; 38(7):966.

127. Greenberg JD, Reddy SM, Schloss SG, et al. Comparison of an in vitro tuberculosis interferon-gamma assay with delayed-type hypersensitivity testing for detection of latent Mycobacterium tuberculosis: a pilot study in rheumatoid arthritis. J Rheumatol 2008;35(5):770.

128. Mazurek GH, Jereb J, Lobue P, et al, Centers for Disease Control Prevention (CDC). Guidelines for using the QuantiFERON-TB Gold test for detecting

Mycobacterium tuberculosis infection, United States. MMWR Recomm Rep 2005;54(RR-15):49.

129. American Thoracic Society (ATS) and the Centers for Disease Control Prevention (CDC). Targeted tuberculin testing and treatment of latent tuberculosis infection. This official statement of the American Thoracic Society was adopted by the ATS Board of Directors, July 1999. This statement was endorsed by the Council of the Infectious Diseases Society of America. (IDSA), September 1999. Am J Respir Crit Care Med 2000;161:S221.

130. Furst DE, Keystone EC, Kirkham B, et al. Updated consensus statement on biological agents for the treatment of rheumatic diseases, 2008. Ann Rheum Dis 2008;67(Suppl 3):iii2–25.

131. Garcia Vidal C, Rodríguez Fernández S, Martínez Lacasa J, et al. Paradoxical response to antituberculous therapy in infliximab-treated patients with disseminated tuberculosis. Clin Infect Dis 2005;40(5):756.

132. Wallis RS, van Vuuren C, Potgieter S. Adalimumab treatment of life-threatening tuberculosis. Clin Infect Dis 2009;48(10):1429–32.

133. Winthrop KL, Yamashita S, Beekmann SE, et al. Infectious Diseases Society of America Emerging Infections Network. Mycobacterial and other serious infections in patients receiving anti-tumor necrosis factor and other newly approved biologic therapies: case finding through the Emerging Infections Network. Clin Infect Dis 2008;46(11):1738.

134. Winthrop KL, Chang E, Yamashita S, et al. Nontuberculous mycobacteria infections and anti-tumor necrosis factor-alpha therapy. Emerg Infect Dis 2009; 15(10):1556.

135. Lowrie DB, Tascon RE, Bonato VL, et al. Therapy of tuberculosis vaccine in mice by DNA vaccination. Nature 1999;400(6741):269–71.

136. Cardona PJ. RUTI: a new chance to shorten the treatment of latent tuberculosis infection. Tuberculosis (Edinb) 2006;86(3–4):273–89.

137. Nuermberger E, Tyagi S, Williams KN, et al. Rifapentine, moxifloxacin, or DNA vaccine improves treatment of latent tuberculosis in a mouse model. Am J Respir Crit Care Med 2005;172(11):1452–6.

138. Hernández-Pando R, Orozco-Esteves H, Maldonado HA, et al. A combination of a transforming growth factor-beta antagonist and an inhibitor of cyclooxygenase is an effective treatment for murine pulmonary tuberculosis. Clin Exp Immunol 2006;144(2):264–72.

139. Roy E, Stavropoulos E, Brennan J, et al. Therapeutic efficacy of high-dose intravenous immunoglobulin in *Mycobacterium tuberculosis* infection in mice. Infect Immun 2005;73(9):6101–9.

140. Dlugovitzky D, Stanford C, Stanford J. Immunological basis for the introduction of immunotherapy with *Mycobacterium vaccae* into the routine treatment of TB. Immunotherapy 2011;3(4):557–68.

141. Skinner MA, Yuan S, Prestidge R, et al. Immunization with heat-killed *Mycobacterium vaccae* stimulates CD8+ cytotoxic T cells specific for macrophages infected with *Mycobacterium tuberculosis*. Infect Immun 1997;65(11):4525–30.

142. Stanford J, Stanford C, Grange J. Immunotherapy with *Mycobacterium vaccae* in the treatment of tuberculosis [review]. Front Biosci 2004;9:1701–19.

143. Immunotherapy with *Mycobacterium vaccae* in patients with newly diagnosed pulmonary tuberculosis: a randomised controlled trial. Durban Immunotherapy Trial Group. Lancet 1999;354(9173):116–9.

144. Johnson JL, Kamya RM, Okwera A, et al. Randomized controlled trial of *Mycobacterium vaccae* immunotherapy in non-human immunodeficiency virus-infected

Ugandan adults with newly diagnosed pulmonary tuberculosis. The Uganda-Case Western Reserve University Research Collaboration. J Infect Dis 2000; 181(4):1304–12.

145. Grahmann PR, Braun RK. A new protocol for multiple inhalation of IFN-gamma successfully treats MDR-TB: a case study. The international journal of tuberculosis and lung disease : the official journal of the International Union against Tuberculosis and Lung Disease. Int J Tuberc Lung Dis 2008;12(6):636–44.

146. Assefa A, Bahr G, Rosa Brunet L. Report of the expert consultation on immunotherapeutic interventions for tuberculosis. Meeting report. Geneva, January 29–31, 2007.

147. Giosué S, Casarini M, Alemanno L, et al. Effects of aerosolized interferon-alpha in patients with pulmonary tuberculosis. Am J Respir Crit Care Med 1998;158(4): 1156–62.

148. Condos R, Rom WN, Schluger NW. Treatment of multidrug-resistant pulmonary tuberculosis with interferon-gamma via aerosol. Lancet 1997;349(9064):1513–5.

149. Park SK, Cho S, Lee IH, et al. Subcutaneously administered interferon-gamma for the treatment of multidrug-resistant pulmonary tuberculosis. Int J Infect Dis 2007;11(5):434–40.

150. Johnson JL, Ssekasanvu E, Okwera A, et al. Randomized trial of adjunctive interleukin-2 in adults with pulmonary tuberculosis. Am J Respir Crit Care Med 2003;168(2):185–91.

151. Katoch K, Singh P, Adhikari T, et al. Potential of Mw as a prophylactic vaccine against pulmonary tuberculosis. Vaccine 2008;26(9):1228–34.

152. Patel N, Deshpande MM, Shah M. Effect of an immunomodulator containing Mycobacterium w on sputum conversion in pulmonary tuberculosis. J Indian Med Assoc 2002;100(3):191–3.

153. Tsenova L, Bergtold A, Freedman VH, et al. Tumor necrosis factor alpha is a determinant of pathogenesis and disease progression in mycobacterial infection in the central nervous system. Proc Natl Acad Sci U S A 1999;96(10):5657–62.

154. Moreira AL, Tsenova-Berkova L, Wang J, et al. Effect of cytokine modulation by thalidomide on the granulomatous response in murine tuberculosis. Tuber Lung Dis 1997;78(1):47–55.

155. Fu LM, Fu-Liu CS. Thalidomide and tuberculosis. Int J Tuberc Lung Dis 2002; 6(7):569–72.

156. Schoeman JF, Andronikou S, Stefan DC, et al. Tuberculous meningitis-related optic neuritis: recovery of vision with thalidomide in 4 consecutive cases. J Child Neurol 2010;25(7):822–8.

157. Schoeman JF, Fieggen G, Seller N, et al. Intractable intracranial tuberculous infection responsive to thalidomide: report of four cases. J Child Neurol 2006; 21(4):301–8.

158. Schoeman JF, Springer P, van Rensburg AJ, et al. Adjunctive thalidomide therapy for childhood tuberculous meningitis: results of a randomized study. J Child Neurol 2004;19(4):250–7.

159. Lu HZ, Li BQ. Effect of HMG Co A reductase inhibitors on activation of human $\gamma\delta$ T cells induced by Mycobacterium tuberculosis antigens. Immunopharmacol Immunotoxicol 2009;31(3):485–91.

160. Alzeer AH, FitzGerald JM. Corticosteroids and tuberculosis: risks and use as adjunct therapy. Tuber Lung Dis 1993;74(1):6–11.

161. Martineau AR, Timms PM, Bothamley GH, et al. High dose vitamin D3 during intensive-phase antimicrobial treatment for pulmonary tuberculosis: a double-blind randomized controlled trial. Lancet 2011;377:242–50.

162. Lawson L, Thacher TD, Yassin MA, et al. Randomized controlled trial of zinc and vitamin A as co-adjuvants for the treatment of pulmonary tuberculosis. Trop Med Int Health 2010;15(12):1481–90.

163. Visset ME, Grewal HM, Swart EC, et al. The effect of vitamin A and zinc supplementation on treatment outcomes in pulmonary tuberculosis: a randomized controlled trial. Am J Clin Nutr 2011;93(1):93–100.

164. Tarallo MB, Urquiola C, Monge A, et al. Design of novel iron compounds as potential therapeutic agents against tuberculosis. J Inorg Biochem 2010;104(11): 1164–70.

Biologics and Infections: Lessons from Tumor Necrosis Factor Blocking Agents

Robert S. Wallis, MD

KEYWORDS

- Tumor necrosis factor-α • Granulomatous infection
- Granulomatous inflammation • Tuberculosis

In the decade since tumor necrosis factor α (TNF-α) antagonists were first approved for clinical use, they have proven invaluable for the treatment of specific types of chronic inflammation. Currently licensed TNF blockers fall into two classes, monoclonal antibody (or antibody fragments) and soluble receptor. Although they are equally effective in rheumatoid arthritis (RA) and psoriasis, important differences have emerged with regard to efficacy in granulomatous inflammation and risks of granulomatous infections, particularly tuberculosis (TB). This review focuses on recent studies that inform prevention and management of infections in this susceptible patient population.

TNF ANTAGONISTS

Four monoclonal anti-TNF antibodies are presently in clinical use: infliximab, adalimumab, golimumab, and certolizumab pegol (**Fig. 1**). Infliximab, the first to be approved, is a chimeric mouse/human protein, whereas the others contain only fully human amino acid sequences. Certolizumab pegol, the most recently approved, differs in that it is a pegylated, humanized Fab' fragment. All are approved for treatment of RA; all but certolizumab are also approved for psoriatic arthritis, psoriasis, and ankylosing spondylitis. Infliximab, adalimumab, and certolizumab are approved for treatment of Crohn disease (CD).[1,2] Infliximab is also approved for ulcerative colitis, and may be effective in sarcoidosis.[3–5] Infliximab is administered by intravenous infusion, whereas adalimumab, certolizumab, and golimumab are administered by subcutaneous injection.

Etanercept is the only soluble TNF receptor presently in clinical use. It comprises two extracellular domains of human TNF-R2 fused to the Fc fragment of human

Department of Specialty Care, Pfizer, 445 Eastern Point Road, Groton, CT 06340, USA
E-mail address: robert.wallis@pfizer.com

Infect Dis Clin N Am 25 (2011) 895–910
doi:10.1016/j.idc.2011.08.002
0891-5520/11/$ – see front matter © 2011 Elsevier Inc. All rights reserved.

id.theclinics.com

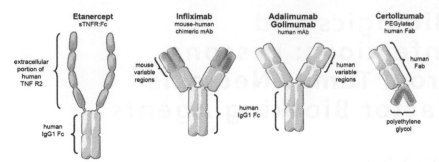

Fig. 1. Structures of the TNF antagonists. (*Adapted from* Wallis RS. Tumor necrosis factor antagonists: structure, function, and tuberculosis risks. Lancet Infect Dis 2008;8(10): 602; with permission.)

IgG1 (hTNFRII:hFc). It binds both TNF and lymphotoxin. Etanercept is approved for the treatment of RA, psoriatic arthritis, psoriasis, and ankylosing spondylitis.[6] Etanercept appears to be equally as effective as TNF antibodies for the treatment of RA. It is somewhat less effective in the treatment of psoriasis, although response rates approach those for infliximab as the duration of treatment is extended.[7] Etanercept is ineffective against granulomatous inflammatory conditions such as CD and sarcoidosis.[8,9] It is administered by subcutaneous injection.

INFECTION SURVEILLANCE: METHODS AND CHALLENGES

Clinical studies of the infectious complications of biologic therapies face several important limitations. Some types of infections are relatively uncommon in the United States and the European Union. As a result, their incidence may not be adequately appreciated at the time of licensing. Infection risks may change post licensing, reflecting the shift from research to clinical patient populations. In the United States, postlicensing surveillance of adverse events is conducted by the Food and Drug Administration (FDA) using a voluntary adverse event reporting system (AERS). It is anticipated that only a fraction of adverse events is captured. Duplication of reports, or submission of incomplete or inaccurate reports also may occur. Some studies have been conducted using prescription databases prepared by insurers or pharmacies, based on specific combinations of diagnosis codes and treatments. However, these may have limited ability to differentiate true treatment of an infectious complication from prophylactic or brief empiric therapy. In the European Union, the collection of postlicensing safety surveillance data has been substantially enhanced by the creation of national biologics registries, which are more complete and accurate than voluntary reporting systems. However, even in this circumstance, event frequencies can be unduly influenced by the nonrandom assignment of patients to specific therapies, particularly when infection risk and disease status are associated independently of treatment, as they are in RA.[10-13] Two strategies may be considered to account for this potential confounding effect. Risks may be adjusted based on patient demographic risk factors and disease activity scores, if available. Alternatively, adjustment may not be required if risks are compared among patients treated with agents considered to be equally efficacious. Studies summarized here have used one or both of these strategies.

SERIOUS INFECTIONS

Two studies have described the overall risk of serious infections posed by TNF blockers. In the first, Listing and colleagues[14] reported infectious complications for 512 German patients receiving etanercept, 346 receiving infliximab, and 601 control patients treated with disease-modifying antirheumatic drugs (DMARDs). After adjustment for disease-associated infection risks using a propensity score, the relative risks of serious infectious adverse events were 2.2 (95% confidence interval [CI] 0.9–5.4) for patients receiving etanercept and 2.1 (95% CI 0.8–5.5) for patients receiving infliximab, compared with controls. Bacterial infections of the lung, skin and soft tissue, and bone and joint, which are common in RA patients, predominated in this report. A recent, larger report based on British biologics registry data compared the risk of serious infection between 11,798 anti-TNF-treated patients and 3598 nonbiologic DMARD controls.[15] A total of 1808 patients had at least one serious infection. Crude incidence rates were 42 (95% CI 40–44) and 32 (95% CI 28–36) per 1000 patient-years for anti-TNF and control patients, respectively. Risks were adjusted based on disease activity and demographic characteristics. The adjusted hazard ratio for serious infection in the anti-TNF cohort was 1.2 (95% CI 1.1–1.5), and did not differ significantly among adalimumab, etanercept, and infliximab. The adjusted risk was highest during the first 6 months of therapy (1.8), after which it declined. Together, these studies appear to indicate that for most pathogens, sufficient redundancies exist in human host defenses against infection to substantially compensate for the loss of TNF signaling.

GRANULOMATOUS INFECTIONS: TUBERCULOSIS, HISTOPLASMOSIS, AND COCCICIDIOIDOMYCOSIS

A different, and possibly more illuminating, story emerges if one focuses on granulomatous infections, in which a critical role for TNF is better appreciated. These studies are summarized in **Table 1**. In 2004, the author and colleagues published a study of granulomatous infections associated with infliximab or etanercept reported to FDA AERS from January 1998 through September 2002.[16] The report was corrected shortly thereafter to remove European TB cases attributable to infliximab.[17] Compared with etanercept, infliximab was associated with significantly greater risks (2–7 fold) of TB, coccidioidomycosis, and histoplasmosis. In addition, a shorter time to TB onset (17 vs 48 weeks), and a higher proportion of TB cases with disseminated or extrapulmonary disease (25% vs 10%) were also observed. The findings with regard to coccidioidomycosis were confirmed by a retrospective study conducted in the US Southwest, which found a fivefold higher rate due to infliximab than other antirheumatic drugs (P<.01).[18]

A large prospective study of TB using the French RATIO registry identified 69 cases in patients treated with TNF blockers over 3 years.[19] The sex-adjusted and age-adjusted TB incidence rate was 1.17 per 1000 patient-years, 12.2 times that of the general population. Nearly all of the excess risk was due to infliximab (standardized incidence ratio [SIR] = 18.6, 95% CI 13.4–25.8) and adalimumab (SIR = 29.3, 95% CI 20.2–42.4) rather than etanercept (SIR = 1.8, 95% CI 0.7–4.3). A similar conclusion was reached by a Portuguese biologics registry study of 13 TB cases that found the TB risk of TNF antibodies 6.4-fold greater than with etanercept.[20]

One additional study, by Brassard and colleagues,[21] used prescriptions for isoniazid in a large pharmaceutical claims database to identify TB cases occurring in patients with a diagnosis of RA. The added risk attributable to TNF blockade in this study appeared small; however, TB rates in the entire RA cohort were greater than 5 times

Table 1
Tuberculosis, coccidioidomycosis, and histoplasmosis risks of TNF blockers

Disease Country	Data Source	Data Type	Years	Total Cases	INFL	ADAL	ETAN
						Case Rate Ratio	
Tuberculosis							
USA[17]	FDA	Voluntary reports	1998–2002	138	1.9		1
France[19]	RATIO	Biologics registry	2004–2007	69	13.3	17.1	1
USA[21]	Pharmetrics	Prescription database	1998–2003	51	1.3		1
UK[95]	BSRBR	Biologics registry	2001–2008	40	3.1	4.2	1
Sweden[96]	ARTIS	Biologics registry	1999–2004	13	1.8		1
Portugal[20]	GEAR	Biologics registry	1999–2005	13	5.8	7.7	1
Coccidioidomycosis							
USA[17]	FDA	Voluntary reports	1998–2002	12	6		1
USA[18]	Clinic	Patient records	1998–2003	13	5		1
Histoplasmosis							
USA[17]	FDA	Voluntary reports	1998–2002	40	7		1

Case rate ratios are expressed relative to etanercept.
Abbreviations: ADAL, adalimumab; ETAN, etanercept; FDA, Food and Drug Administration; INFL, infliximab

that expected. It is likely that the study findings were confounded by the misclassification of latent TB infection (LTBI) as active TB.[22,23]

REACTIVATION OF LATENT INFECTION VERSUS PROGRESSION OF NEW INFECTION

The twin observations of increased risk and shorter time to onset provide important clues as to the etiology of TB caused by TNF antibody, as early clustering of excess cases is consistent with reactivation. By contrast, TB due to progression of new infection occurs at random over time; such cases would be expected to occur uniformly over time after initiation of anti-TNF treatment. A study by the author systematically examined these issues using hidden Markov modeling, which describes transitions among clinical states.[24] The study revealed that more than 20% of LTBIs are reactivated each month by infliximab, 12.1-fold greater than with etanercept ($P<.001$). However, the analysis also revealed that both drugs caused a high proportion of new infections to progress directly to active disease. The findings were consistent with the reported effects of soluble murine TNF receptor (mTNFRII:mFc) and anti-mouse TNF antibody in acutely and chronically TB-infected mice.[25] Mice pretreated with either anti-TNF agent were unable to contain aerosol challenge with *Mycobacterium tuberculosis*; all rapidly succumbed. However, in chronically TB-infected mice, in which the infection is stable due to containment by granulomas, only anti-TNF antibody treatment resulted in disease progression and death.

Thus, in both humans and mice, only TNF antibody (and not soluble receptor) appears to affect the integrity of established granulomas. This observation appears to be consistent both in granulomas of infectious origin (TB, histoplasmosis, and coccidioidomycosis) and in those of unknown cause (CD and sarcoidosis), if one considers both the efficacy and infection profiles of these agents.

OTHER GRANULOMATOUS INFECTIONS

A survey of Infection Disease physicians in the United States revealed that disease due to nontuberculous mycobacteria (NTM) may surpass TB in patients treated with biologic therapies, in part due to increased awareness and screening for LTBI.[26] TNF antibodies and soluble receptor appear to pose equal risks of NTM infections.[17,26] Aspergillosis, candidiasis, and cryptococcosis similarly appear to have equal incidence in TNF antibody and etanercept-treated patients.[17,26,27] It is likely that this reflects a reduced role for latency and reactivation—and a corresponding increase in the role of progression of new infection—in the pathogenesis of these infections compared with TB.

VIRAL INFECTIONS

A study by Strangfeld and colleagues[28] used the German biologics registry to examine the impact of TNF blockers on herpes zoster. The study identified 86 episodes in 5040 patients. After adjusting for age, RA severity, and glucocorticoid use, a small but significantly increased risk was observed for treatment with the monoclonal antibodies (hazard ratio [HR] 1.82; 95% CI 1.05–3.15) but not for etanercept (HR 1.36; 95% CI 0.73–2.55). The risks posed by TNF antibodies were greater when the analysis was restricted to ophthalmic and multidermatomal disease, or when a within-subjects analysis was conducted in patients who had been treated with multiple agents. Eighteen cases of severe herpes infection were similarly identified among 45 non-TB opportunistic infections in anti-TNF–treated patients in the French RATIO registry.[29] All but 1 case occurred in patients treated with anti-TNF antibodies. Other infections in that report included bacterial, fungal, and parasitic infections. Risk factors for opportunistic infections were treatment with infliximab (odds ratio [OR] = 17.6, 95% CI 4.3–72.9; $P<.0001$) or adalimumab (OR = 10.0, 95% CI 2.3–44.4; $P = .002$) versus etanercept, and oral steroid use greater than 10 mg/d or intravenous boluses during the previous year (OR = 6.3, 95% CI 2.0–20.0; $P = .002$). Lastly, a retrospective study of RA patients in a large cohort of United States veterans also found an increased risk of zoster in association with infliximab treatment.[30] Latency and reactivation are central to the pathogenesis of herpesvirus infections.

Reactivation of hepatitis B virus (HBV) infection has also been attributed to anti-TNF therapy, although this literature is limited to individual case reports and small retrospective series.[31–38] A small retrospective study suggests HBV reactivation may be prevented by concurrent antiviral therapy.[39] By contrast, hepatitis C infection appears relatively unaffected by TNF blockers of either class.[40,41]

STRUCTURE-FUNCTION RELATIONSHIP

The differences in biologic activity and infection risks of the two classes of TNF blockers have been attributed to their molecular structures.[42] Most research in this area has focused on the ability of anti-TNF antibodies to cross-link transmembrane TNF and thereby induce apoptosis in TNF-expressing T cells. This activity can be demonstrated in vitro using reporter cell constructs and, in vivo, in T cells infiltrating the gut of CD patients.[43–48] Other studies have examined complement-mediated lysis of TNF-expressing T cells. A recent study by Bruns and colleagues,[49] for example, found that numbers of circulating effector memory CD8 T cells were reduced by infliximab treatment.

However, experience with the Fab' TNF antibody fragment certolizumab pegol calls into question the significance of these observations. With only one TNF binding region and without Fc, certolizumab can neither cross-link tmTNF nor activate complement; it can cause neither cell lysis nor apoptosis. Nonetheless, two phase 3 placebo-controlled trials of certolizumab in RA (RAPID 1 and 2) reported TB rates of 8.5 and 12.5 cases per 1000 patient-years of certolizumab exposure, with no cases in controls.[50–52] Certolizumab is also highly effective as therapy for CD.[53,54] These findings indicate that despite its structural differences, certolizumab shares with other TNF antibodies efficacy against granulomatous inflammation and efficiency in reactivating LTBI. Other properties not involving cell death, such as binding avidity and inhibition of cell activation, must therefore be more important in defining the structure-function relationship.[55–57]

LATENT TUBERCULOSIS: DIAGNOSIS AND TREATMENT

Strategies to reduce TB risk due to TNF blockade emphasize detection and treatment of LTBI. Although the largest experience for LTBI diagnosis exists for the tuberculin skin test (TST), its specificity is reduced by antigens shared by *Mycobacterium bovis* bacille Calmette-Guérin (BCG) and other NTM. BCG vaccination is performed in infants in more than 100 countries. BCG is not administered in the United States, due to concerns that it interferes with the TST. However, TST reactions due to BCG decline rapidly in adults and infants.[58,59] Large reactions in adults are unlikely to be caused solely by vaccination in infancy.

The specificity of testing for LTBI can be improved by the use of the antigens ESAT-6 and CFP-10, which are encoded by genes absent from all BCG strains.[60] T-cell responses to these antigens are detected by in vitro assays as the release of inter-feron-γ (IGRA), either by enzyme-linked immunosorbent assay (ELISA) or enzyme-linked immunosorbent spot assay. Some studies have reported reduced sensitivity of testing with ESAT-6 and CFP-10 compared with purified protein derivative,[61] although others have not.[62] Studies in India and Peru indicate that most TST reactivity in regions of high TB prevalence is indeed due to *M tuberculosis* infection rather than merely BCG sensitization.[62,63] No studies have yet reported outcomes when IGRA testing is used rather than TST to identify persons with LTBI before starting anti-TNF therapy, nor have any studies compared IGRA with boosted (2-step) TST. Such studies are needed if the trend toward preference for IGRA versus TST is to be based on science rather than convenience.

TST responses are reduced in RA.[64–66] TST sensitivity may be increased by repeated testing 7 to 10 days after a negative test (boosting), at the cost of reduced specificity.[67,68] The sensitivity of screening can be further improved by chest radiography to identify regional scarring and hilar lymphadenopathy. The effectiveness of screening using a boosted (2-step) TST has been documented by the Spanish BIOBADASER registry, initiated in 2000. Thirty-two cases of TB were reported among the first 1648 patients treated with infliximab, a rate 23 times the general population. Beginning in 2002, recommendations were implemented requiring patients to be screened by chest radiography and 2-step TST using a 5-mm threshold. Persons with evidence of LTBI were required to receive at least the first of 9 months' treatment with isoniazid before initiating anti-TNF therapy. TB rates in infliximab-treated patients declined by 74%.[69] Isoniazid was well tolerated. Elevated transaminases were reported in 7 of 324 isoniazid-treated patients, with no deaths or hospitalizations.

Boosted TST appears to be critical for successful LTBI detection in RA. A follow-up study reported by BIOBADASER found that the probability of developing TB after starting a TNF blocker was more than sevenfold greater if recommendations were not explicitly followed.[70] Lack of boosted testing was the main failure in complying with recommendations. This finding is consistent with the experience in the French RATIO registry, in which only a single TST was used. Of the 69 TB cases in the RATIO study, 45 had undergone TST screening and 30 had been found negative (<5 mm).[19] No TB cases occurred in patients who had been prescribed and were compliant with appropriate LTBI treatment, indicating the failure was one of diagnosis rather than therapy. No studies have yet been reported examining the effectiveness of IGRA-based screening programs.

No studies (either prospective or retrospective) have examined the required duration of LTBI treatment before starting anti-TNF treatment. Most authorities recommend that isoniazid be given alone for at least 1 month to ascertain its safety and tolerability in any given patient, but that the remaining 5 to 8 months may be given concurrently with a TNF blocker. Studies conducted in the 1970s indicated that a 52-week regimen of isoniazid was 75% effective in preventing active TB.[71,72] This level of efficacy is consistent with that observed in the Spanish cohort cited earlier. Thus, concurrent TNF blockade does not appear to interfere with the efficacy of LTBI treatment with isoniazid. However, it is of interest that the same historical isoniazid trials showed that shorter durations of treatment of 24 and 12 weeks were only 65% and 21% effective, respectively.[71,72] It is therefore highly unlikely that 1 month of isoniazid treatment is sufficient to eradicate LTBI. This finding indicates that eradication of LTBI before starting TNF blockade is not required, but merely that preventive treatment has been initiated and continues concurrently.

In other settings, larger TST or interferon-γ responses have been linked to higher TB risk.[73–76] The significance of large reactions in patients with RA or CD is not yet known. Patients being switched from etanercept to antibody should be tested and treated for LTBI if this had not been done previously. Periodic retesting should be considered for patients who may have acquired LTBI since their first screening.[77] TB due to progression of new infection will not be affected by LTBI treatment, except, presumably, during the time the treatment is administered. Alternative strategies, such as life-long preventive therapy, may be required as the use of biologics increases in TB-endemic regions where ongoing transmission of new infection is more likely to occur.

MANAGEMENT OF INCIDENT TUBERCULOSIS CASES

Many questions remain regarding optimal management of patients who develop TB due to TNF blockade. Although the RATIO database describes 2 TB patients who were continued on anti-TNF therapy without apparent ill effect, most guidelines recommend halting anti-TNF therapy until a response to anti-TB therapy is evident. These recommendations place patients at risk of disease exacerbation, due to recovery of TNF-dependent inflammation. Such cases, termed paradoxic reactions (PR), are marked by worsening inflammation despite microbiologic improvement. Such cases are most likely to occur in patients who develop disseminated or extrapulmonary TB attributable to treatment with anti-TNF antibody and in whom that treatment is stopped.[20,78–82] The most common case definition for this syndrome requires an initial clinical response before subsequent deterioration. However, this definition may fail to identify cases due to withdrawal of the short-acting TNF antibodies adalimumab and certolizumab, in which progressive exacerbation may occur without initial improvement. The syndrome is therefore likely underrecognized.

Two cases have been recently reported in which anti-TNF antibodies were used to treat life-threatening TB. In one, a South African RA patient developed extensive bilateral lower lobe TB 8 months into treatment with adalimumab.[83] Adalimumab was withdrawn and standard TB therapy started. Culture and molecular testing revealed fully susceptible *M tuberculosis* at diagnosis that was appropriately cleared by treatment. Nonetheless, signs and symptoms worsened during the following 3 weeks, ultimately requiring ventilatory support and lung biopsy. Improvement did not occur until adalimumab was resumed at the dose for initial treatment of CD (**Fig. 2**). A delayed, contributing role of corticosteroid cannot be excluded in this case. However, other studies of prednisolone given in substantially greater doses in TB have not shown comparable levels of effectiveness.[84] This may be due to induction of hepatic enzymes by rifampin, which reduces methylprednisolone exposure and effect by 66%.[85] In the second case, infliximab was successfully used to treat an intractable paradoxic reaction of the central nervous system (CNS) in a patient with multiple tuberculomas that had failed to respond to high-dose corticosteroids.[86] In a third case, adalimumab was used to treat recurrent immune reconstitution inflammatory syndrome in an AIDS patient with CNS cryptococcoma.[87] All 3 cases were remarkable for the rapidity of the radiographic and clinical responses to anti-TNF therapy. Further studies are warranted to confirm these observations.

ADJUNCTIVE ANTI-TNF THERAPY IN TUBERCULOSIS

Early resumption of anti-TNF therapy in patients who develop TB has generally not been recommended because of the concern that this might interfere with TB treatment. However, in neither of the aforementioned cases was the microbiologic response to therapy compromised. More significantly, two controlled clinical trials have prospectively examined the effects of potent immunosuppressive and/or anti-TNF therapies on microbiologic outcomes in TB. Both were conducted in human immunodeficiency virus (HIV)-1–infected TB cases with relatively preserved TB immune responses (based on the presence of high CD4 counts and cavitary lung disease). The studies shared a single control arm (TB therapy only). Their main

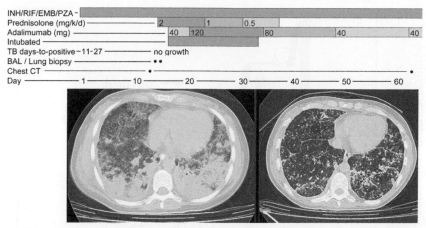

Fig. 2. Adalimumab treatment of life-threatening tuberculosis (TB). Day 1 indicates start of anti-TB therapy. Clearance of viable mycobacteria during the first 2 weeks of chemotherapy was accompanied by progressive clinical exacerbation attributed to withdrawal of the TNF antibody adalimumab. Clinical improvement was delayed until after day 20, when the patient received the full adalimumab dose recommended for initial treatment of Crohn disease (160 mg). BAL, bronchoalveolar lavage; EMB, ethambutol; INH, isoniazid; PZA, pyrazinamide; RIF, rifampin. (*Adapted from* Wallis RS, van Vuuren C, Potgieter S. Adalimumab treatment of life-threatening tuberculosis. Clin Infect Dis 2009;48(10):1430; with permission.)

objective was to examine the role of TNF in the acceleration of HIV disease progression due to TB; as such, their main end points were CD4 cell count and plasma HIV RNA load. However, both studies prospectively collected clinical and microbiologic data as indicators of safety. In both instances, these end points proved more interesting than the main study end points (which showed neither benefit nor harm).

One small prospective trial examined the effects of etanercept, 25 mg given subcutaneously twice weekly for 8 doses to 16 subjects, starting on day 4 of TB treatment.[88] Responses were compared with 42 CD4-matched controls. Sputum culture conversion occurred a median of 7 days earlier in the etanercept arm ($P = .04$) (filled triangles in **Fig. 3**). Etanercept was well tolerated. There were no serious opportunistic infections. CD4 cell counts rose by 96 cells/μL after 1 month of etanercept treatment ($P = .1$ compared with controls). The etanercept arm also showed trends toward superior resolution of lung infiltrates, closure of lung cavities, improvement in performance score, and weight gain; these approached statistical significance despite the small number of treated subjects.

A substantially greater microbiologic effect was observed in a phase 2 study in which 189 subjects were treated with prednisolone, 2.75 mg/kg/d or placebo for the first month of standard TB therapy.[84] The prednisolone dose had been selected based on a pilot study indicating this dose was required to reduce TB-stimulated TNF production ex vivo by half. The daily dose was tapered to zero during the second month; the average subject received a cumulative dose of more than 6500 mg. Although there is extensive experience in the use of corticosteroids to ameliorate symptoms in TB, no previous studies have examined the microbiologic effects of doses of this magnitude. Half of the prednisolone-treated subjects in this study converted to sputum culture negative after 1 month of treatment (open triangles in **Fig. 3**), versus 10% in the placebo arm ($P = .001$). The end point is important, as accelerated

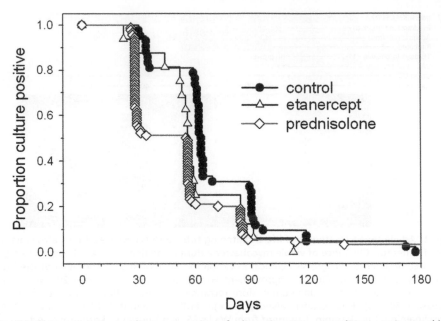

Fig. 3. Effects on sputum culture conversion of adjunctive etanercept (25 mg twice weekly) and high-dose methylprednisolone (2.75 mg/kg/d) during the first month of treatment of pulmonary tuberculosis. (*Reprinted from* Wallis RS. Reconsidering adjuvant immunotherapy for tuberculosis. Clin Infect Dis 2005;41(2):204; with permission.)

sputum culture conversion is strongly associated with accelerated tissue sterilization and reduced relapse risk.[89] The magnitude of this effect is striking, as the increment was superior to that observed in the landmark studies of rifampin, a key component of modern short-course TB therapy.[90] The effect of prednisolone was not caused by reduced sputum production, which declined similarly during treatment in both arms. There were no serious opportunistic infections. However, prednisolone-treated subjects were more likely to experience other early serious adverse events, including edema, hyperglycemia, electrolyte disturbances, and severe hypertension. Two other prospective randomized trials of adjunctive corticosteroids administered at lower doses have observed similar, albeit smaller, effects on the kinetics of sputum culture conversion.[91,92] A third found no effect.[93] There have been no reports of deleterious effects of corticosteroids on microbiologic outcomes in TB.

These findings support the concept that adjunctive therapy targeting granulomatous inflammation may accelerate the clinical and microbiologic response to treatment in TB, potentially hastening resolution of symptoms and shortening the required duration of treatment.[94] Anti-TNF antibodies, with their greater efficiency in reactivating LTBI, and greater efficacy in treatment of granulomatous inflammation, would be the logical candidates for such a trial. Such adjunctive treatment could potentially produce the same beneficial responses observed with high-dose corticosteroids without the harmful mineralocorticoid and glucocorticoid effects.

SUMMARY

Biologic anti-TNF therapies specifically increase the risk of granulomatous infections both by interfering with new granuloma formation and by weakening the integrity of established granulomas. The latter risk is greatest with anti-TNF antibodies. The risks of reactivation of latent TB infection can be substantially reduced in patients starting anti-TNF therapy by careful screening and treatment of LTBI. Although granulomas are an essential part of host defenses against mycobacterial infection, they appear paradoxically to protect *M tuberculosis* bacilli during TB therapy. Further research is needed to investigate the potential role of anti-TNF antibody to accelerate and shorten TB chemotherapy.

REFERENCES

1. Humira prescribing information. Abbott Park (IL): Abbott Laboratories; 2007. Available at: http://www.rxabbott.com/pdf/humira.pdf. Last Accessed November 22, 2007.
2. Infliximab (Remicade®) prescribing information. Malvern (PA): Centocor; 2008. Available at: http://www.remicade.com/remicade/assets/HCP_PPI.pdf. Last Accessed November 22, 2007.
3. Baughman RP, Drent M, Kavuru M, et al. Infliximab therapy in patients with chronic sarcoidosis and pulmonary involvement. Am J Respir Crit Care Med 2006;174(7):795–802.
4. Saleh S, Ghodsian S, Yakimova V, et al. Effectiveness of infliximab in treating selected patients with sarcoidosis. Respir Med 2006;100(11):2053–9.
5. Rossman MD, Newman LS, Baughman RP, et al. A double-blinded, randomized, placebo-controlled trial of infliximab in subjects with active pulmonary sarcoidosis. Sarcoidosis Vasc Diffuse Lung Dis 2006;23(3):201–8.
6. Enbrel prescribing information. Thousand Oaks (CA) and Madison (NJ): Amgen and Wyeth Pharmaceuticals; 2008. Available at: http://www.enbrel.com/prescribing-information.jsp. Last Accessed November 22, 2007.
7. Leonardi CL, Powers JL, Matheson RT, et al. Etanercept as monotherapy in patients with psoriasis. N Engl J Med 2003;349(21):2014–22.
8. Sandborn WJ, Hanauer SB, Katz S, et al. Etanercept for active Crohn's disease: a randomized, double-blind, placebo-controlled trial. Gastroenterology 2001; 121(5):1088–94.
9. Utz JP, Limper AH, Kalra S, et al. Etanercept for the treatment of stage II and III progressive pulmonary sarcoidosis. Chest 2003;124(1):177–85.
10. Au K, Reed G, Curtis JR, et al. Extended report: high disease activity is associated with an increased risk of infection in patients with rheumatoid arthritis. Ann Rheum Dis 2011;70(5):785–91.
11. Yamada T, Nakajima A, Inoue E, et al. Increased risk of tuberculosis in patients with rheumatoid arthritis in Japan. Ann Rheum Dis 2006;65(12):1661–3.
12. Seong SS, Choi CB, Woo JH, et al. Incidence of tuberculosis in Korean patients with rheumatoid arthritis (RA): effects of RA itself and of tumor necrosis factor blockers. J Rheumatol 2007;34(4):706–11.
13. Carmona L, Hernandez-Garcia C, Vadillo C, et al. Increased risk of tuberculosis in patients with rheumatoid arthritis. J Rheumatol 2003;30(7):1436–9.
14. Listing J, Strangfeld A, Kary S, et al. Infections in patients with rheumatoid arthritis treated with biologic agents. Arthritis Rheum 2005;52(11):3403–12.
15. Galloway JB, Hyrich KL, Mercer LK, et al. Anti-TNF therapy is associated with an increased risk of serious infections in patients with rheumatoid arthritis especially in the first 6 months of treatment: updated results from the British Society for Rheumatology Biologics Register with special emphasis on risks in the elderly. Rheumatology (Oxford) 2011;50(1):124–31.

16. Wallis RS, Broder MS, Wong JY, et al. Granulomatous infectious diseases associated with TNF antagonists. Clin Infect Dis 2004;38(9):1261–5.
17. Wallis RS, Broder MS, Wong JY, et al. Granulomatous infections due to tumor necrosis factor blockade: correction. Clin Infect Dis 2004;39:1254–6.
18. Bergstrom L, Yocum DE, Ampel NM, et al. Increased risk of coccidioidomycosis in patients treated with TNF antagonists. Arthritis Rheum 2004;50(6):1959–66.
19. Tubach F, Salmon D, Ravaud P, et al. Risk of tuberculosis is higher with anti-tumor necrosis factor monoclonal antibody therapy than with soluble tumor necrosis factor receptor therapy: the three-year prospective French research axed on tolerance of biotherapies registry. Arthitis Rheum 2009;60(7):1884–94.
20. Fonseca JE, Canhao H, Silva C, et al. Tuberculosis in rheumatic patients treated with tumour necrosis factor alpha antagonists: the Portuguese experience. Acta Reumatol Port 2006;31(3):247–53 [in Portuguese].
21. Brassard P, Kezouh A, Suissa S. Antirheumatic drugs and the risk of tuberculosis. Clin Infect Dis 2006;43(6):717–22.
22. Mines D, Novelli L. Antirheumatic drugs and the risk of tuberculosis. Clin Infect Dis 2007;44(4):619–20.
23. Subramanyan GS, Yokoe DS, Sharnprapai S, et al. Using automated pharmacy records to assess the management of tuberculosis. Emerg Infect Dis 1999; 5(6):788–91.
24. Wallis RS. Mathematical modeling of the cause of tuberculosis during tumor necrosis factor blockade. Arthritis Rheum 2008;58(4):947–52.
25. Plessner HL, Lin PL, Kohno T, et al. Neutralization of tumor necrosis factor (TNF) by antibody but not TNF receptor fusion molecule exacerbates chronic murine tuberculosis. J Infect Dis 2007;195(11):1643–50.
26. Winthrop KL, Yamashita S, Beekmann SE, et al. Mycobacterial and other serious infections in patients receiving anti-tumor necrosis factor and other newly approved biologic therapies: case finding through the Emerging Infections Network. Clin Infect Dis 2008;46(11):1738–40.
27. Tsiodras S, Samonis G, Boumpas DT, et al. Fungal infections complicating tumor necrosis factor alpha blockade therapy. Mayo Clin Proc 2008;83(2):181–94.
28. Strangfeld A, Listing J, Herzer P, et al. Risk of herpes zoster in patients with rheumatoid arthritis treated with Anti–TNF-a agents. JAMA 2009;301(7):737–44.
29. Salmon-Ceron D, Tubach F, Lortholary O, et al. Drug-specific risk of non-tuberculosis opportunistic infections in patients receiving anti-TNF therapy reported to the 3-year prospective French RATIO registry. Ann Rheum Dis 2011; 70(4):616–23.
30. McDonald JR, Zeringue AL, Caplan L, et al. Herpes zoster risk factors in a national cohort of veterans with rheumatoid arthritis. Clin Infect Dis 2009; 48(10):1364–71.
31. Wendling D, Auge B, Bettinger D, et al. Reactivation of a latent precore mutant hepatitis B virus related chronic hepatitis during infliximab treatment for severe spondyloarthropathy. Ann Rheum Dis 2005;64(5):788–9.
32. Ueno Y, Tanaka S, Shimamoto M, et al. Infliximab therapy for Crohn's disease in a patient with chronic hepatitis B. Dig Dis Sci 2005;50(1):163–6.
33. Ostuni P, Botsios C, Punzi L, et al. Hepatitis B reactivation in a chronic hepatitis B surface antigen carrier with rheumatoid arthritis treated with infliximab and low dose methotrexate. Ann Rheum Dis 2003;62(7):686–7.
34. Michel M, Duvoux C, Hezode C, et al. Fulminant hepatitis after infliximab in a patient with hepatitis B virus treated for an adult onset still's disease. J Rheumatol 2003;30(7):1624–5.

35. Esteve M, Saro C, Gonzalez-Huix F, et al. Chronic hepatitis B reactivation following infliximab therapy in Crohn's disease patients: need for primary prophylaxis. Gut 2004;53(9):1363–5.

36. Sakellariou GT, Chatzigiannis I. Long-term anti-TNFalpha therapy for ankylosing spondylitis in two patients with chronic HBV infection. Clin Rheumatol 2007; 26(6):950–2.

37. Vassilopoulos D, Apostolopoulou A, Hadziyannis E, et al. Long-term safety of anti-TNF treatment in patients with rheumatic diseases and chronic or resolved hepatitis B virus infection. Ann Rheum Dis 2010;69(7):1352–5.

38. Caporali R, Bobbio-Pallavicini F, Atzeni F, et al. Safety of tumor necrosis factor alpha blockers in hepatitis B virus occult carriers (hepatitis B surface antigen negative/anti-hepatitis B core antigen positive) with rheumatic diseases. Arthritis Care Res (Hoboken) 2010;62(6):749–54.

39. Roux CH, Brocq O, Breuil V, et al. Safety of anti-TNF-alpha therapy in rheumatoid arthritis and spondylarthropathies with concurrent B or C chronic hepatitis. Rheumatology (Oxford) 2006;45(10):1294–7.

40. Oniankitan O, Duvoux C, Challine D, et al. Infliximab therapy for rheumatic diseases in patients with chronic hepatitis B or C. J Rheumatol 2004;31(1):107–9.

41. Ferri C, Ferraccioli G, Ferrari D, et al. Safety of anti-tumor necrosis factor-alpha therapy in patients with rheumatoid arthritis and chronic hepatitis C virus infection. J Rheumatol 2008;35(10):1944–9.

42. Wallis RS. Tumor necrosis factor antagonists: structure, function, and tuberculosis risks. Lancet Infect Dis 2008;8(10):601–11.

43. ten Hove T, van Montfrans C, Peppelenbosch MP, et al. Infliximab treatment induces apoptosis of lamina propria T lymphocytes in Crohn's disease. Gut 2002;50(2):206–11.

44. Van den Brande JM, Braat H, van den Brink GR, et al. Infliximab but not etanercept induces apoptosis in lamina propria T-lymphocytes from patients with Crohn's disease. Gastroenterology 2003;124(7):1774–85.

45. Di Sabatino A, Ciccocioppo R, Cinque B, et al. Defective mucosal T cell death is sustainably reverted by infliximab in a caspase dependent pathway in Crohn's disease. Gut 2004;53(1):70–7.

46. Van den Brande JM, Koehler TC, Zelinkova Z, et al. Prediction of antitumour necrosis factor clinical efficacy by real-time visualisation of apoptosis in patients with Crohn's disease. Gut 2007;56(4):509–17.

47. Shen C, Assche GV, Colpaert S, et al. Adalimumab induces apoptosis of human monocytes: a comparative study with infliximab and etanercept. Aliment Pharmacol Ther 2005;21(3):251–8.

48. Kirchner S, Holler E, Haffner S, et al. Effect of different tumor necrosis factor (TNF) reactive agents on reverse signaling of membrane integrated TNF in monocytes. Cytokine 2004;28(2):67–74.

49. Bruns H, Meinken C, Schauenberg P, et al. Anti-TNF immunotherapy reduces CD8+ T cell-mediated antimicrobial activity against *Mycobacterium tuberculosis* in humans. J Clin Invest 2009;119(5):1167–77.

50. Keystone E, Heijde D, Mason D Jr, et al. Certolizumab pegol plus methotrexate is significantly more effective than placebo plus methotrexate in active rheumatoid arthritis: findings of a fifty-two-week, phase III, multicenter, randomized, double-blind, placebo-controlled, parallel-group study. Arthritis Rheum 2008;58(11): 3319–29.

51. Smolen J, Brezezicki J, Mason D, et al. Efficacy and safety of certolizumab pegol in combination with methotrexate (MTX) in patients with active rheumatoid

arthritis despite MTX therapy: results from the RAPID 2 study. Ann Rheum Dis 2007;66(Suppl II): Ref Type: Abstract.

52. Keystone EC. Certolizumab. OP0016. Barcelona (Spain): Annual European Congress of Rheumatology; 2007. Ref Type: Abstract.

53. Nesbitt A, Fossati G, Bergin M, et al. Mechanism of action of certolizumab pegol (CDP870): in vitro comparison with other anti-tumor necrosis factor alpha agents. Inflamm Bowel Dis 2007;13(11):1323–32.

54. Sandborn WJ, Feagan BG, Stoinov S, et al. Certolizumab pegol for the treatment of Crohn's disease. N Engl J Med 2007;357(3):228–38.

55. Scallon B, Cai A, Solowski N, et al. Binding and functional comparisons of two types of tumor necrosis factor antagonists. J Pharmacol Exp Ther 2002;301(2):418–26.

56. Saliu O, Sofer C, Stein DS, et al. Tumor necrosis factor blockers: differential effects on mycobacterial immunity. J Infect Dis 2006;194:486–92.

57. Bourne T, Fossati G, Nesbitt A. A PEGylated Fab' fragment against tumor necrosis factor for the treatment of Crohn disease: exploring a new mechanism of action. BioDrugs 2008;22(5):331–7.

58. Brewer MA, Edwards KM, Palmer PS, et al. Bacille Calmette-Guerin immunization in normal healthy adults. J Infect Dis 1994;170:476–9.

59. Mudido PM, Guwatudde D, Nakakeeto MK, et al. The effect of bacille Calmette-Guerin vaccination at birth on tuberculin skin test reactivity in Ugandan children. Int J Tuberc Lung Dis 1999;3(10):891–5.

60. Behr MA, Wilson MA, Gill WP, et al. Comparative genomics of BCG vaccines by whole-genome DNA microarray. Science 1999;284(5419):1520–3.

61. Brock I, Weldingh K, Leyten EM, et al. Specific T-cell epitopes for immunoassay-based diagnosis of *Mycobacterium tuberculosis* infection. J Clin Microbiol 2004;42(6):2379–87.

62. Ponce de Leon D, Cevedo-Vasquez E, Alvizuri S, et al. Comparison of an interferon-gamma assay with tuberculin skin testing for detection of tuberculosis (TB) infection in patients with rheumatoid arthritis in a TB-endemic population. J Rheumatol 2008;35(5):776–81.

63. Lalvani A, Nagvenkar P, Udwadia Z, et al. Enumeration of T cells specific for RD1-encoded antigens suggests a high prevalence of latent *Mycobacterium tuberculosis* infection in healthy urban Indians. J Infect Dis 2001;183(3):469–77.

64. Ponce de Leon D, Cevedo-Vasquez E, Sanchez-Torres A, et al. Attenuated response to purified protein derivative in patients with rheumatoid arthritis: study in a population with a high prevalence of tuberculosis. Ann Rheum Dis 2005;64(9):1360–1.

65. Coaccioli S, Di Cato L, Marioli D, et al. Impaired cutaneous cell-mediated immunity in newly diagnosed rheumatoid arthritis. Panminerva Med 2000;42(4):263–6.

66. Paimela L, Johansson-Stephansson EA, Koskimies S, et al. Depressed cutaneous cell-mediated immunity in early rheumatoid arthritis. Clin Exp Rheumatol 1990;8(5):433–7.

67. Richards NM, Nelson KE, Batt MD, et al. Tuberculin test conversion during repeated skin testing, associated with sensitivity to nontuberculous mycobacteria. Am Rev Respir Dis 1979;120(1):59–65.

68. Thompson NJ, Glassroth JL, Snider DEJ, et al. The booster phenomenon in serial tuberculin testing. Am Rev Respir Dis 1979;119(4):587–97.

69. Carmona L, Gomez-Reino JJ, Rodriguez-Valverde V, et al. Effectiveness of recommendations to prevent reactivation of latent tuberculosis infection in

patients treated with tumor necrosis factor antagonists. Arthritis Rheum 2005; 52(6):1766–72.

70. Gomez-Reino JJ, Carmona L, Angel DM. Risk of tuberculosis in patients treated with tumor necrosis factor antagonists due to incomplete prevention of reactivation of latent infection. Arthritis Rheum 2007;57(5):756–61.

71. Comstock GW, Baum C, Snider DE Jr. Isoniazid prophylaxis among Alaskan Eskimos: a final report of the Bethel isoniazid studies. Am Rev Respir Dis 1979; 119(5):827–30.

72. IUAT Committee on Prophylaxis. Efficacy of various durations of isoniazid preventive therapy for tuberculosis: five years of follow-up in the IUAT trial. International Union Against Tuberculosis Committee on Prophylaxis. Bull World Health Organ 1982;60(4):555–64.

73. Higuchi K, Harada N, Fukazawa K, et al. Relationship between whole-blood interferon-gamma responses and the risk of active tuberculosis. Tuberculosis (Edinb) 2008;88(3):244–8.

74. Edwards LB, Acquaviva FA, Livesay VT. Identification of tuberculous infected: dual tests and density of reaction. Am Rev Respir Dis 1973;108:1334–9.

75. Diel R, Loddenkemper R, Meywald-Walter K, et al. Predictive value of a whole blood IFN-gamma assay for the development of active tuberculosis disease after recent infection with Mycobacterium tuberculosis. Am J Respir Crit Care Med 2008;177(10):1164–70.

76. Diel R, Loddenkemper R, Niemann S, et al. Value of a whole-blood interferon-(gamma) release assay for developing active tuberculosis: an update. Am J Respir Crit Care Med 2011;183(1):88–95.

77. Cooray DV, Moran R, Khanna D, et al. Screening, re-screening and treatment of PPD positivity in patients on anti-TNF-a therapy. Arthitis Rheum 2008;58: S546–547 Ref Type: Abstract.

78. Belknap R, Reves R, Burman W. Immune reconstitution to Mycobacterium tuberculosis after discontinuing infliximab. Int J Tuberc Lung Dis 2005;9(9):1057–8.

79. Arend SM, Leyten EM, Franken WP, et al. A patient with de novo tuberculosis during anti-tumor necrosis factor-alpha therapy illustrating diagnostic pitfalls and paradoxical response to treatment. Clin Infect Dis 2007;45(11):1470–5.

80. Strady C, Brochot P, Alnine K, et al. Tuberculosis during treatment by TNFalpha-inhibitors. Presse Med 2006;35(11 Pt 2):1765–72 [in French].

81. Garcia-Vidal C, Rodriguez FS, Martinez LJ, et al. Paradoxical response to antituberculous therapy in infliximab-treated patients with disseminated tuberculosis. Clin Infect Dis 2005;40(5):756–9.

82. Hess S, Hospach T, Nossal R, et al. Life threatening disseminated tuberculosis as a complication of TNF blockade in an adolescent. Eur J Pediatr 2011. [Epub ahead of print].

83. Wallis RS, van Vuuren C, Potgieter S. Adalimumab treatment of life-threatening tuberculosis. Clin Infect Dis 2009;48(10):1429–32.

84. Mayanja-Kizza H, Jones-Lopez EC, Okwera A, et al. Immunoadjuvant therapy for HIV-associated tuberculosis with prednisolone: a phase II clinical trial in Uganda. J Infect Dis 2005;191(6):856–65.

85. McAllister WA, Thompson PJ, Al-Habet SM, et al. Rifampicin reduces effectiveness and bioavailability of prednisolone. Br Med J (Clin Res Ed) 1983;286(6369): 923–5.

86. Blackmore TK, Manning L, Taylor W, et al. Therapeutic use of infliximab in tuberculosis to control severe paradoxical reaction involving the brain, lung, and lymph nodes. Clin Infect Dis 2008;47(10):e79–82.

87. Sitapati AM, Kao CL, Cachay ER, et al. Treatment of HIV-related inflammatory cerebral cryptococcoma using adalimumab. Clin Infect Dis 2009;50(2):e7–10.
88. Wallis RS, Kyambadde P, Johnson JL, et al. A study of the safety, immunology, virology, and microbiology of adjunctive etanercept in HIV-1-associated tuberculosis. AIDS 2004;18(2):257–64.
89. Wallis RS, Wang C, Doherty TM, et al. Biomarkers for tuberculosis disease activity, cure, and relapse. Lancet Infect Dis 2010;10(2):68–9.
90. East African-British Medical Research Councils. Controlled clinical trial of four short-course (6-month) regimens of chemotherapy for treatment of pulmonary tuberculosis. Third report. Lancet 1974;2(7875):237–40.
91. Bilaceroglu S, Perim K, Buyuksirin M, et al. Prednisolone: a beneficial and safe adjunct to antituberculosis treatment? a randomized controlled trial. Int J Tuberc Lung Dis 1999;3(1):47–54.
92. Horne NW. Prednisolone in treatment of pulmonary tuberculosis: a controlled trial. Final report to the Research Committee of the Tuberculosis Society of Scotland. Br Med J 1960;5215:1751–6.
93. Tripathy SP, Ramakrishnan CV, Nazareth O, et al. Study of chemotherapy regimens of 5 and 7 months' duration and the role of corticosteroids in the treatment of sputum-positive patients with pulmonary tuberculosis in South India. Tubercle 1983;64:73–91.
94. Wallis RS. Reconsidering adjuvant immunotherapy for tuberculosis. Clin Infect Dis 2005;41(2):201–8.
95. Dixon WG, Hyrich KL, Watson KD, et al. Drug-specific risk of tuberculosis in patients with rheumatoid arthritis treated with anti-TNF therapy: results from the British Society for Rheumatology Biologics Register (BSRBR). Ann Rheum Dis 2009;69(3):522–8.
96. Askling J, Fored CM, Brandt L, et al. Risk and case characteristics of tuberculosis in rheumatoid arthritis associated with tumor necrosis factor antagonists in Sweden. Arthritis Rheum 2005;52(7):1986–92.

Index

Note: Page numbers of article titles are in **boldface** type.

A

Adaptive immune response
   biologic response modifiers and, 735–737
S-Adenosylmethionine (SAMe)
   for hepatitis, 825–826
Albinterferon
   for hepatitis, 824
Anti-ID mAbs. *See* Anti-infectious disease (anti-ID) monoclonal antibodies (mAbs)
Anti-infectious disease (anti-ID) monoclonal antibodies (mAbs)
   scientific and technological basis for generation of, 789–791
Anti-inflammatory mediators, 841–842
Anti-TNF therapy
   adjuvant
      in tuberculosis, 900–902
Antibody(ies)
   monoclonal
      in infectious diseases, **789–802**. *See also* Monoclonal antibodies
Antimicrobial peptides
   in infectious diseases, 729
Arthritis
   rheumatoid
      vaccines in, 762–763
ASIA (autoimmune/inflammatory syndrome)
   adjuvants and, 856–858
Autoimmune diseases
   vaccines in, 762–764
Autoimmunity
   described, 746–747

B

Bacillus Calmette-Guérin (BCG) vaccine
   as biologic response modifier, 759–761
Bacterial infections
   biologic response modifiers' role in, 740–741
   polyclonal immunoglobulins and hyperimmune globulins in management and prevention
      of, 774–777
BCG vaccine. *See* Bacillus Calmette-Guérin (BCG) vaccine
Biologic response modifiers, **865–892**
   adaptive immune response and, 735–737
   described, 733–734
   endogenous

Infect Dis Clin N Am 25 (2011) 911–921
doi:10.1016/S0891-5520(11)00096-1
0891-5520/11/$ – see front matter © 2011 Elsevier Inc. All rights reserved.

id.theclinics.com

United States Postal Service

Statement of Ownership, Management, and Circulation
(All Periodicals Publications Except Requestor Publications)

1. Publication Title
Infectious Disease Clinics of North America

2. Publication Number
0 0 1 1 - 5 5 1 6

3. Filing Date
9/16/11

4. Issue Frequency
Mar, Jun, Sep, Dec

5. Number of Issues Published Annually
4

6. Annual Subscription Price
$251.00

7. Complete Mailing Address of Known Office of Publication (Not printer) (Street, city, county, state, and ZIP+4®)
Elsevier Inc.
360 Park Avenue South
New York, NY 10010-1710

Contact Person
Stephen Bushing

Telephone (Include area code)
215-235-3688

8. Complete Mailing Address of Headquarters or General Business Office of Publisher (Not printer)
Elsevier Inc., 360 Park Avenue South, New York, NY 10010-1710

9. Full Names and Complete Mailing Addresses of Publisher, Editor, and Managing Editor (Do not leave blank)

Publisher (Name and complete mailing address)
Kim Murphy, Elsevier, Inc., 1600 John F. Kennedy Blvd. Suite 1800, Philadelphia, PA 19103-2899

Editor (Name and complete mailing address)
Stephanie Donley, Elsevier, Inc., 1600 John F. Kennedy Blvd. Suite 1800, Philadelphia, PA 19103-2899

Managing Editor (Name and complete mailing address)
Barton Dudlick, Elsevier, Inc., 1600 John F. Kennedy Blvd. Suite 1800, Philadelphia, PA 19103-2899

10. Owner (Do not leave blank. If the publication is owned by a corporation, give the name and address of the corporation immediately followed by the names and addresses of all stockholders owning or holding 1 percent or more of the total amount of stock. If not owned by a corporation, give the names and addresses of the individual owners. If owned by a partnership or other unincorporated firm, give its name and address as well as those of each individual owner. If the publication is published by a nonprofit organization, give its name and address.)

Full Name	Complete Mailing Address
Wholly owned subsidiary of	4520 East-West Highway
Reed/Elsevier, US holdings	Bethesda, MD 20814

11. Known Bondholders, Mortgagees, and Other Security Holders Owning or Holding 1 Percent or More of Total Amount of Bonds, Mortgages, or Other Securities. If none, check box ► ☐ None

Full Name	Complete Mailing Address
N/A	

12. Tax Status (For completion by nonprofit organizations authorized to mail at nonprofit rates) (Check one)
The purpose, function, and nonprofit status of this organization and the exempt status for federal income tax purposes:
☐ Has Not Changed During Preceding 12 Months
☐ Has Changed During Preceding 12 Months (Publisher must submit explanation of change with this statement)

PS Form 3526, September 2007 (Page 1 of 3 (Instructions Page 3)) PSN 7530-01-000-9931 PRIVACY NOTICE: See our Privacy policy in www.usps.com

---

13. Publication Title
Infectious Disease Clinics of North America

14. Issue Date for Circulation Data Below
September 2011

15. Extent and Nature of Circulation

		Average No. Copies Each Issue During Preceding 12 Months	No. Copies of Single Issue Published Nearest to Filing Date
a. Total Number of Copies (Net press run)		1377	1143
b. Paid Circulation (By Mail and Outside the Mail)	(1) Mailed Outside-County Paid Subscriptions Stated on PS Form 3541. (Include paid distribution above nominal rate, advertiser's proof copies, and exchange copies)	735	661
	(2) Mailed In-County Paid Subscriptions Stated on PS Form 3541 (Include paid distribution above nominal rate, advertiser's proof copies, and exchange copies)		
	(3) Paid Distribution Outside the Mails Including Sales Through Dealers and Carriers, Street Vendors, Counter Sales, and Other Paid Distribution Outside USPS®	212	211
	(4) Paid Distribution by Other Classes Mailed Through the USPS (e.g. First-Class Mail®)		
c. Total Paid Distribution (Sum of 15b (1), (2), (3), and (4)) ►		947	872
d. Free or Nominal Rate Distribution (By Mail and Outside the Mail)	(1) Free or Nominal Rate Outside-County Copies Included on PS Form 3541	70	62
	(2) Free or Nominal Rate In-County Copies Included on PS Form 3541		
	(3) Free or Nominal Rate Copies Mailed at Other Classes Through the USPS (e.g. First-Class Mail)		
	(4) Free or Nominal Rate Distribution Outside the Mail (Carriers or other means)		
e. Total Free or Nominal Rate Distribution (Sum of 15d (1), (2), (3) and (4)) ►		70	62
f. Total Distribution (Sum of 15c and 15e) ►		1017	934
g. Copies not Distributed (See instructions to publishers #4 (page #3)) ►		360	209
h. Total (Sum of 15f and g) ►		1377	1143
i. Percent Paid (15c divided by 15f times 100)		93.12%	93.36%

16. Publication of Statement of Ownership
☐ If the publication is a general publication, publication of this statement is required. Will be printed in the **December 2011** issue of this publication. ☐ Publication not required.

17. Signature and Title of Editor, Publisher, Business Manager, or Owner

Stephen R. Bushing
Stephen R. Bushing –Inventory Distribution Coordinator

Date
September 16, 2011

I certify that all information furnished on this form is true and complete. I understand that anyone who furnishes false or misleading information on this form or who omits material or information requested on the form may be subject to criminal sanctions (including fines and imprisonment) and/or civil sanctions (including civil penalties).

PS Form 3526, September 2007 (Page 2 of 3)

Moving?

Make sure your subscription moves with you!

To notify us of your new address, find your **Clinics Account Number** (located on your mailing label above your name), and contact customer service at:

Email: journalscustomerservice-usa@elsevier.com

800-654-2452 (subscribers in the U.S. & Canada)
314-447-8871 (subscribers outside of the U.S. & Canada)

Fax number: 314-447-8029

Elsevier Health Sciences Division
Subscription Customer Service
3251 Riverport Lane
Maryland Heights, MO 63043

*To ensure uninterrupted delivery of your subscription, please notify us at least 4 weeks in advance of move.

Printed and bound by CPI Group (UK) Ltd, Croydon, CR0 4YY

03/10/2024

01040447-0001